CONTENTS

INTRODUCTION

The Ninja Foodi Grill is a tabletop multi-function appliance that can grill, roast, bake, air crisp, and even dehydrate.It makes use of their cyclonic grilling technology that utilizes rapidly circulating hot air to cook and sea food. The Ninja Foodi grill is an electric grill, air fryer, convection oven, oven toaster, and dehydrator all rolled into one.

The Benefits of The Ninja Foodi Grill

Whether it is a trend or the general convenience of it, more people are appreciating smaller and more portable indoor cookers due to a number of benefits from owning one.

Easy to clean and operate – Indoor grills are plug and play appliances making them user-friendly to a wider demographic. The cooking components are coated with a non-stick ceramic material that can be effortlessly taken apart and cleaned using a standard dishwasher.

Smokeless – This is probably one of the best things about indoor electric grills. People who do not have any access to open areas can still enjoy grilling since it does not produce smoke like standard grillers.

Multi-function – Most indoor cookers come with various functionalities giving you more value for your money. It can also eliminate the need to purchase other appliances and save you essential kitchen space.

Compact – Electric grills are small enough to fit most kitchen counters and tables. It is also portable enough to be easily transported or moved around.

Capable of high temperatures – A wide range of temperature settings let you cook a variety of foods from char-grilled vegetables to restaurant-level steaks. Unlike other tabletop cookers, the Ninja Grill will let you cook frozen foods without the need to defrost. It can also get as hot as 500 to 510 degrees Fahrenheit.

Browns and crisps food – Indoor grills like the Ninja Foodi use the circulating hot air to cook the food thoroughly. This creates delectable flavors through a browning process called the Maillard reaction. Similar to convection ovens and toasters, the Ninja Foodi is excellent at making food crunchy when you need it to be.

Grill marks - Like traditional outdoor grills, indoor grills can also give meat and other foods those appetizing grill marks. Although, the Ninja Foodi's grill marks are curved, unlike the typical straight markings you get from regular outdoor grills.

Using Your Ninja Foodi Grill

When you are cooking for the first time with your Foodi grill, you must first wash the detachable cooking parts with warm soapy water to remove any oil and debris. Let it air dry and put them back inside once you are ready to cook. An easy-to-follow instruction guide comes with each unit, so make sure to go over it prior to cooking.

Position your grill on a level and secure surface. Leave at least 6 inches of space around it, especially at the back where the air intake vent and air socket are located. Ensure that the splatter guard is installed whenever the grill is in use. This is a wire mesh that covers the heating element on the inside of the lid.

For Grilling

Plug your unit into an outlet and power on the grill.

Use the grill grate over the cooking pot and choose the grill function. This has four default temperature settings of low at 400 degrees F, medium at 450 degrees F, high at 500 degrees F, and max at 510 degrees F.

Set the time needed to cook. You may check the grilling cheat sheet that comes with your unit to guide you with the time and temperature settings. It is best to check the food regularly depending on the doneness you prefer and to avoid overcooking.

Once the required settings are selected, press start and wait for the digital display to show 'add food'. The unit will start to preheat similar to an oven and will show the progress through the display. This step takes about 8 minutes.

If you need to check the food or flip it, the timer will pause and resume once the lid is closed.

The screen will show 'Done' once the timer and cooking has completed. Turn off the unit and unplug the device. Leave the hood open to let the unit cool faster.

For Roasting

Remove the grill grates and use the cooking pot that comes with the unit. You may also purchase their roasting rack for this purpose.

Press the roast option and set the timer between 1 to 4 hours depending on the recipe requirements. The Foodi will preheat for 3 minutes regardless of the time you have set.

Once ready, place the meat directly on the roasting pot or rack.

Check occasionally for doneness. A meat thermometer is another useful tool to get your meats perfectly cooked.

For Baking

Remove the grates and use the cooking pot.

Choose the bake setting and set your preferred temperature and time. Preheating will take about 3 minutes.

Once done with preheating, you may put the ingredients directly on the cooking pot, or you may use your regular baking tray. An 8-inch baking tray can fit inside as well as similar-sized oven-safe containers.

For Air Frying / Air Crisping

Put the crisper basket in and close the lid.

Press the air crisp or air fry option then the start button. The default temperature is set at 390° F and will preheat at about 3 minutes. You can adjust the temperature and time by pressing the buttons beside these options.

If you do not need to preheat, just press the air crisp button a second time and the display will show you the 'add food' message.

Put the food inside and shake or turn every 10 minutes. Use oven mitts or tongs with silicone tips when doing this.

For Dehydrating

Place the first layer of food directly on the cooking pot.

Add the crisper basket and add one more layer.

Choose the dehydrate setting and set the timer between 7 to 10 hours.

You may check the progress from time to time.

For cooking frozen foods:

Choose the medium heat, which is 450° F using the grill option. You may also use the air crisp option if you are cooking fries, vegetables, and other frozen foods.

Set the time needed for your recipe. Add a few minutes to compensate for the thawing.

Flip or shake after a few minutes to cook the food evenly.

Cleaning and Maintenance

Components are dishwasher-safe and are fabricated with a non-stick ceramic coating, to make clean-up and maintenance easier. Plus, the grill conveniently comes with a plastic cleaning brush with a scraper at the other end.

Cleaning Tips

Let the grill cool down completely and ensure that it is unplugged from the power outlet before trying to clean the unit.

Take out the splatter guard, grill grates and cooking pot and soak in soapy water for a few hours to let the debris soften and make cleaning easier. Wash only the removable parts.

Gently brush off dirt and debris using the plastic brush that comes with your grill. Use the other end of the brush to dislodge food in hard-to-reach areas.

Let the parts dry thoroughly.

Clean the insides and exterior of the unit with a clean damp cloth.

Maintenance Tips

Always keep your unit clean, especially before putting in a new batch for cooking. You should clean the parts and the unit after each use.

Never use cleaning instruments or chemicals that are too harsh and can damage the coating.

Keep the electrical cords away from children and any traffic in your kitchen.

Avoid getting the unit and electrical components wet and place it away from areas that constantly get soaked or damp.

At all times, unplug the unit when not in use.

BREAKFAST RECIPES

1. Breakfast Bell Peppers

Servings: 2
Cooking Time: 15 Minutes
Ingredients:
- 4 eggs, beaten
- 1 large bell pepper, sliced in half
- 1 teaspoon olive oil
- Salt and pepper to taste

Directions:
1. Brush the bell pepper halves with oil.
2. Pour eggs into the bell pepper.
3. Sprinkle with salt and pepper.
4. Place these in the air fryer basket.
5. Set the Ninja Foodi Grill to air fry.
6. Cook at 390 degrees F for 15 minutes.

2. Quiche

Servings: 4
Cooking Time: 15 Minutes
Ingredients:
- 6 eggs
- ¾ cup heavy cream
- Salt and pepper to taste
- 1 pre-made pie crust
- 1 cup cheddar cheese, shredded

Directions:
1. Beat the eggs in a bowl.
2. Stir in the cream, salt and pepper.
3. Pour mixture into the pie crust.
4. Sprinkle cheese on top.
5. Press air crisp.
6. Set it to 320 degrees F.
7. Cook for 12 to 15 minutes.

3. Roasted Garlic Potatoes

Servings: 4
Cooking Time: 20 Minutes
Ingredients:
- 2 lb. baby potatoes, sliced into wedges
- 2 tablespoons olive oil
- 2 teaspoons garlic salt

Directions:
1. Toss the potatoes in olive oil and garlic salt. Add the potatoes to the Ninja Foodi basket. Seal the crisping lid. Set it to air crisp. Cook at 390 degrees F for 20 minutes.

4. Sausage & Veggies Casserole

Servings: 8
Cooking Time: 7 Hours 3 Minutes
Ingredients:
- 2½ cups cauliflower florets
- 12 organic eggs
- ¾ cup unsweetened almond milk
- 1 teaspoon dried oregano, crushed
- ¾ teaspoon paprika
- Salt, as required
- 1 red ringer pepper, seeded and cleaved finely
- 1 lb. gluten-free cooked sausages, cut into slices
- 1½ cups cheddar cheese, grated

Directions:
1. In an enormous pot of bubbling water, cook cauliflower for about 2-3 minutes.
2. Expel from the warmth and channel the cauliflower completely. Set aside to cool.
3. In a bowl, add the eggs, almond milk, and oregano, paprika, and salt and beat until well combined.
4. In the greased pot of the Ninja Foodi, place the cauliflower followed by the bell pepper, sausage slices, and cheddar cheese.
5. Top with the egg mixture evenly.
6. Close the Ninja Foodi with the crisping lid and select Slow Cooker.
7. Set on Low for 6-7 hours.
8. Press Start/Stop to begin cooking.
9. Cut into equal-sized wedges and serve hot.
- **Nutrition Info:** Calories: 389 Fats: 30.1 g Net Carbs: 2.8 g Carbs: 4 g Fiber: 1.2 g Sugar: 2.2 g Proteins: 25.2 g Sodium: 695 mg

5. Bacon And Tomato Omelet

Servings: 4
Cooking Time: 20 Minutes
Ingredients:
- 1 tablespoon cheddar, grated
- ¼ pound bacon, cooked and chopped
- 4 tomatoes, cubed
- 1 tablespoon parsley, chopped
- 1 tablespoon olive oil
- Salt and pepper to taste

Directions:
1. Take a small pan and place it over medium heat, add bacon and Sauté for 2 minutes until crisp
2. Take a bowl and add bacon, add remaining ingredients, and gently stir. Sprinkle cheese on top
3. Preheat Ninja Foodi by pressing the "BAKE" option and setting it to "400 Degrees F" and timer to 10 minutes
4. Let it preheat until you hear a beep
5. Pour mixture into a baking dish and transfer baking dish inside Ninja Foodi Grill, let it bake for 8 minutes
6. Serve and enjoy!

6. Buttermilk Pancake

Servings: 12
Cooking Time: 10 Minutes
Ingredients:
- 2 cups all-purpose flour

- 2 teaspoons baking powder
- 2 tablespoons sugar
- Pinch salt
- 2 eggs, beaten
- ¼ cup milk
- 2 cups buttermilk
- ¼ butter, melted

Directions:
1. Combine the flour, baking powder, sugar and salt.
2. Stir in the eggs and remaining ingredients.
3. Spray the air fryer tray with oil.
4. Pour the batter into the tray.
5. Select air crisp.
6. Cook at 320 degrees F for 5 minutes.
7. Flip and cook for another 5 minutes.

7. Cheesy Broccoli Quiche

Servings: 8
Cooking Time: 40 Minutes
Ingredients:
- 1 cup water
- 2 cups broccoli florets
- 1 carrot, chopped
- 1 cup cheddar cheese, grated
- ¼ cup Feta cheese, crumbled
- ¼ cup milk
- 2 eggs
- 1 teaspoon parsley
- 1 teaspoon thyme
- Salt and pepper to taste

Directions:
1. Pour the water inside the Ninja Foodi. Place the basket inside.
2. Put the carrots and broccoli on the basket. Cover the pot.
3. Set it to pressure. Cook at high pressure for 2 minutes.
4. Release the pressure quickly. Crack the eggs into a bowl and beat.
5. Season with the salt, pepper, parsley, and thyme. Put the vegetables on a small baking pan. Layer with the cheese and pour in the beaten eggs. Place on the basket.
6. Choose the Air Crisp function. Seal the crisping lid. Cook at 350°F for 20 minutes.
7. serving Suggestions:
8. Garnish with chopped parsley or chives.
- **Nutrition Info:** Calories: 401 Total Fat: 28 g Saturated Fat: 16.5 g Cholesterol: 242 mg Sodium: 688 mg Total Carbohydrate: 12.8 g Dietary Fiber: 3.3 g Total Sugars: 5.8 g Protein: 26.2 g Potassium: 537 mg

8. Eggs In Avocado Cups

Servings: 2
Cooking Time: 10 Minutes
Ingredients:
- avocado halved and pitted

- large eggs
- Salt and ground black pepper, as required
- cooked bacon slices, crumbled

Directions:
1. Carefully, scoop out about 2 teaspoons of flesh from each avocado half.
2. Crack 1 egg in each avocado half and sprinkle with salt and black pepper.
3. Press the "Power Button" of Air Fry Oven and turn the dial to select the "Air Roast" mode.
4. Press the Time button and again turn the dial to set the cooking time to 10 minutes.
5. Now push the Temp button and rotate the dial to set the temperature at 375 degrees F.
6. Press the "Start/Pause" button to start.
7. When the unit beeps to show that it is preheated, open the lid and line the "Sheet Pan" with a lightly, grease piece of foil.
8. Arrange avocado halves into the "Sheet Pan" and insert it in the oven.
9. Top each avocado half with bacon pieces and serve.

9. Cinnamon French Toast

Servings: 2
Cooking Time: 6 Minutes
Ingredients:
- 2 eggs
- ¼ cup whole milk
- 3 tablespoons sugar
- 2 teaspoons olive oil
- 1/8 teaspoon vanilla extract
- 1/8 teaspoon ground cinnamon
- 4 bread slices

Directions:
1. In a large bowl, mix all the ingredients except bread slices.
2. Coat the bread slices with egg mixture evenly.
3. Press the "Power Button" of Air Fry Oven and turn the dial to select the "Air Fry" mode.
4. Press the Time button and again turn the dial to set the cooking time to 6 minutes.
5. Now push the Temp button and rotate the dial to set the temperature at 390 degrees F.
6. Press the "Start/Pause" button to start.
7. When the unit beeps to show that it is preheated, open the lid and lightly grease the sheet pan.
8. Arrange the bread slices into "Air Fry Basket" and insert it in the oven.
9. Flip the bread slices once halfway through.
10. Serve warm.

10. French Toast

Servings: 4
Cooking Time: 10 Minutes
Ingredients:

- 6 eggs
- 1 cup milk
- Cooking spray
- 1 loaf French bread, sliced
- 1 teaspoon honey
- 1 cup heavy cream
- 1/2 cup sugar
- 1/2 cup butter

Directions:
1. Beat the eggs in a bowl.
2. Stir in milk, cream and honey.
3. Dip the bread slices into the mixture.
4. Add to the grill basket inside the Ninja Foodi Grill.
5. Spread some butter and sprinkle sugar on top of the bread slices.
6. Seal the pot and air fry at 350 degrees F for 5 to 10 minutes.

11. Tater Tot Egg Bake

Servings: 4
Cooking Time: 25 Minutes
Ingredients:
- 5 eggs
- ¼ cup milk
- Salt and pepper to taste
- Cooking spray
- 2 sausages, cooked and sliced
- 1 cup cheddar cheese, shredded
- 1 lb. frozen tater tots

Directions:
1. Preheat your unit by pressing bake.
2. Set it to 390 degrees F for 3 minutes.
3. In a bowl, beat the eggs and milk.
4. Season with salt and pepper.
5. Spray a small baking pan with oil.
6. Add egg mixture to the pan.
7. Add to the unit.
8. Cook for 5 minutes.
9. Place the sausages on top of the eggs.
10. Sprinkle cheese on top.
11. Press bake and set it to 390 degrees F.
12. Cook for 20 minutes.

12. Pumpkin Porridge

Servings: 8
Cooking Time: 5 Hours
Ingredients:
- 1 cup unsweetened almond milk, divided
- 2 pounds pumpkin, peeled and cubed into ½-inch pieces
- 6-8 drops liquid Stevia
- ½ teaspoon ground allspice
- 1 tablespoon ground cinnamon
- 1 teaspoon ground nutmeg
- ¼ teaspoon ground cloves

Directions:

1. In the pot of Ninja Foodi, place ½ cup of almond milk and remaining ingredients and stir to combine.
2. Close the Ninja Foodi with the crisping lid and select Slow Cooker.
3. Set on Low for 4-5 hours.
4. Press Start/Stop to begin cooking.
5. Stir in the remaining almond milk and with a potato masher, mash the mixture completely.
6. Serve warm.
- **Nutrition Info:** Calories: 48 Fats: 0.9 g Net Carbs: 6 g Carbs: 10 g Fiber: 4 g Sugar: 3.8 g Proteins: 1.4 g Sodium: 29 mg

13. French Toast Sticks

Servings: 12
Cooking Time: 10 Minutes
Ingredients:
- 5 eggs
- 1 cup almond milk
- 1 teaspoon vanilla extract
- 1/4 cup sugar
- 4 tablespoons melted butter
- 4 bread slices, sliced into 12 sticks

Directions:
1. Beat the eggs in a bowl.
2. Stir in milk, sugar, vanilla and butter.
3. Dip the bread sticks into the mixture.
4. Add these to the air fryer basket and place inside the Ninja Foodi Grill.
5. Air fry at 350 degrees F for 8 to 10 minutes.

14. Egg & Turkey Sausage Cups

Servings: 8
Cooking Time: 30 Minutes
Ingredients:
- 8 tablespoons turkey sausage, cooked and crumbled, divided
- 8 tablespoons frozen spinach, chopped and divided
- 8 teaspoons shredded cheddar cheese, divided
- 4 eggs

Directions:
1. Add a layer of the sausage, spinach, and cheese to each muffin cup.
2. Crack the egg open on top. Seal the crisping lid. Set it to Air Crisp.
3. Cook at 330°F for 10 minutes.
- **Nutrition Info:** Calories: 171 Total Fat: 13.3 g Saturated Fat: 4.7 g Cholesterol: 190 mg Sodium: 289 mg Total Carbohydrate: 0.5 g Dietary Fiber: 0.1 g Total Sugars: 0.4 g Protein: 11.9 g Potassium: 161 mg

15. Nuts Granola

Servings: 12
Cooking Time: 1½ Hours

Ingredients:
- 1 cup raw pecans
- 1 cup raw almonds
- 1 cup raw walnuts
- 1½ teaspoons ground cinnamon
- ¼ cup Erythritol

Directions:
1. In the greased pot of Ninja Foodie, add all the ingredients and mix until well combined.
2. Close the Ninja Foodi with a crisping lid and select "Slow Cooker".
3. Set on "Low" for 1½-2 hours.
4. Press "Start/Stop" to begin cooking.
5. Move the granola onto an enormous heating sheet and set aside to cool completely before serving.

16. Roasted Breakfast Potatoes

Servings: 4
Cooking Time: 25 Minutes
Ingredients:
- 3 large potatoes, diced
- Garlic salt and pepper to taste
- 1 tablespoon butter
- 3 sprigs thyme
- 1 tablespoon olive oil
- 2 sprigs rosemary

Directions:
1. Add potatoes to the Ninja Foodi Grill pot.
2. Toss in olive oil and butter.
3. Season with garlic salt and pepper.
4. Top with the herb sprigs.
5. Seal the pot.
6. Set it to air fry.
7. Cook at 375 degrees F for 25 minutes.

17. Breakfast Omelette

Servings: 6
Cooking Time: 10 Minutes
Ingredients:
- 6 eggs
- 1 white onion, diced
- 2 slices ham, chopped and cooked
- 1 cup cheddar cheese, shredded
- 1 red bell pepper, diced
- 6 mushrooms, chopped
- Salt and pepper to taste

Directions:
1. Beat eggs in a bowl.
2. Stir in the rest of the ingredients.
3. Set your Ninja Foodi Grill to air fry.
4. Pour the egg mixture into the pot.
5. Cook at 390 degrees F for 10 minutes, stirring halfway through.

18. Elegant Pineapple Toast

Servings: 4
Cooking Time: 15 Minutes
Ingredients:

- Cooking spray as needed
- ½ cup cooking flakes
- 10 slices pineapple
- 1 cup of coconut milk
- 3 large whole egg
- ¼ cup milk
- ¼ cup of sugar
- 10 bread slices

Directions:
1. Take a medium-sized bowl and whisk in eggs, coconut milk, sugar and stir well
2. Dip your pineapple slices into the mixture and let them sit for 2 minutes
3. Pre-heat your Ninja Foodi Grill in MED settings, giving timer to 15 minutes
4. Transfer prepared slices to Grill and cook for 2 minutes, flip and cook for 2 minutes more
5. Repeat with all the slices
- **Nutrition Info:** Calories: 202 Fat: 15 g Saturated Fat: 3 g Carbohydrates: 49 g Fiber: 3 g Sodium: 524 mg Protein: 8 g

19. Breakfast Burrito

Servings: 12
Cooking Time: 30 Minutes
Ingredients:
- 1 teaspoon olive oil
- 1 lb. breakfast sausage
- 10 eggs, beaten
- 3 cups cheddar cheese, shredded
- 2 cups potatoes, diced
- Salt and pepper to taste
- 12 tortillas

Directions:
1. Pour olive oil into a pan over medium heat.
2. Cook potatoes and sausage for 7 to 10 minutes, stirring frequently.
3. Spread this mixture on the bottom of the Ninja Foodi Grill pot.
4. Season with salt and pepper.
5. Pour the eggs and cheese on top.
6. Select bake setting.
7. Cook at 325 degrees F for 20 minutes.
8. Top the tortilla with the cooked mixture and roll.
9. Sprinkle cheese on the top side.
10. Add the air fryer basket to the Ninja Foodi Grill.
11. Air fry the burrito at 375 degrees F for 10 minutes.

20. Simple Zucchini Egg Muffins

Servings: 4
Cooking Time: 7 Minutes
Ingredients:
- 4 whole eggs
- 2 tablespoons almond flour
- 1 zucchini, grated

- 1 teaspoon butter
- ½ teaspoon salt

Directions:
1. Take a small-sized bowl and add almond flour, salt, zucchini. Mix well
2. Take muffin molds and grease them gently, add the zucchini mix
3. Arrange your molds in Ninja Foodi Grill and cook on "AIR CRISP" mode for 7 minutes at a temperature of 375 degrees F
4. Serve and enjoy the meal once complete!
- **Nutrition Info:** Calories: 94 Fat: 8 g Saturated Fat: 1.5 g Carbohydrates: 2 g Fiber: 0.5 g Sodium: 209 mg Protein: 7 g

21. Omelet

Servings: 8
Cooking Time: 40 Minutes
Ingredients:
- 2 eggs
- ¼ cup milk
- 1 tablespoon red bell pepper, chopped
- 1 slice ham, diced
- 1 tablespoon mushroom, chopped
- Salt to taste
- ¼ cup cheese, shredded

Directions:
1. Whisk the eggs and milk in a bowl. Add the ham and vegetables. Season with the salt.
2. Pour the mixture into a small pan. Place the pan inside the Ninja Foodi basket.
3. Seal the crisping lid. Set it to Air Crisp. Cook at 350°F for 8 minutes.
4. Before it is fully cooked, sprinkle the cheese on top.
5. Coat the beef cubes with the salt and pickling spice.
6. In a skillet over medium heat, pour in the olive oil.
7. serving Suggestions
8. Garnish with chopped green onion.
- **Nutrition Info:** Calories: 177 Total Fat: 11 g Saturated Fat: 5.1 g Cholesterol: 189 mg Sodium: 425 mg Total Carbohydrate: 7.1 g Dietary Fiber: 1 g Total Sugars: 4.8 g Protein: 13.1 g Potassium: 249 mg

22. Cheesy Baked Eggs

Servings: 1
Cooking Time: 5 Minutes
Ingredients:
- 2 eggs, beaten
- 2 tablespoons heavy cream
- 2 tablespoons cheddar cheese, shredded
- 1 teaspoon Parmesan cheese, grated
- Salt and pepper to taste

Directions:
1. Beat the eggs and cream in a bowl.
2. Stir in the rest of the ingredients.

3. Pour mixture into a ramekin.
4. Add the ramekin to the unit.
5. Choose air crisp setting.
6. Cook at 330 degrees F for 5 minutes.

23. Hearty Ninja Food Bean

Servings: 4
Cooking Time: 10 Minutes
Ingredients:
- Fresh ground black pepper
- Flaky sea salt
- Pinch of pepper
- 1 lemon, juiced
- 2 tablespoon oil
- 1-pound green bean, trimmed

Directions:
1. Take a medium bowl and add the green bean
2. Mix and stir well
3. Preheat your Ninja Foodi Grill to MAX and set the timer to 10 minutes
4. Wait until you hear a beep
5. Transfer beans to the grill grate, cook for 8-10 minutes
6. Toss well to ensure that all sides cooked evenly
7. Squeeze a bit of lemon juice on top
8. Season with salt, pepper and pepper flakes according to your taste
9. Enjoy!
- **Nutrition Info:** Calories: 100 Fat: 7 g Saturated Fat: 1 g Carbohydrates: 10 g Fiber: 4 g Sodium: 30 mg Protein: 2 g

24. Sausage & Bacon Omelet

Servings: 2
Cooking Time: 10 Minutes
Ingredients:
- 4 eggs
- Ground black pepper, as required
- 1 bacon slice, chopped
- 2 sausages, chopped
- 1 onion, chopped
- 1 teaspoon fresh parsley, minced

Directions:
1. In a bowl, crack the eggs and black pepper and beat well.
2. Add the remaining ingredients and gently stir to combine.
3. Place the mixture into a baking pan.
4. Arrange the drip pan at the bottom of the Instant Ninja Foodi Plus Air Fryer Oven cooking chamber.
5. Select "Air Dry" and then adjust the temperature to 320 degrees F.
6. Set the timer for 10 minutes and press the "Start."
7. When the display shows "Add Food," place the baking pan over the drip pan.

8. When the display shows "Turn Food," do nothing.
9. When cooking time is complete, remove the pan from the Ninja Foodi and serve warm.

25. Healthy Potato Pancakes

Servings: 4
Cooking Time: 24 Minutes
Ingredients:
- Salt and pepper to taste
- 3 tablespoons flour
- ¼ teaspoon salt
- ½ teaspoon garlic powder
- 2 tablespoons unsalted butter
- ¼ cup milk
- 1 egg, beaten
- 1 medium onion, chopped
- 4 medium potatoes, peeled and cleaned

Directions:
1. Take your potatoes and peel them. Shred the potatoes and soak the shredded potatoes under cold water.
2. Drain your potatoes in a colander.
3. In a separate bowl, add milk, eggs, butter, garlic powder, pepper, and salt. Add flour and mix the whole mixture well.
4. Add shredded potatoes.
5. Preheat your Ninja Foodi to Air Crisp mode with a temperature of 390°F, setting the timer to 24 minutes.
6. Once you hear the beep, add ¼ cup of potato pancake batter to the cooking basket.
7. Cook for 12 minutes until you have a nice golden texture.
8. Repeat with remaining batter.
9. Serve once done, enjoy!
- **Nutrition Info:** Calories: 240 Fat: 11 g Saturated Fat: 3 g Carbohydrates: 33 g Fiber: 4 g Sodium: 259 mg Protein: 6 g

26. Sausage Patties

Servings: 6-8
Cooking Time: 10 Minutes
Ingredients:
- 1 pack sausage patties

Directions:
1. Add sausage patties to the air fryer tray.
2. Select air crisp.
3. Set it to 400 degrees F.
4. Cook for 5 minutes per side.

27. Carrot Bread

Servings: 12
Cooking Time: 3 Hours
Ingredients:
- 1 cup almond flour
- 1/3 cup coconut flour
- 1½ teaspoons organic baking powder
- 1 teaspoon ground cinnamon

- ¼ teaspoon ground cloves
- ¼ teaspoon ground nutmeg
- ¼ teaspoon salt
- 1 cup Erythritol
- 1/3 cup coconut oil, softened
- 3 organic eggs
- 1 teaspoon organic vanilla extract
- ½ teaspoon organic almond extract
- 2 cups plus 2 tablespoons carrots, peeled and shredded

Directions:
1. In a bowl, add the flours, baking powder, baking soda, spices, and salt and mix well.
2. In another large bowl, add the Erythritol, coconut oil, eggs, and both extracts and beat until well combined.
3. Add the flour mixture and mix until just combined.
4. Fold in the carrots.
5. Place the mixture into a greased 8x4-inch silicone bread pan.
6. Arrange a "Reversible Rack" in the pot of Ninja Foodi.
7. Place the pan over the "Reversible Rack".
8. Close the Ninja Foodi with a crisping lid and select "Slow Cooker".
9. Set on "Low" for 3 hours.
10. Press "Start/Stop" to begin cooking.
11. Place the bread pan onto a wire rack for about 5-10 minutes.
12. Carefully, remove the bread from the pan and place it onto the wire rack to cool completely before slicing.
13. Cut the bread into desired-sized slices and serve.

28. Avocado Toast

Servings: 1
Cooking Time: 3 Minutes
Ingredients:
- 1 avocado, mashed
- 1 clove garlic, minced
- 1 teaspoon lemon juice
- Salt to taste
- 2 slices bread
- ¼ cup tomato, chopped

Directions:
1. Mix the avocado, garlic, lemon juice, salt and pepper.
2. Spread mixture on top of bread slices.
3. Sprinkle tomato on top.
4. Add to the grill grate.
5. Press grill setting.
6. Grill at 350 degrees F for 2 to 3 minutes.

29. Early Morning Kale And Sausage Delight

Servings: 4
Cooking Time: 10 Minutes

Ingredients:
- Olive oil as needed
- 1 cup mushrooms
- 2 cups kale,e chopped
- 4 sausage links
- 4 medium eggs
- 1 medium yellow onion, sweet

Directions:
1. Open the lid of your Ninja Foodi Grill and arrange the Grill Grate
2. Pre-heat your Ninja Foodi Grill to HIGH and set the timer to 5 minutes
3. Once you hear the beeping sound, arrange sausages over the grill grate
4. Cook for 2 minutes, flip and cook for 3 minutes more
5. Take a baking pan and spread out the kale, onion, mushroom, sausage and crack an egg on top
6. Cook on BAKE mode on 350 degrees F for about 5 minutes more
7. Serve and enjoy!
- **Nutrition Info:** Calories: 236 Fat: 12 g Saturated Fat: 2 g Carbohydrates: 17 g Fiber: 4 g Sodium: 369 mg Protein: 18 g

30. Prosciutto Egg Panini

Servings: 8
Cooking Time: 30 Min
Ingredients:
- 3 - large eggs
- 2 - large egg whites
- 6 - Tbsp fat-free milk
- 1 - green onion, thinly sliced
- 1 - Tbsp Dijon mustard
- 1 - Tbsp maple syrup
- 8 - slices sourdough bread
- 8 - thin slices prosciutto or deli ham
- ½ cup shredded sharp cheddar cheese
- 8 - Tsp butter

Directions:
1. In a little bowl, whisk the eggs, egg whites, milk, and onion. Coat an enormous skillet with cooking splash and spot over medium warmth. Include egg blend; cook and mix over medium warmth until totally set.
2. Join mustard and syrup; spread more than 4 bread cuts. Layer with fried eggs, prosciutto, and cheddar; top with outstanding bread. Spread exterior of sandwiches.
3. Cook on a Panini producer or indoor Ninja Foodi oven broil for 3-4MIN or until bread is seared and cheddar is liquefied. Cut every Panini down the middle to serve.
- **Nutrition Info:** Calories 228, fat 10g, carbohydrate 21g, protein 13g.

31. Chocolate Granola

Servings: 20

Cooking Time: 2 Hours
Ingredients:
- 5 cups unsweetened coconut, shredded 1 cup almonds, chopped
- 1/3 cups sunflower seeds
- 1/3 cups pumpkin seeds
- ¼ cup cacao nibs
- 2½ ounces coconut oil, melted
- 3 tablespoons Erythritol
- 4 tablespoons cocoa powder unsweetened 1 tablespoon lemon zest, grated finely

Directions:
1. In the pot of Ninja Foodi, add all ingredients and mix well.
2. Close the Ninja Foodi with a crisping lid and select "Slow Cooker".
3. Set on "High" for 2 hours.
4. Press "Start/Stop" to begin cooking.
5. Stir the mixture after every 15 minutes.
6. Move the granola onto an enormous heating sheet and set aside to cool completely before serving.

32. Eggs & Veggie Burrito

Servings: 4
Cooking Time: 25 Minutes
Ingredients:
- 3 eggs, beaten
- Salt and pepper to taste
- Cooking spray
- 8 tortillas
- 2 red bell peppers, sliced into strips
- 1 onion, sliced thinly

Directions:
1. Beat the eggs in a bowl. Season with the salt and pepper. Set aside.
2. Choose the Sauté mode in the Ninja Foodi. Spray with the oil. Cook the vegetables until soft. Remove and set aside. Pour in the eggs to the pot. Cook until firm.
3. Wrap the eggs and veggies with a tortilla.
4. serving Suggestions
5. Sprinkle top part with cheese.
- **Nutrition Info:** Calories: 92 Total Fat: 2.5 g Saturated Fat: 0.6 g Cholesterol: 61 mg Sodium: 35 mg Total Carbohydrate: 14.4 g Dietary Fiber: 2.2 g Total Sugars: 2.4 g Protein: 3.9 g Potassium: 143 mg

33. Sweet Spiced Toast

Servings: 3
Cooking Time: 4 Minutes
Ingredients:
- ¼ cup of sugar
- ½ teaspoon ground cinnamon
- 1/8 teaspoon ground cloves
- 1/8 teaspoon ground ginger
- ½ teaspoons vanilla extract
- ¼ cup salted butter softened

- 6 bread slices

Directions:
1. In a bowl, add the sugar, vanilla, cinnamon, pepper, and butter. Mix until smooth.
2. Spread the butter mixture evenly over each bread slice.
3. Press the "Power Button" of Air Fry Oven and turn the dial to select the "Air Fry" mode.
4. Press the Time button and again turn the dial to set the cooking time to 4 minutes.
5. Now push the Temp button and rotate the dial to set the temperature at 400 degrees F.
6. Press the "Start/Pause" button to start.
7. When the unit beeps to show that it is preheated, open the lid and lightly grease the sheet pan.
8. Arrange the bread slices into "Air Fry Basket" buttered side up and insert in the oven.
9. Serve warm.

34. Breakfast Omelet

Servings: 6
Cooking Time: 10 Minutes
Ingredients:
- 6 eggs
- 1 white onion, diced
- 1 red bell pepper, diced
- 6 mushrooms, chopped
- 2 slices ham, chopped and cooked
- 1 cup cheddar cheese, shredded
- Salt and pepper to taste

Directions:
1. Beat eggs in a bowl.
2. Stir in the rest of the ingredients.
3. Set your Ninja Foodi Grill to air fry.
4. Pour the egg mixture into the pot.
5. Cook at 390 degrees F for 10 minutes, stirring halfway through.

35. Breakfast Casserole

Servings: 8
Cooking Time: 15 Minutes
Ingredients:
- ¼ cup white onion, diced
- 1/2 cup Colby Jack cheese, shredded
- 8 eggs, beaten
- 1 green bell pepper, diced
- 1 lb. ground sausage, cooked
- Garlic salt to taste

Directions:
1. Add white onion, bell pepper and ground sausage to your Ninja Foodi Grill pot.
2. Spread cheese and then the eggs on top.
3. Season with garlic salt.
4. Set to air fry and cook at 390 degrees F for 15 minutes.

36. Herb & Cheese Frittata

Servings: 4
Cooking Time: 25 Minutes
Ingredients:
- 4 eggs
- ½ cup half and half
- 2 tablespoons parsley, chopped
- 2 tablespoons chives, chopped
- ¼ cup shredded cheddar cheese
- Salt and pepper to taste

Directions:
1. Beat the eggs in a bowl. Add the rest of the ingredients and stir well.
2. Pour the mixture into a small baking pan.
3. Place the pan on top of the Ninja Foodi basket.
4. Seal the crisping lid. Set it to Air Crisp. Cook at 330°F for 15 minutes.
5. serving Suggestions:
6. Garnish with fresh cilantro.
- **Nutrition Info:** Calories: 132 Total Fat: 10.2 g Saturated Fat: 5 g Cholesterol: 182 mg Sodium: 119 mg Total Carbohydrate: 1. 9g Dietary Fiber: 0.1 g Total Sugars: 0.5 g Protein: 8.3 g Potassium: 121 mg

37. Bacon

Servings: 3
Cooking Time: 10 Minutes
Ingredients:
- 2 tablespoons water
- 6 slices bacon

Directions:
1. Pour water to the bottom of the Ninja Foodi Grill pot.
2. Place the grill rack inside.
3. Put the bacon slices on the grill rack.
4. Select air fry function.
5. Cook at 350 degrees F for 5 minutes per side or until golden and crispy.

38. Exciting Tomato Bacon Omelet

Servings: 4
Cooking Time: 10 Minutes
Ingredients:
- Salt and pepper to taste
- 1 tablespoon olive oil
- 1 tablespoon parsley, chopped
- 4 tomatoes, cubed
- ¼ pound bacon, cooked and chopped
- 4 whole eggs, whisked

Directions:
1. Take a small-sized pan and place it over medium level heat, add bacon and Sauté for about 2 minutes until finely crisped
2. Take another bowl and add the Sautéed bowl and add rest of the listed ingredients, sprinkle cheese and stir

3. Pre-heat your Ninja Foodi Grill using BAKE option to a temperature of 400 degrees F for about 10 minutes
4. Wait until you hear a beep
5. Transfer the prepared mixture into your baking dish and transfer to your Grill, bake for 8 minutes
6. Serve once done, enjoy!
- **Nutrition Info:** Calories: 311 Fat: 16g Saturated Fat: 4 g Carbohydrates: 23 g Fiber: 2 g Sodium: 149 mg Protein: 22 g

39. Pecan & Coconut Porridge

Servings: 4
Cooking Time: 1 Hour
Ingredients:
- 1 cup pecan halves
- ½ cup unsweetened dried coconut shreds
- ¼ cup pumpkin seeds, shelled
- 1 cup water
- 2 teaspoons butter, melted
- 4-6 drops liquid Stevia

Directions:
1. In a food processor, add the walnuts, coconut, and pumpkin seeds, and pulse for about 30 seconds.
2. In the pot of the Ninja Foodi, place the pecan mixture and remaining ingredients, and stir to combine.
3. Close the Ninja Foodi with the crisping lid and select Slow Cooker.
4. Set on High for 1 hour.
5. Press Start/Stop to begin cooking.
6. Serve warm.
- **Nutrition Info:** Calories: 317 Fats: 31.5 g Net Carbs: 2.9 g Carbs: 7.5 g Fiber: 4.6 g Sugar: 1.8 g Proteins: 5.8 g Sodium: 19 mg

40. Eggs & Avocado

Servings: 2
Cooking Time: 15 Minutes
Ingredients:
- 2 eggs
- 1 avocado, sliced in half and pitted
- Salt and pepper to taste
- Cheddar cheese, shredded

Directions:
1. Scoop out about a tablespoon of avocado flesh to make a hole.
2. Crack egg on top of the avocado.
3. Season with salt and pepper.
4. Sprinkle with cheese.
5. Air fry at 390 degrees F for 12 to 15 minutes.

41. French Toast(1)

Servings: 4
Cooking Time: 10 Minutes

Ingredients:
- 6 eggs
- 1 cup milk
- 1 cup heavy cream
- 1 teaspoon honey
- Cooking spray
- 1 loaf French bread, sliced
- ½ cup butter
- ½ cup sugar

Directions:
1. Beat the eggs in a bowl.
2. Stir in milk, cream, and honey.
3. Dip the bread slices into the mixture.
4. Add to the grill basket inside the Ninja Foodi Grill.
5. Spread some butter and sprinkle sugar on top of the bread slices.
6. Seal the pot and air fry at 350°F for 5-10 minutes.
7. serving Suggestions
8. Serve with maple syrup.
9. preparation/Cooking Tips
10. It's a good idea to use day-old bread for this recipe.
- **Nutrition Info:** Calories: 72 Fats: 3.3 g Net Carbs: 2.9 g Carbs: 5.9 g Fiber: 3 g Sugar: 1.5 g Proteins: 5.2 g Sodium: 104 mg

42. Completely Stuffed Up Bacon And Pepper

Servings: 4
Cooking Time: 15 Minutes
Ingredients:
- Chopped parsley, for garnish
- Salt and pepper to taste
- 4 whole large eggs
- 4 bell pepper, seeded and tops removed
- 4 slices bacon, cooked and chopped
- 1 cup cheddar cheese, shredded

Directions:
1. Take the bell pepper and divide the cheese and bacon evenly between them.
2. Crack eggs into each of the bell pepper.
3. Season the bell pepper with salt and pepper.
4. Preheat your Ninja Food Grill in Air Crisp mode with temperature to 390°F.
5. Set timer to 15 minutes.
6. Once you hear the beep, transfer the bell pepper to the cooking basket.
7. Transfer your prepared pepper to Ninja Foodi Grill and cook for 10-15 minutes until the eggs are cooked, and the yolks are just slightly runny.
8. Garnish with a bit of parsley.
9. Enjoy!

- **Nutrition Info:** Calories: 326 Fat: 23 g Saturated Fat: 10 g Carbohydrates: 10 g Fiber: 2 g Sodium: 781 mg Protein: 22 g

43. Spinach Quiche

Servings: 4
Cooking Time: 4 Hours
Ingredients:
- 10 ounces frozen chopped spinach, thawed and squeezed
- 4 ounces' feta cheese, shredded
- 2 cups unsweetened almond milk
- 4 organic eggs
- ¼ teaspoon red pepper flakes, crushed
- Salt and ground black pepper, as required

Directions:
1. In the pot of Ninja Foodie, add all the ingredients and mix until well combined.
2. Close the Ninja Foodi with a crisping lid and select "Slow Cooker".
3. Set on "Low" for 4 hours.
4. Press "Start/Stop" to begin cooking.
5. Cut into equal-sized wedges and serve hot.

44. Buttered Up Garlic And Fennel

Servings: 4
Cooking Time: 2.5 Minutes
Ingredients:
- 1 and ½ pounds fennel bulbs, cut into wedges
- ¼ teaspoon dried dill weed
- 1/3 cup dry white wine
- ½ stick butter
- 2 garlic cloves, sliced
- ½ teaspoon cayenne
- 2/3 cup stock
- ½ teaspoon salt
- ¼ teaspoon ground black pepper

Directions:
1. Set your Ninja Foodi on Sauté mode
2. Then add butter, let it heat up
3. Add garlic and cook for 30 seconds
4. Add rest of the ingredients
5. Close the lid and cook on LOW pressure for 2 minutes
6. Remove the lid once done
7. Serve and enjoy!

45. Breakfast Potatoes

Servings: 4
Cooking Time: 55 Minutes
Ingredients:
- 4 potatoes
- 2 cups cheddar cheese, shredded
- 8 slices bacon, cooked crispy and chopped
- 1 1/4 cups sour cream

- 4 teaspoons butter

Directions:
1. Take out the grill gate and crisper basket.
2. Set Ninja Foodi Grill to bake.
3. Set it to 390 degrees F.
4. Preheat by selecting "start".
5. Add the potatoes inside.
6. Seal and cook for 45 minutes.
7. Let cool.
8. Make slices on top of the potatoes.
9. Create a small hole.
10. Top with butter and cheese.
11. Put the potatoes back to the pot.
12. Bake at 375 degrees F for 10 minutes.
13. Top with sour cream and bacon before serving.

46. Ham & Cheese Casserole

Servings: 8
Cooking Time: 20 Minutes
Ingredients:
- 1 lb. ham, chopped and cooked
- 1 red bell pepper, chopped
- 1 white onion, chopped
- 1 yellow bell pepper, chopped
- 2 cups Colby Jack cheese, shredded
- 8 eggs, beaten
- Salt and pepper to taste

Directions:
1. Line the air fryer basket with foil.
2. Spread ham on the bottom of the basket.
3. Top with the cheese, onion, bell peppers and eggs.
4. Sprinkle with salt and pepper.
5. Choose air fry function.
6. Cook at 390 degrees F for 15 to 20 minutes.

47. Bacon & Scrambled Eggs

Servings: 4
Cooking Time: 25 Minutes
Ingredients:
- 4 strips bacon
- 2 eggs
- 1 tablespoon milk
- Salt and pepper to taste

Directions:
1. Place the bacon inside the Ninja Foodi. Set it to Air Crisp.
2. Cover the crisping lid. Cook at 390°F for 3 minutes.
3. Flip the bacon and cook for another 2 minutes. Remove the bacon and set aside.
4. Whisk the eggs and milk in a bowl. Season with the salt and pepper.
5. Set the Ninja Foodi to Sauté. Add the eggs and cook until firm.

6. serving Suggestions:
7. Serve with toasted bread.
- **Nutrition Info:** Calories: 272 Total Fat: 20.4 g Saturated Fat: 6.7 g Cholesterol: 206 mg Sodium: 943 mg Total Carbohydrate: 1.3 g Dietary Fiber: 0 g Total Sugars: 0.7 g Protein: 19.9 g Potassium: 279 mg

48. Sausage Casserole

Servings: 4
Cooking Time: 20 Minutes
Ingredients:
- 1 lb. hash browns
- 2 red bell peppers, chopped
- 1 white onion, chopped
- 4 eggs, beaten
- 1 lb. ground breakfast sausage, cooked
- Salt and pepper to taste

Directions:
1. Line the air fryer basket with foil.
2. Add hash browns at the bottom part.
3. Spread sausage, onion and bell peppers on top.
4. Air fry at 355 degrees F for 10 minutes.
5. Pour eggs on top and cook for another 10 minutes.
6. Season with salt and pepper.

49. Eclairs On The Grill

Servings: 6
Cooking Time: 5 Min
Ingredients:
- Wooden dowel (5/8-inch diameter and 24 inches long)
- 1 - tube (8 ounces) refrigerated seamless crescent dough sheet
- 3 - snack-size cups (3- ¼ ounces each) vanilla or chocolate pudding
- ½ cup chocolate frosting
- Whipped cream in a can

Directions:
1. Set up an open-air fire or Ninja Foodi oven broil for high warmth. Wrap one finish of a stick or wooden dowel with foil. Unroll sickle mixture and cut into six 4-in. squares. Fold one bit of mixture over the readied stick; squeeze end and crease to seal.
2. Cook over open-air fire or Ninja Foodi oven broil 5-7MIN or until brilliant earthy colored, turning at times. At the point when the mixture is sufficiently cool to deal with, expel from the stick. Get done with cooling. Rehash with residual batter.
3. Spot pudding in a resealable plastic pack; cut a little opening in one corner. Crush

pack to squeeze blend into each shell. Spread with icing; top with whipped cream.
- **Nutrition Info:** Calories 293, fat 12g, carbohydrate 43g, protein 4g.

50. French Toast(2)

Servings: 4
Cooking Time: 35 Minutes
Ingredients:
- 2 eggs, beaten
- ¼ cup milk
- ¼ cup brown sugar
- 1 tablespoon honey
- 1 teaspoon cinnamon
- ¼ teaspoon nutmeg
- 4 slices wholemeal bread, sliced into strips

Directions:
1. In a bowl, combine all the ingredients except the bread. Mix well.
2. Dip each strip in the mixture. Place the bread strips in the Ninja Foodi basket.
3. Place basket inside the pot. Cover with the crisping lid. Set it to Air Crisp.
4. Cook at 320°F for 10 minutes.
5. serving Suggestions:
6. Dust with confectioners' sugar.
- **Nutrition Info:** Calories: 295 Total Fat: 6.1 g Saturated Fat: 2.1 g Cholesterol: 166 mg Sodium: 332 mg Total Carbohydrate: 49.8 g Dietary Fiber: 3.9 g Total Sugars: 29.4 g Protein: 11.9 g Potassium: 112 mg

51. Hash Browns

Servings: 4
Cooking Time: 20 Minutes
Ingredients:
- 6 potatoes, grated
- 1 bell pepper, chopped
- 2 teaspoons olive oil
- 1 onion, chopped
- Salt and pepper to taste

Directions:
1. Toss the grated potatoes, onion and bell pepper separately in oil.
2. Season with salt and pepper.
3. Add potatoes to the air fryer.
4. Air fry at 400 degrees F for 10 minutes.
5. Shake and stir in onion and pepper.
6. Cook for another 10 minutes.

52. Crispy Garlic Potatoes

Servings: 8
Cooking Time: 20 Minutes
Ingredients:
- 1 teaspoon garlic powder
- 1 1/2 lb. potatoes, diced

- 1 tablespoon avocado oil
- Salt and pepper to taste

Directions:
1. Toss the potatoes in oil.
2. Season with garlic powder, salt and pepper.
3. Add the air fryer basket to the Ninja Foodi Grill.
4. Select air fry setting.
5. Cook at 400 degrees F for 20 minutes, tossing halfway through.

53. Bacon Stuffed Pepper

Servings: 4
Cooking Time: 15 Minutes
Ingredients:
- 4 slices bacon, cooked and chopped
- 4 large eggs
- 1 cup cheddar cheese, shredded
- 4 bell peppers, seeded and tops removed
- Salt and pepper to taste
- Chopped parsley, for garnish

Directions:
1. Take your bell peppers and divide cheese and bacon between them.
2. Crack an egg into each of the bell peppers. Season them with salt and pepper.
3. Preheat your Ninja Foodi by pressing the Air Crisp option and setting it to 390°F.
4. Set your timer to 15 minutes.
5. Allow it to preheat until it beeps.
6. Transfer bell pepper to your cooking basket and transfer to Foodi Grill.
7. Lock the lid and cook for 10-15 minutes until egg whites are cooked well until the yolks are slightly runny.
8. Remove peppers from the basket and garnish with parsley.
9. Serve and enjoy!
- **Nutrition Info:** Calories: 326 Fat: 23 g Saturated Fat: 10 g Carbohydrates: 10 g Fiber: 2 g Sodium: 781 mg Protein: 22 g

54. Low-carb Breakfast Casserole

Servings: 8
Cooking Time: 15min
Ingredients:
- 1 - LB Ground Sausage
- ¼ Cup Diced White Onion
- 1 - Diced Green Bell Pepper
- 8 - Whole Eggs, Beaten
- ½ Cup Shredded Colby Jack Cheese
- 1 - Tsp Fennel Seed
- ½ Tsp Garlic Salt

Directions:
1. On the off threat that you are utilizing the Ninja Foodi, utilize the sauté potential to

brown the frankfurter inside the pot of the foodi. In the occasion that you are utilizing a Ninja Foodi, you could make use of a skillet to do that.
2. Include the onion and pepper and prepare dinner along with the ground wiener until the vegetables are sensitive and the hotdog is cooked.
3. Utilizing the 8.75-inch container or the Air Fryer skillet, splash it with a non-stick cooking bathe.
4. Spot the floor wiener mixture on the base of the skillet.
5. Top uniformly with cheddar.
6. Pour the crushed eggs uniformly over the cheddar and frankfurter.
7. Include fennel seed and garlic salt uniformly over the eggs.
8. Spot the rack within the low state of affairs within the Ninja Foodi, and in a while region the box on the pinnacle.
9. Set to Air Crisp for 15MIN at 390 levels.
10. In the occasion which you are using an air fryer, place the dish legitimately into the bin of the air fryer and cook for 15MIN at 390 tiers.
11. Cautiously expel and serve.
- **Nutrition Info:** CALORIES: 282 FAT: 23g CARBOHYDRATES: 3g SUGAR: 2g PROTEIN: 15g

55. Cast-iron Scrambled Eggs

Servings: 6
Cooking Time: 25 Min
Ingredients:
- 12 - large eggs
- 2 - Tbsp water
- ¼ teaspoon salt
- ¼ teaspoon pepper
- 2/3 - cup finely chopped sweet onion
- 1 - jalapeno pepper, seeded and chopped
- 2 - Tbsp butter
- 1 - log (4 ounces) fresh goat cheese, crumbled
- 3 - Tbsp Minced chives

Directions:
1. In an enormous bowl, whisk the eggs, water, salt and pepper; put in a safe spot.
2. Spot a 10-in. cast-iron skillet on Ninja Foodi oven broil rack over medium-hot warmth. In the skillet, sauté onion and jalapeno in margarine until delicate. Include egg blend; cook and mix until nearly set. Mix in cheddar and chives; cook and mix until eggs are totally set.

- **Nutrition Info:** Calories 217, fat 16g, carbohydrate 3g, protein 15g.

56. Nuts & Seeds Granola

Servings: 12
Cooking Time: 2 Hours
Ingredients:
- 1/3 cup unsalted butter
- 1 teaspoon liquid stevia
- 1 teaspoon organic vanilla extract
- 1½ cups pumpkin seeds
- 1½ cups sunflower seeds
- ½ cup raw pecans, chopped roughly
- ½ cup raw hazelnuts, chopped roughly
- ½ cup raw walnuts, chopped roughly
- ½ cup raw almonds, chopped roughly
- 1 teaspoon ground cinnamon

Directions:
1. Select the "Sauté/Sear" setting of Ninja Foodi and place the butter into the pot.
2. Press "Start/Stop" to begin cooking and heat for about 2-3 minutes.
3. Include the fluid stevia and vanilla concentrate and mix to combine.
4. Immediately, press "Start/Stop" to stop cooking
5. Now, add the remaining ingredients and stir to combine.
6. Close the Ninja Foodi with a crisping lid and select "Slow Cooker".
7. Set on "Low" for 2 hours, stirring after every 30 minutes.
8. Press "Start/Stop" to begin cooking.
9. Move the granola onto an enormous heating sheet and set aside to cool completely before serving.

57. Breakfast Tart

Servings: 4
Cooking Time: 14 Minutes
Ingredients:
- 4 oz. cream cheese
- 3 tablespoons confectioners' sugar
- ¼ cup blueberry preserves
- 8 oz. crescent roll dough (refrigerated)
- Cooking spray

Directions:
1. Blend the cream cheese, sugar and blueberry preserves in a bowl using a hand mixer.
2. Slice the dough into 4 portions.
3. Roll out each portion until flattened.
4. Spread the cream cheese mixture on top of the dough portions.
5. Roll up the dough and seal.
6. Add these to the unit.

7. Press air crisp.
8. Preheat at 325 degrees F for 3 minutes.
9. Add the rolls to the unit.
10. Cook for 14 minutes.

58. Zucchini & Coconut Bread

Servings: 10
Cooking Time: 3 Hours
Ingredients:
- 2½ cups zucchini, shredded
- ½ teaspoon salt
- 1 1/3 cups almond flour
- 2/3 cup coconut, shredded
- 2 teaspoons ground cinnamon
- ½ teaspoon ground ginger
- ¼ teaspoon ground nutmeg
- 3 large organic eggs
- ¼ cup butter, melted
- ¼ cup water
- ½ teaspoon organic vanilla extract
- ½ cup walnuts, chopped

Directions:
1. Arrange a large sieve in a sink.
2. Place the zucchini in a sieve and sprinkle with salt. Set aside to drain for about 1 hour.
3. With your hands, squeeze out the moisture from zucchini.
4. In a large bowl, add the almond flour, coconut, Erythritol, protein powder, baking powder, and spices and mix well.
5. Add the zucchini, eggs, coconut oil, water, and vanilla extract and mix until well combined.
6. Fold in the walnuts.
7. At the bottom of a greased Ninja Foodie, place the mixture.
8. Close the Ninja Foodi with a crisping lid and select "Slow Cooker".
9. Set on "Low" for 2½-3 hours.
10. Press "Start/Stop" to begin cooking.
11. Keep the bread inside for about 5-10 minutes.
12. Carefully, remove the bread from the pot and place onto a wire rack to cool completely before slicing.
13. Cut the bread into desired-sized slices and serve.

59. Ginger-glazed Grilled Honeydew

Servings: 6
Cooking Time: 25 Min
Ingredients:
- ¼ cup peach preserves
- 1 - Tbsp lemon juice
- 1 - Tbsp finely chopped crystallized ginger
- 2 - Tsp grated lemon zest

- 1/8 - teaspoon ground cloves
- 1 - medium honeydew melon, cut into 2-inch cubes

Directions:

1. In a little bowl, join the initial 5 fixings. String honeydew onto 6 metal or drenched wooden sticks; brush with a large portion of the coating.
2. On a gently oiled rack, barbecue honeydew, secured, over medium-high warmth or sear 4 in. from the warmth just until melon starts to mollify and brown, 4 to 6MIN, turning and seasoning oftentimes with residual coating.
- **Nutrition Info:** Calories 101, fat 0, carbohydrate 26g, protein 1g.

60. Savory Cauliflower Bread

Servings: 8
Cooking Time: 4 Hours
Ingredients:

- 12 ounces cauliflower florets
- 2 large organic eggs
- 2 cups mozzarella cheese, shredded and divided
- 3 tablespoons coconut flour
- Salt and ground black pepper, as required
- 2 garlic cloves, minced

Directions:

1. In a food processor, include cauliflower and heartbeat until a rice-like consistency is achieved.
2. Transfer the cauliflower rice into a large bowl.
3. Add 1 cup of the cheese, eggs, coconut flour, salt, and black pepper, and mix until well combined.
4. In the greased pot of the Ninja Foodi, place the cauliflower mixture and press firmly.
5. Sprinkle with garlic and remaining cheese evenly.
6. Close the Ninja Foodi with the crisping lid and select Slow Cooker.
7. Set on High for 2-4 hours.
8. Press Start/Stop to begin cooking.
9. Keep the bread inside for about 5-10 minutes.
10. Carefully, remove the bread from the pot and place onto a platter.
11. Cut the bread into desired-sized slices and serve warm.
- **Nutrition Info:** Calories: 72 Fats: 3.3 g Net Carbs: 2.9 g Carbs: 5.9 g Fiber: 3 g Sugar: 1.5 g Proteins: 5.2 g Sodium: 104 mg

FISH & SEAFOOD RECIPES

61. Grilled Coconut Shrimp With Shishito Peppers

Servings: 4
Cooking Time:25min
Ingredients:
- 6 - garlic cloves, finely grated
- 1 - Tbsp. finely grated lime zest
- ¼ cup low-sodium
- ¼ cup grape seed or vegetable oil
- 1 lb. large shrimp, peeled, deveined
- ½ cup toasted unsweetened shredded coconut
- 8 - oz. shish to peppers
- ½ cup basil leaves
- ¼ cup fresh lime juice
- Flaky sea salt

Directions:
1. Mix together garlic, lime get-up-and-go, soy sauce, and ¼ cup oil in a medium bowl. Add shrimp and hurl to cover. Include ½ cup coconut and hurl again to cover. Let sit while the Ninja Foodi oven broil warms, in any event, 5MIN and up to 30MIN.
2. Set up a Ninja Foodi oven broil for high warmth, delicately oil grind.
3. Cautiously organize shrimp in an even layer on the mesh. Ninja Foodi oven broil, cautiously turning part of the way through, until hazy and daintily singed, about 2MIN. A portion of the coconuts will tumble off all the while, and that is alright. Move to a serving platter.
4. Ninja Foodi oven broil peppers, turning every so often and being mindful so as not to let them fall through the mesh until delicately roasted all over about 6MIN. Move to platter with shrimp.
5. Top shrimp and peppers with basil, shower with a lime squeeze, and sprinkle with ocean salt and more coconut.
- **Nutrition Info:** Calories 82, fat 7g, carbohydrate 4g, Protein 2g.

62. Crusted Flounder Fillets

Servings: 2
Cooking Time: 12 Minutes
Ingredients:
- 2 flounder fillets
- 1 egg
- 1/2 teaspoon worcestershire sauce
- 1/4 cup coconut flour
- 1/4 cup almond flour
- 1/2 teaspoon lemon pepper
- 1/2 teaspoon coarse sea salt
- 1/4 teaspoon chili powder

Directions:
1. Rinse and pat dry the flounder fillets.
2. Whisk the egg and worcestershire sauce in a shallow bowl. In a separate bowl, mix the coconut flour, almond flour, lemon pepper, salt, and chili powder.
3. Then, dip the fillets into the egg mixture. Lastly, coat the fish fillets with the coconut flour mixture until they are coated on all sides.
4. Spritz with cooking spray and transfer to the air fryer basket. Cook at 390 degrees for 7 minutes.
5. Turn them over, spritz with cooking spray on the other side, and cook another 5 minutes.
- **Nutrition Info:** 325 calories; 18.3g fat; 6.1g carbs; 34.4g protein; 2.2g sugars; 1.7g fiber

63. Tuna Burger

Servings: 4
Cooking Time: 10 Minutes
Ingredients:
- Cooking spray
- Tuna patties
- 6 oz. tuna flakes
- 1 tablespoon lemon juice
- 1 teaspoon lemon zest
- 1 teaspoon Dijon mustard
- 1 egg, beaten
- 1 tablespoon Italian seasoning
- ½ cup breadcrumbs
- Burger
- 4 burger buns
- Lettuce leaves
- 1 tomato, sliced

Directions:
1. Mix tuna patty ingredients in a bowl.
2. Form 4 patties from the mixture.
3. Spray the patties with oil.
4. Place these in the air crisp tray.
5. Choose air crisp setting.
6. Air fry 360 degrees F for 5 minutes per side.
7. Serve in burger buns with tomato and lettuce.

64. Shrimp Boil

Servings: 6
Cooking Time: 15 Minutes
Ingredients:
- 12 oz. shrimp, peeled and deveined
- 14 oz. smoked sausage, sliced
- 4 corn on cobs, sliced into 4
- 3 cups potatoes, sliced in half and boiled
- 1/8 cup Old Bay seasoning
- ¼ cup white onion, diced
- Cooking spray

Directions:

1. Mix all the ingredients in the inner pot of the Ninja Foodi Grill.
2. Spray mixture with oil.
3. Set the unit to Air Fry.
4. Air fry at 390°F for 5-7 minutes.
5. Stir and cook for another 6 minutes.
6. serving Suggestionss:
7. Sprinkle with dried herbs before serving.
8. preparation/Cooking Tips:
9. Check the dish halfway through cooking to see if it's cooking evenly.
- **Nutrition Info:** Calories: 267 Fat: 23 g Carbohydrates: 10 g Protein: 22 g

65. The Rich Guy Lobster And Butter

Servings: 8
Cooking Time: 20 Minutes
Ingredients:
- 6 lobster tails
- 4 garlic cloves,
- ¼ cup butter

Directions:
1. Preheat the Ninja Foodi to 400°F at first.
2. Open the lobster tails gently by using kitchen scissors.
3. Remove the lobster meat gently from the shells but keep it inside the shells.
4. Take a plate and place it.
5. Add some butter to a pan and allow it melt.
6. Put some garlic cloves in it and heat it over medium-low heat.
7. Pour the garlic butter mixture all over the lobster tail meat.
8. Let the fryer to broil the lobster at 130°F.
9. Remove the lobster meat from Ninja Foodi and set aside.
10. Use a fork to pull out the lobster meat from the shells entirely.
11. Pour some garlic butter over it if needed. Serve and enjoy!
- **Nutrition Info:** Calories: 160 Fat: 1 g Carbohydrates: 1 g Protein: 20 g

66. Crispy Fish Sandwich

Servings: 2
Cooking Time: 12 Minutes
Ingredients:
- Tartar Sauce
- 1/4 cup mayonnaise
- 1 teaspoon pickle juice
- 2 tablespoons dill pickles, chopped
- Fish Sandwiches
- 2 white fish fillets
- 2 teaspoons Old Bay Seasoning
- 2 tablespoons flour
- 1 egg, beaten
- 1/2 cup breadcrumbs
- 2 slices low-fat cheese slices
- 2 burger buns

Directions:
1. Mix mayo, pickle juice and dill pickles in a bowl.
2. Cover and place inside the refrigerator.
3. Add seasoning and flour in a dish.
4. Beat egg in a bowl.
5. Put breadcrumbs in the third bowl.
6. Coat fish fillets with flour mixture.
7. Dip in egg and then dredge with breadcrumbs.
8. Add fish fillets to the air fryer basket.
9. Set Ninja Foodi Grill to air fry.
10. Cook at 350 degrees F for 10 to 12 minutes.
11. Add crispy fish to burger buns.
12. Top with tartar sauce and cheese.

67. Cheesy Fish Gratin

Servings: 4
Cooking Time: 20 Minutes
Ingredients:
- 1 tablespoon avocado oil
- 1 pound hake fillets
- 1 teaspoon garlic powder
- Sea salt and ground white pepper, to taste
- 2 tablespoons shallots, chopped
- 1 bell pepper, seeded and chopped
- 1/2 cup cottage cheese
- 1/2 cup sour cream
- 1 egg, well whisked
- 1 teaspoon yellow mustard
- 1 tablespoon lime juice
- 1/2 cup swiss cheese, shredded

Directions:
1. Brush the bottom and sides of a casserole dish with avocado oil. Add the hake fillets to the casserole dish and sprinkle with garlic powder, salt, and pepper.
2. Add the chopped shallots and bell peppers.
3. In a mixing bowl, thoroughly combine the cottage cheese, sour cream, egg, mustard, and lime juice. Pour the mixture over fish and spread evenly.
4. Cook in the preheated air fryer at 370 degrees f for 10 minutes.
5. Top with the swiss cheese and cook an additional 7 minutes. Let it rest for 10 minutes before slicing and serving.
- **Nutrition Info:** 335 calories; 18.1g fat; 7.8g carbs; 33.7g protein; 2.6g sugars; 0.6g fiber

68. Grilled Shrimp

Servings: 8
Cooking Time: 10 Minutes
Ingredients:
- 2 lb. shrimp, de-veined
- 2 tablespoons olive oil
- 1 tablespoon Old Bay seasoning
- Garlic salt to taste

Directions:

1. Preheat your grill to medium.
2. Brush shrimp with olive oil.
3. Season with Old Bay seasoning and garlic salt.
4. Cook for 3-5 minutes per side.
5. serving Suggestionss:
6. Serve with grilled corn.
7. preparation/Cooking Tips:
8. Add cayenne pepper if you want your shrimp spicier.
- **Nutrition Info:** Calories: 234 Fat: 45 g Carbohydrates: 6 g Protein: 23 g

69. Shrimp Tempura

Servings: 6
Cooking Time: 10 Minutes
Ingredients:
- 1 pack frozen shrimp tempura

Directions:
1. Preheat the air fryer to 390 degrees F for 5 minutes.
2. Arrange the frozen tempura on a single layer on your air crisp basket.
3. Cook the shrimp for 5 minutes per side.

70. Easy Fish Stew

Servings: 4
Cooking Time: 20 Minutes
Ingredients:
- 1 pound white fish fillets, chopped
- 1 cup broccoli, chopped
- 3 cups fish stock
- 1 onion, diced
- 2 cups celery stalks, chopped
- 1 cup heavy cream
- 1 bay leaf
- 1½ cups cauliflower, diced
- 1 carrot, sliced
- 2 tablespoons butter
- ¼ teaspoon garlic powder
- ½ teaspoon salt
- ¼ teaspoon pepper

Directions:
1. Set your Ninja Foodi to Sauté.
2. Add butter, and let it melt.
3. Add onion and carrots, cook for 3 minutes.
4. Stir in remaining ingredients.
5. Close the lid.
6. Cook for 4 minutes on High.
7. Release the pressure naturally over 10 minutes.
8. Remove the bay leave once cooked.
9. Serve and enjoy!
- **Nutrition Info:** Calories: 298 g Fat: 18 g Saturated Fat: 3 g Carbohydrates: 6 g Fiber: 2 g Sodium: 846 mg Protein: 24 g

71. Tangy Cod Fillets

Servings: 2

Cooking Time: 15 Minutes
Ingredients:
- 1 ½ tablespoons sesame oil
- 1/2 heaping teaspoon dried parsley flakes
- 1/3 teaspoon fresh lemon zest, finely grated
- 2 medium-sized cod fillets
- 1 teaspoon sea salt flakes
- A pinch of salt and pepper
- 1/3 teaspoon ground black pepper, or more to savor
- 1/2 tablespoon fresh lemon juice

Directions:
1. Set the air fryer to cook at 375 degrees f. Season each cod fillet with sea salt flakes, black pepper and dried parsley flakes. Now, drizzle them with sesame oil.
2. Place the seasoned cod fillets in a single layer at the bottom of the cooking basket; air-fry approximately 10 minutes.
3. While the fillets are cooking, prepare the sauce by mixing the other ingredients. Serve cod fillets on four individual plates garnished with the creamy citrus sauce.
- **Nutrition Info:** 291 calories; 11.1g fat; 2.7g carbs; 41.6g protein; 1.2g sugars; 0.5g fiber

72. Pecan Crusted Tilapia

Servings: 5
Cooking Time: 15 Minutes
Ingredients:
- 2 tablespoons ground flaxseeds
- 1 teaspoon paprika
- Sea salt and white pepper, to taste
- 1 teaspoon garlic paste
- 2 tablespoons extra-virgin olive oil
- 1/2 cup pecans, ground
- 5 tilapia fillets, slice into halves

Directions:
1. Combine the ground flaxseeds, paprika, salt, white pepper, garlic paste, olive oil, and ground pecans in a ziploc bag. Add the fish fillets and shake to coat well.
2. Spritz the air fryer basket with cooking spray. Cook in the preheated air fryer at 400 degrees f for 10 minutes; turn them over and cook for 6 minutes more. Work in batches.
3. Serve with lemon wedges, if desired.
- **Nutrition Info:** 264 calories; 17.1g fat; 3.9g carbs; 25.5g protein; 1g sugars; 2g fiber

73. Herbed Salmon

Servings: 2
Cooking Time: 10 Minutes
Ingredients:
- 2 salmon fillets
- 2 tablespoons olive oil
- 1 teaspoon Herbes de Provence
- 1/4 teaspoon smoked paprika

- Salt and pepper to taste
- 1 tablespoon butter
- 1/2 teaspoon lemon juice

Directions:
1. Coat the salmon with olive oil.
2. Sprinkle with herbs, paprika, salt and pepper.
3. Insert grill grate to the Ninja Foodi Grill.
4. Set it to high. Set it to 10 minutes.
5. Press start to preheat.
6. Add fish to the grill.
7. Grill for 3 to 5 minutes per side.
8. Top the fish with the butter and drizzle with lemon juice before serving.

74. Lovely Air Fried Scallops(2)

Servings: 4
Cooking Time: 5 Minutes
Ingredients:
- 12 scallops
- 3 tablespoons olive oil
- Salt and pepper, to taste

Directions:
1. Rub the scallops with salt, pepper, and olive oil.
2. Transfer it to the Ninja Foodi.
3. Place the insert in your Ninja Foodi.
4. Close the air crisping lid.
5. Cook for 4 minutes at 390°F.
6. Flip them after 2 minutes.
7. Serve and enjoy!
- **Nutrition Info:** Calories: 372 g Fat: 11 g Saturated Fat: 3 g Carbohydrates: 0.9 g Fiber: 0 g Sodium: 750 mg Protein: 63 g

75. Fish And Cauliflower Cakes

Servings: 4
Cooking Time: 13 Minutes
Ingredients:
- 1/2 pound cauliflower florets
- 1/2 teaspoon english mustard
- 2 tablespoons butter, room temperature
- 1/2 tablespoon cilantro, minced
- 2 tablespoons sour cream
- 2 ½ cups cooked white fish
- Salt and freshly cracked black pepper, to savor

Directions:
1. Boil the cauliflower until tender. Then, purée the cauliflower in your blender. Transfer to a mixing dish.
2. Now, stir in the fish, cilantro, salt, and black pepper.
3. Add the sour cream, english mustard, and butter; mix until everything's well incorporated. Using your hands, shape into patties.

4. Place in the refrigerator for about 2 hours. Cook for 13 minutes at 395 degrees f. Serve with some extra english mustard.
- **Nutrition Info:** 285 calories; 15.1g fat; 4.3g carbs; 31.1g protein; 1.6g sugars; 1.3g fiber

76. Ninja Foodi Cedar-plank Salmon

Servings: 6
Cooking Time:2½ Hr
Ingredients:
- 2 - Tbsp grainy mustard
- 2 - Tbsp mild honey or pure maple syrup
- 1 - teaspoon Minced rosemary
- 1 - Tbsp grated lemon zest
- 1 (2-pounds) salmon fillet with skin (1½ inches thick)

Directions:
1. Splash cedar Ninja Foodi oven broiling board in water to cover 2 HRS, keeping it inundated.
2. Plan barbecue for direct-heat cooking over medium-hot charcoal. Open vents on the base and top of a charcoal Ninja Foodi oven broil.
3. Mix together mustard, nectar, rosemary, pizzazz, and½ teaspoon every one of salt and pepper. Spread blends on the substance side of salmon and let remain at room temperature 15MIN.
4. Put salmon on board, skin side down. Barbecue, secured with a cover, until salmon is simply cooked through and edges are seared, 13 to 15MIN. Let salmon remain on board 5MIN before serving.
- **Nutrition Info:** Calories 240, fat 15g, carbohydrate 0g, Protein 23g.

77. Fried Clams

Servings: 4
Cooking Time: 5 Minutes
Ingredients:
- 1 pack frozen clams

Directions:
1. Preheat your unit to 400 degrees F for 5 minutes.
2. Add clams to the air crisp tray.
3. Cook for 5 minutes.
4. Check to see if they are done. If not, cook for another 3 to 5 minutes.

78. Tuna Patties(2)

Servings: 2
Cooking Time:x
Ingredients:
- 1 teaspoon garlic powder
- 1 tablespoon lemon juice
- 2 cans tuna flakes
- 1 tablespoon mayo
- 1/2 tablespoon almond flour

- 1/2 teaspoon onion powder
- 1 teaspoon dried dill
- Salt and pepper to taste

Directions:
1. Mix all the ingredients in a bowl. Form patties. Set the tuna patties on the Ninja Foodi basket. Seal the crisping lid. Set it to air crisp.
2. Cook at 400 degrees for 10 minutes. Flip and cook for 5 more minutes.
- **Nutrition Info:** Calories 141, Total Fat 6.4g, Saturated Fat 0.7g, Cholesterol 17mg, Sodium 148mg, Total Carbohydrate 5.2g, Dietary Fiber 1g, Total Sugars 1.2g, Protein 17g, Potassium 48mg

79. French-style Sea Bass

Servings: 2
Cooking Time: 10 Minutes
Ingredients:
- 1 tablespoon olive oil
- 2 sea bass fillets
- Sauce:
- 1/2 cup mayonnaise
- 1 tablespoon capers, drained and chopped
- 1 tablespoon gherkins, drained and chopped
- 2 tablespoons scallions, finely chopped
- 2 tablespoons lemon juice

Directions:
1. Start by preheating your air fryer to 395 degrees f. Drizzle olive oil all over the fish fillets.
2. Cook the sea bass in the preheated air fryer for 10 minutes, flipping them halfway through the cooking time.
3. Meanwhile, make the sauce by whisking the remaining ingredients until everything is well incorporated. Place in the refrigerator until ready to serve.
- **Nutrition Info:** 384 calories; 28.5g fat; 3.5g carbs; 27.6g protein; 1g sugars; 1g fiber

80. Mesmerizing Parmesan Fish

Servings: 3
Cooking Time: 13 Minutes
Ingredients:
- ¼ teaspoon salt
- ¾ cup breadcrumbs
- ¼ cup parmesan cheese, grated
- 1-pound haddock fillets
- ¼ teaspoon ground dried thyme
- ¼ cup butter, melted
- ¾ cup milk

Directions:
1. Coat fish fillets in milk, season with salt and keep it on the side
2. Take a mixing bowl and add breadcrumbs, parmesan, cheese, thyme and combine well

3. Coat fillets in bread crumb mixture
4. Pre-heat Ninja Foodi by pressing the "BAKE" option and setting it to "325 Degrees F" and timer to 13 minutes
5. Let it pre-heat until you hear a beep
6. Arrange fish fillets directly over Grill Grate, lock lid and cook for 8 minutes, flip and cook for the remaining time
7. Serve and enjoy!
- **Nutrition Info:** Calories: 450, Fat: 27 g, Saturated Fat: 12 g, Carbohydrates: 16 g, Fiber: 3 g, Sodium: 1056 mg, Protein: 44 g

81. Clams With Spicy Tomato Broth And Garlic Mayo

Servings: 4
Cooking Time:50 Min
Ingredients:
- ½ lemon
- 5 - garlic cloves, 1 whole, 4 thinly sliced
- ½ cup mayonnaise
- Kosher salt
- ¼ cup plus 3 Tbsp. extra-virgin olive oil
- 2 - large shallots, thinly sliced
- 1 - red Chile (such as Holland or Fresno), thinly sliced, or½ tsp. crushed red pepper flakes
- 2 - Tbsp. tomato paste
- 2 - cups cherry tomatoes
- 1 - cup dry white wine
- 36 - littleneck clams, scrubbed
- 6 - Tbsp. unsalted butter, cut into pieces
- 3 - Tbsp. finely chopped chives
- 4 - thick slices country-style bread

Directions:
1. Set up a Ninja Foodi oven broil for medium warmth. Finely grind the get-up-and-go from lemon half into a little bowl, at that point crush in the juice. Finely grind entire garlic clove into a bowl and blend in mayonnaise. Season garlic mayo with salt and put in a safe spot.
2. Spot a huge cast-iron skillet on the Ninja Foodi oven broil and warmth ¼ cup oil in a skillet. Include cut garlic, shallots, and Chile and cook, mixing regularly, until simply mollified, about 2MIN. Include tomato glue and cook, mixing frequently, until glue obscures somewhat, around 1 MIN. Include tomatoes and a touch of salt and cook, mixing every so often, until tomatoes mellow and discharge their juices, about 4MIN. Include wine and cook until it is nearly decreased considerably and no longer scents boozy about 3MIN.
3. Add shellfishes and margarine to the skillet and spread. Cook until shellfishes have opened, 6–10MIN, contingent upon the size of mollusks and warmth level. Expel skillet

28

from Ninja Foodi oven broil; dispose of any mollusks that don't open. Sprinkle with chives.

4. In the interim, shower bread with the staying 3 Tbsp. oil and season softly with salt. Barbecue until brilliant earthy colored and fresh, about 3MIN per side.
5. Serve mollusks with toasted bread and saved garlic mayo.
- **Nutrition Info:** Calories 282, fat 10g, carbohydrate 0g, Protein 20g.

82. Spicy Shrimp Kebab

Servings: 4
Cooking Time: 20 Minutes
Ingredients:
- 1 ½ pounds jumbo shrimp, cleaned, shelled and deveined
- 1 pound cherry tomatoes
- 2 tablespoons butter, melted
- 1 tablespoons sriracha sauce
- Sea salt and ground black pepper, to taste
- 1/2 teaspoon dried oregano
- 1/2 teaspoon dried basil
- 1 teaspoon dried parsley flakes
- 1/2 teaspoon marjoram
- 1/2 teaspoon mustard seeds

Directions:
1. Toss all ingredients in a mixing bowl until the shrimp and tomatoes are covered on all sides.
2. Soak the wooden skewers in water for 15 minutes.
3. Thread the jumbo shrimp and cherry tomatoes onto skewers. Cook in the preheated air fryer at 400 degrees f for 5 minutes, working with batches.
- **Nutrition Info:** 247 calories; 8.4g fat; 6g carbs; 36.4g protein; 3.5g sugars; 1.8g fiber

83. Garlicky Grilled Shrimp

Servings: 4
Cooking Time: 5 Minutes
Ingredients:
- 18 shrimps, shelled and deveined
- 2 tablespoons freshly squeezed lemon juice
- 1/2 teaspoon hot paprika
- 1/2 teaspoon salt
- 1 teaspoon lemon-pepper seasoning
- 2 tablespoons extra-virgin olive oil
- 2 garlic cloves, peeled and minced
- 1 teaspoon onion powder
- 1/4 teaspoon cumin powder
- 1/2 cup fresh parsley, coarsely chopped

Directions:
1. Place all the ingredients in a mixing dish; gently stir, cover and let it marinate for 30 minutes in the refrigerator.

2. Air-fry in the preheated air fryer at 400 degrees f for 5 minutes or until the shrimps turn pink.
- **Nutrition Info:** 188 calories; 8.9g fat; 3.5g carbs; 23.1g protein; 0g sugars; 0.5g fiber

84. Crispy Fish Fillet

Servings: 6
Cooking Time: 5 Minutes
Ingredients:
- 6 fish fillets
- 1 egg, beaten
- 2 tablespoons Old Bay seasoning
- 1 cup breadcrumbs
- Cooking spray

Directions:
1. Set the Ninja Foodi Grill to air fry.
2. Dip the fish fillets in egg.
3. Mix the seasoning and breadcrumbs.
4. Add the fish to the air fryer basket.
5. Cook at 400 degrees F for 5 minutes.

85. Packets Of Lemon And Dill Cod

Servings: 8
Cooking Time: 5-10 Minutes
Ingredients:
- 2 tilapia cod fillets
- Salt, pepper, and garlic powder to taste
- 2 sprigs fresh dill
- 4 slices lemon
- 2 tablespoons butter

Directions:
1. Lay out two large squares of parchment paper.
2. Place fillet in center of each parchment square and season with salt, pepper, and garlic powder.
3. On each fillet, place 1 sprig of dill, 2 lemon slices, and 1 tablespoon butter.
4. Place trivet at the bottom of your Ninja Foodi. Add 1 cup water into the pot.
5. Close parchment paper around fillets and fold to make a nice seal.
6. Place both packets in your pot. Lock the lid and cook on high pressure for 5 minutes.
7. Quickly release the pressure. Serve and enjoy!
- **Nutrition Info:** Calories: 259 Fat: 11 g Carbohydrates: 8 g Protein: 20 g

86. Authentic Garlic Salmon Meal

Servings: 3
Cooking Time: 12 Minutes
Ingredients:
- 2 salmon fillet, 6 ounces each
- 1 garlic cloves, minced
- ¼ teaspoon salt
- ¼ teaspoon fresh rosemary, minced
- 1 teaspoon lemon zest, grated

- ¼ teaspoon pepper

Directions:
1. Take a bowl and add listed ingredients except for your salmon. Mix the whole mixture well
2. Add salmon to the mix and let the fish sit in the marinade for 15 minutes
3. Pre-heat your Ninja Foodi in MED mode with the timer set to 6 minutes
4. Once you hear the beep, transfer prepared salmon over the grill grate
5. Cook for 3 minutes, flip and cook for 3 minutes more
6. Serve and enjoy once ready!
- **Nutrition Info:** Calories: 250 Fat: 8 g Saturated Fat: 3g Carbohydrates: 22 g Fiber: 3 g Sodium: 370 mg Protein: 36 g

87. Buttery Scallops

Servings: 4
Cooking Time: 5 Minutes
Ingredients:
- 2 pounds sea scallops
- ½ cup butter
- 4 garlic cloves, minced
- 4 tablespoons rosemary, chopped
- Salt and pepper to taste

Directions:
1. Set your Ninja Foodi to Sauté.
2. Add rosemary, garlic, and butter. Sauté for 1 minute.
3. Add scallops, salt, and pepper. Sauté for 2 minutes.
4. Close the crisping lid.
5. Cook for 3 minutes to 350°F.
6. Serve and enjoy!
- **Nutrition Info:** Calories: 278 g Fat: 15 g Saturated Fat: 4 g Carbohydrates: 5 g Fiber: 2 g Sodium: 502 mg Protein: 25 g

88. Garlic And Lemon Prawn Delight

Servings: 8
Cooking Time: 5 Minutes
Ingredients:
- 2 tablespoons olive oil
- 1 pound prawns
- 2 tablespoons garlic, minced
- 2/3 cup fish stock
- 1 tablespoon butter
- 2 tablespoons lemon juice
- 1 tablespoon lemon zest
- Salt and pepper to taste

Directions:
1. Set your Ninja Foodi to Sauté mode and add butter and oil. Let it heat up.
2. Stir in remaining ingredients. Lock the lid and cook on low pressure for 5 minutes.
3. Quick-release the pressure. Serve and enjoy!

- **Nutrition Info:** Calories: 236 Fat: 12 g Carbohydrates: 2 g Protein: 27 g

89. Salmon Paprika

Servings: 4
Cooking Time: 7 Minutes
Ingredients:
- 2 wild-caught salmon fillets, 1 to 1 and ½ inches thick
- 2 teaspoons paprika
- 2 teaspoons avocado oil
- Green herbs, to garnish
- Salt and pepper to taste

Directions:
1. Season salmon fillets with salt, pepper, paprika, and olive oil
2. Place Crisping basket in your Ninja Foodi
3. Preheat your Ninja Foodie at 390 degrees F
4. Place insert insider your Food and place the fillet in the insert
5. Seal the Air Crisping lid and cook for 7 minutes
6. Add herbs on top
7. Serve and enjoy!

90. Tuna Patties(1)

Servings: 2
Cooking Time:x
Ingredients:
- 2 cans tuna flakes
- 1 tablespoon mayo
- 1 teaspoon garlic powder
- 1/2 teaspoon onion powder
- 1/2 tablespoon almond flour
- 1 teaspoon dried dill
- Salt and pepper to taste
- 1 tablespoon lemon juice

Directions:
1. Mix all the ingredients in a bowl. Form patties. Set the tuna patties on the Ninja Foodi basket. Seal the crisping lid. Set it to air crisp.
2. Cook at 400 degrees for 10 minutes. Flip and cook for 5 more minutes.
- **Nutrition Info:** Calories 141, Total Fat 6.4g, Saturated Fat 0.7g, Cholesterol 17mg, Sodium 148mg, Total Carbohydrate 5.2g, Dietary Fiber 1g, Total Sugars 1.2g, Protein 17g, Potassium 48mg

91. Grilled Paprika Salmon

Servings: 2
Cooking Time: 10 Minutes
Ingredients:
- 2 salmon fillets
- Pinch paprika
- Salt and pepper to taste

Directions:
1. Insert grill grate to the Ninja Foodi Grill.

2. Choose grill function.
3. Set it to high and preheat for 10 minutes.
4. Season salmon with paprika, salt and pepper.
5. Add salmon to the grill.
6. Cook for 5 minutes per side.

92. Lemon Garlic Shrimp

Servings: 4
Cooking Time: 40 Minutes
Ingredients:
- 1 lb. shrimp, peeled and deveined
- 4 cloves garlic, minced
- 1 tablespoon lemon juice
- 1 tablespoon olive oil
- Salt to taste

Directions:
1. Mix the olive oil, salt, lemon juice, and garlic. Toss shrimp in the mixture.
2. Marinate for 15 minutes. Place the shrimp in the Ninja Foodi basket.
3. Seal the crisping lid. Select the crisp air setting.
4. Cook at 350 degrees for 8 minutes. Flip and cook for 2 more minutes.
- **Nutrition Info:** Calories 170, Total Fat 5.5g, Saturated Fat 1.1g, Cholesterol 239mg, Sodium 317mg, Total Carbohydrate 2.8g, Dietary Fiber 0.1g, Total Sugars 0.1g, Protein 26.1g, Potassium 209mg

93. Grilled Spiced Snapper With Mango And Red Onion Salad

Servings: 4
Cooking Time:30 Min
Ingredients:
- 1 (5-lb.) or 2 (2½-lb.) head-on whole fish, cleaned
- Kosher salt
- 1/3 - cup chaat masala, vadouvan, or tandoori spice
- 1/3 - cup vegetable oil, plus more for grill
- 1 - ripe but firm mango, peeled, cut into irregular 1½" pieces
- 1 - small red onion, thinly sliced, rinsed
- 1 - bunch cilantro, coarsely chopped
- 3 - Tbsp. fresh lime juice
- Extra-virgin olive oil
- Lime wedges (for serving)

Directions:
1. Spot fish on a cutting board and pat dry altogether with paper towels. With a sharp blade, make slices across on an askew along the body each 2" on the two sides, chopping right down to the bones. Season fish liberally all around with salt. Coat fish with flavor blend, pressing on more if necessary. Let sit at room temperature 20MIN.

2. In the interim, set up a Ninja Foodi oven broil for medium-high warmth. Clean and oil grind.
3. Shower the two sides of fish with staying 1/3 cup vegetable oil to cover. Ninja Foodi oven broil fish undisturbed, 10MIN. Lift up somewhat from one edge to check whether the skin is puffed and softly roasted and effectively discharges from the mesh. If not exactly prepared, take off alone for another MIN or somewhere in the vicinity and attempt once more. When it is prepared, delicately slide 2 huge metal spatulas underneath and turn over. Barbecue fish until the opposite side is daintily roasted and skin is puffed, 8–12MIN, contingent upon the size of the fish. Move to a platter.
4. Sling mango, onion, cilantro, lime juice, and a major spot of salt in a medium bowl. Sprinkle with a touch of olive oil and sling again to cover. Disperse mango plate of mixed greens over fish and present with lime wedges for pressing over.
- **Nutrition Info:** Calories 224, fat 9g, carbohydrate 17g, Protein 24g.

94. Heartfelt Sesame Fish

Servings: 8
Cooking Time: 8 Minutes
Ingredients:
- 1½ pound salmon fillet
- 1 teaspoon sesame seeds
- 1 teaspoon butter, melted
- ½ teaspoon salt
- 1 tablespoon apple cider vinegar
- ¼ teaspoon rosemary, dried

Directions:
1. Take apple cider vinegar and spray it onto the salmon fillets.
2. Then add dried rosemary, sesame seeds, butter, and salt.
3. Mix them well. Take butter sauce and brush the salmon properly.
4. Place the salmon on the rack and lower the air fryer lid. Set to Air Fry mode.
5. Cook the fish for 8 minutes at 360°F. Serve hot and enjoy!
- **Nutrition Info:** Calories: 239 Fat: 11.2 g Carbohydrates: 0.3 g Protein: 33.1 g

95. Swordfish Fillet With Salsa

Servings: 4
Cooking Time: 10 Minutes
Ingredients:
- 4 swordfish fillets
- 1 tablespoon vegetable oil
- Salt and pepper to taste
- Salsa
- 1 onion, chopped

- 2 mangoes, diced
- ½ cup cilantro, chopped
- 2 tablespoons lime juice

Directions:
1. Brush fish with oil.
2. Season both sides with salt and pepper.
3. Marinate for 5 minutes.
4. Place in the air crisp tray.
5. Select air crisp.
6. Cook at 400 degrees F for 5 minutes per side.
7. Mix the salsa ingredients in a bowl.
8. Top the fish with the salsa and serve.

96. Sweet And Sour Fish

Servings: 4
Cooking Time: 6 Minutes
Ingredients:
- 1 pound fish chunks
- 1 tablespoon vinegar
- 2 drops liquid Stevia
- ¼ cup butter
- Salt and pepper to taste

Directions:
1. Set your Ninja Foodi to Sauté.
2. Add butter and melt it.
3. Add fish chunks, sauté for 3 minutes.
4. Add Stevia, salt, pepper, stir it.
5. Close the crisping lid.
6. Cook on Air Crisp mode for 3 minutes at 360°F
7. Serve and enjoy!
- **Nutrition Info:** Calories: 274 g Fat: 15 g Saturated Fat: 4 g Carbohydrates: 2 g Fiber: 0 g Sodium: 896 mg Protein: 33 g

97. Grilled Salmon With Butter And Wine

Servings: 4
Cooking Time: 10 Minutes
Ingredients:
- 2 cloves garlic, minced
- 4 tablespoons butter, melted
- Sea salt and ground black pepper, to taste
- 1 teaspoon smoked paprika
- 1/2 teaspoon onion powder
- 1 tablespoon lime juice
- 1/4 cup dry white wine
- 4 salmon steaks

Directions:
1. Place all ingredients in a large ceramic dish. Cover and let it marinate for 30 minutes in the refrigerator.
2. Arrange the salmon steaks on the grill pan. Bake at 390 degrees for 5 minutes, or until the salmon steaks are easily flaked with a fork.
3. Flip the fish steaks, baste with the reserved marinade, and cook another 5 minutes.

- **Nutrition Info:** 516 calories; 25.6g fat; 2.4g carbs; 65.7g protein; 0.7g sugars; 0.5g fiber

98. Simple Grilled Swordfish

Servings: 4
Cooking Time: 4 Minutes
Ingredients:
- 4 (6-ounce swordfish steaks, about I inch thick
- Juice of ½ lemon
- ½ teaspoon dried oregano
- ¼ cup olive oil

Directions:
1. Rinse the fish and pat dry with paper towels.
2. Combine the olive oil, lemon juice, and oregano in a shallow baking dish large enough to fit all the swordfish steaks. Add the swordfish steaks and marinate for about 15 minutes. Turn the steaks and marinate for another 15 minutes.
3. Insert the Grill Grate and close the hood. Select GRILL, set temperature to HIGH, and set time to 8 minutes. Select START/STOP to begin preheating.
4. Sprinkle the swordfish steaks with the salt and pepper—grill for about 4 minutes. To test for doneness, prod an edge of the swordfish with a fork. The fish should flake easily. Serve immediately.
- **Nutrition Info:** Calories 327, Fat 21 g, Protein 34 g

99. Tuna Patties

Servings: 4
Cooking Time: 10 Minutes
Ingredients:
- 2 cans tuna flakes
- 1/2 tablespoon almond flour
- 1 teaspoon dried dill
- 1 tablespoon mayo
- 1/2 teaspoon onion powder
- 1 teaspoon garlic powder
- Salt and pepper to taste
- 1 tablespoon lemon juice

Directions:
1. Mix all the ingredients in a bowl.
2. Form patties.
3. Set the tuna patties on the Ninja Foodi basket.
4. Seal the crisping lid. Set it to air crisp.
5. Cook at 400 degrees for 5 minutes.
6. Flip and cook for 5 more minutes.

100.Easy Crab Cakes

Servings: 4
Cooking Time: 10 Minutes
Ingredients:
- 8 oz. lump crab
- 2 scallions, finely chopped

- 1 medium red bell pepper, deseeded and diced
- 1 tbsp. Dijon mustard
- 2 tbsp. panko bread crumbs
- 1 tsp. old bay seasoning
- 2 tbsp. mayonnaise
- Olive oil for spraying
- 4 lemon wedges for serving

Directions:
1. Insert the dripping pan in the bottom part of the air fryer and preheat the oven at Bake mode at 370 F for 2 to 3 minutes.
2. Meanwhile, in a medium bowl, mix all the ingredients except for the olive oil and lemon wedges until evenly distributed. From 4 to 6 firm patties from the mixture, arrange on the cooking tray and grease lightly with some olive oil. You may do this in two batches.
3. Fit the cooking tray on the middle rack and close the oven. Set the timer to 10 minutes and cook until the timer reads to the end, and the crab cakes are golden brown and well compacted.
4. Remove the crab cakes from the oven and serve with the lemon wedges.
- **Nutrition Info:** Calories 246, Total Fat 6.19g, Total Carbs 13.65g, Fiber 1.5g, Protein 33.16g

101.Salmon With Coconut Aminos

Servings: 4
Cooking Time: 15 Minutes
Ingredients:
- ½ teaspoon ginger powder
- ½ teaspoon garlic powder
- 1 tablespoon honey
- 4 tablespoons coconut aminos
- Salt and pepper to taste
- 3 salmon fillets

Directions:
1. In a bowl, mix ginger powder, garlic powder, honey, coconut aminos, salt, and pepper in a bowl.
2. Coat the salmon fillets with this mixture.
3. Marinate for 30 minutes, covered in the refrigerator.
4. Add fish to the air fryer basket.
5. Set your Ninja Foodi Grill to Air Fry.
6. Cook at 390°F for 10 to 15 minutes.
7. serving Suggestionss:
8. Garnish with lemon slices.
9. preparation/Cooking Tips:
10. Do not overcrowd the air fryer basket to ensure even cooking. Cook in batches if necessary.
- **Nutrition Info:** Calories: 400 Fat: 23 g Carbohydrates: 6 g Protein: 24 g

102.Marinated Scallops With Butter And Beer

Servings: 4
Cooking Time: 7 Minutes
Ingredients:
- 2 pounds sea scallops
- 1/2 cup beer
- 4 tablespoons butter
- 2 sprigs rosemary, only leaves
- Sea salt and freshly cracked black pepper, to taste

Directions:
1. In a ceramic dish, mix the sea scallops with beer; let it marinate for 1 hour.
2. Meanwhile, preheat your air fryer to 400 degrees f. Melt the butter and add the rosemary leaves. Stir for a few minutes.
3. Discard the marinade and transfer the sea scallops to the air fryer basket. Season with salt and black pepper.
4. Cook the scallops in the preheated air fryer for 7 minutes, shaking the basket halfway through the cooking time. Work in batches.
- **Nutrition Info:** 471 calories; 27.3g fat; 1.9g carbs; 54g protein; 0.2g sugars; 0.1g fiber

103.Shrimp Bang

Servings: 4
Cooking Time: 10 Minutes
Ingredients:
- 1 lb. large shrimp, peeled and deveined
- ¼ cup flour
- 2 eggs, beaten
- 2 cups breadcrumbs
- Sauce
- ¼ cup mayonnaise
- 2 tablespoons sweet chili sauce
- 2 teaspoons sriracha sauce
- 1 tablespoon honey
- 1 teaspoon rice vinegar

Directions:
1. Coat the shrimp with flour.
2. Dip in egg and then dredge with breadcrumbs.
3. Select air crisp setting.
4. Preheat at 250 degrees F for 7 minutes.
5. Add the breaded shrimp to the air crisp tray.
6. Cook at 350 degrees F for 5 minutes per side.
7. Mix the sauce ingredients.
8. Serve shrimp with sauce.

104.Lovely Crab Soup

Servings: 4
Cooking Time: Around 3 Hours
Ingredients:
- 1 cup crab meat, cubed
- 1 tablespoon garlic, minced

- Salt as needed
- Red chili flakes as needed
- 3 cups vegetable broth
- 1 teaspoon salt

Directions:
1. Coat the crab cubes in lime juice and let them sit for a while
2. Add the all ingredients (including marinated crab meat) to your Ninja Foodi and lock the lid
3. Cook on SLOW COOK MODE (MEDIUM) for 3 hours
4. Let it sit for a while
5. Unlock lid and set to Sauté mode, simmer the soup for 5 minutes more on LOW
6. Stir and check to season. Enjoy!

105. Lovely Carb Soup

Servings: 4
Cooking Time: 6-7 Hours
Ingredients:
- 1 cup crab meat, cubed
- 1 tablespoon garlic, minced
- Salt as needed
- Red chili flakes as needed
- 3 cups vegetable broth
- 1 teaspoon salt

Directions:
1. Coat the crab cubes in lime juice and let them sit for a while.
2. Add the all ingredients (including marinated crab meat) to your Ninja Foodi and lock the lid.
3. Cook on Slow Cook mode (medium) for 3 hours.
4. Let it sit for a while.
5. Unlock the lid and set to Sauté mode, simmer the soup for 5 minutes more on Low.
6. Stir and check seasoning. Enjoy!
- **Nutrition Info:** Calories: 201 Fat: 11 g Carbohydrates: 12 g Protein: 13 g

106. Salmon With Lemon & Dill

Servings: 6
Cooking Time: 20 Minutes
Ingredients:
- 6 salmon fillets
- 1 tablespoon vegetable oil
- Salt and pepper to taste
- ¼ cup mayonnaise
- 2 tablespoons Dijon mustard
- 4 tablespoons lemon juice
- 2 tablespoons dill, chopped
- 4 teaspoons garlic, minced

Directions:
1. Choose grill setting in your unit.
2. Set temperature to max.
3. Select fish.

4. Press start to preheat.
5. Brush both sides of salmon with oil.
6. Season with salt and pepper.
7. Add salmon to the grill grate.
8. In a bowl, mix the remaining ingredients.
9. Brush mixture on top side of salmon.
10. Top with lemon slices.
11. Close the unit.
12. Wait for it to beep to signal that cooking is complete.

107. Shrimp Bang Bang

Servings: 4
Cooking Time: 30 Minutes
Ingredients:
- 1/2 cup all-purpose flour
- 2 eggs, beaten
- 2 tablespoons olive oil
- 1 cup breadcrumbs
- Salt and pepper to taste
- 1 teaspoon garlic powder
- 1 lb. shrimp, peeled and deveined
- 1/2 cup mayonnaise
- 1/2 cup sweet chili sauce
- 1 tablespoon lime juice
- 1 tablespoon hot pepper sauce
- Salt to taste
- 2 teaspoons honey

Directions:
1. Add flour to a bowl.
2. Put the eggs in a second bowl.
3. Mix the breadcrumbs, salt, pepper and garlic powder in the third bowl.
4. Coat shrimp with flour and then with egg.
5. Dredge with breadcrumb blend.
6. Set Ninja Foodi Grill to air fry.
7. Cook at 400 degrees F for 15 minutes.
8. Shake and cook for another 15 minutes.
9. Combine the rest of the ingredients in a bowl.
10. Dip the shrimp in this mixture and serve.

108. Awesome Cherry Tomato Mackerel

Servings: 8
Cooking Time: 7 Minutes
Ingredients:
- 4 Mackerel fillets
- ¼ teaspoon onion powder
- ¼ teaspoon lemon powder
- ¼ teaspoon garlic powder
- ½ teaspoon salt
- 2 cups cherry tomatoes
- 3 tablespoons melted butter
- 1½ cups of water
- 1 tablespoon black olives

Directions:
1. Grease baking dish and arrange cherry tomatoes at the bottom of the dish.

2. Top with fillets. Sprinkle all spices. Drizzle melted butter on top.
3. Add water to the lower rack in the Ninja Foodi and place a baking dish on top of the rack.
4. Lock the lid and cook on low pressure for 7 minutes. Quickly release the pressure. Serve and enjoy!
- **Nutrition Info:** Calories: 325 Fat: 24 g Carbohydrates: 2 g Protein: 21 g

109.Grilled Clams With Herb Butter

Servings: 6
Cooking Time:30 Min
Ingredients:
- ½ cup (1 stick) unsalted butter, room temperature
- 1 - Tbsp chopped flat-leaf parsley
- 1 - Tbsp chopped fresh dill
- 1 - Tbsp chopped scallion
- 1 - Tbsp fresh lemon juice
- Kosher salt and freshly ground black pepper
- 24 - littleneck clams, scrubbed
- Lemon wedges

Directions:
1. Blend the initial 5 fixings in a medium bowl until all-around mixed. Season herb margarine to taste with salt and pepper.
2. Manufacture a medium-hot fire in a charcoal Ninja Foodi oven broil, or warmth a gas barbecue to high. Spot mollusks on the barbecue rack and spread Ninja Foodi oven broil with cover. Ninja Foodi oven broil until shellfishes simply open, 6 to 8MIN. Use tongs to move to a platter, being mindful so as to keep however much squeeze in the shells as could reasonably be expected.
3. Speck mollusks with herb margarine; let remain until spread melts. Serve warm with lemon wedges close by for crushing over.
- **Nutrition Info:** Calories 159, fat 12g, carbohydrate 13g, Protein 3g.

110.Teriyaki Coho Glazed Salmon

Servings: 4
Cooking Time: 25 Minutes
Ingredients:
- 1-2 coho salmon filets
- 1 tablespoon honey
- 1 and ½ tablespoons ginger roots, minced
- 2 tablespoons cornstarch
- 1 cup of water
- ¼ cup of soy sauce
- ¼ cup brown sugar
- ½ teaspoon white pepper
- ¼ cup of cold water

Directions:
1. Insert the grill grate and close the hood

2. Pre-heat Ninja Foodi by pressing the "GRILL" option and setting it to "HIGH" for 15 minutes
3. Take a medium saucepan over medium heat, combine sauce ingredients (except salmon, cornstarch and cold water) and bring to a low boil
4. Then add cornstarch and water in another bowl, whisk cornstarch mixture slowly into sauce until it thickens
5. Add one chunk of pecan wood to the hot coal of your grill
6. Brush sauce onto the salmon filet
7. Place on the grill grate, then close the hood
8. Cook for 15 minutes
9. Brush the salmon with another coat of sauce
10. Close the lid and cook for 10 minutes more
11. Serve and enjoy!
- **Nutrition Info:** Calories: 163, Fat: 0 g, Saturated Fat: 0 g, Carbohydrates: 15 g, Fiber: 3 g, Sodium: 456 mg, Protein: 0 g

111.Lovely Air Fried Scallops(1)

Servings: 8
Cooking Time: 5 Minutes
Ingredients:
- 12 scallops
- 3 tablespoons olive oil
- Salt and pepper to taste

Directions:
1. Gently rub scallops with salt, pepper, and oil
2. Transfer to the insert in the Ninja Foodi.
3. Lock the air crisping lid and cook for 4 minutes at 390°F.
4. Half through, make sure to give them a nice flip and keep cooking. Serve warm and enjoy!
- **Nutrition Info:** Calories: 372 Fat: 11 g Carbohydrates: 0.9 g Protein: 63 g

112.Spiced Up Grilled Shrimp

Servings: 4
Cooking Time: 6 Minutes
Ingredients:
- 2 tablespoons brown sugar
- 1 pound jumbo shrimp, peeled and deveined
- 2 tablespoons olive oil
- 1 tablespoon garlic powder
- 1 tablespoon paprika
- ½ teaspoon black pepper
- 1 teaspoon garlic salt

Directions:
1. Take a bowl and add listed ingredients gently mix
2. Let the mixture chill for 30-60 minutes
3. Preheat your Grill in MED mode setting timer to 6 minutes

4. Once you hear the beep, arrange your prepared shrimp over the grill grate
5. Lock and let it cook for 3 minutes
6. Flip and cook for 3 minutes more
7. Once done, serve and enjoy!
- **Nutrition Info:** Calories: 370 Fat: 27 g Saturated Fat: 3 g Carbohydrates: 23 g Fiber: 8 g Sodium: 182 mg Protein: 6 g

113.Coconut Shrimp

Servings: 4
Cooking Time:x
Ingredients:
- 1/2 cup all-purpose flour
- 1/3 cup panko bread crumbs
- 2/3 cup unsweetened coconut flakes
- 1/4 cup honey
- 1-1/2 teaspoons black pepper
- Cooking spray
- 2 eggs
- 12 oz. shrimp, peeled and deveined
- Salt and pepper to taste
- 1/4 cup lime juice

Directions:
1. Mix the flour and black pepper in a bowl. In another bowl, beat the egg.
2. In the third bowl, mix the bread crumbs and coconut flakes.
3. Dip each of the shrimp in the first, second, and third bowls.
4. Place in the Ninja Foodi basket. Set it to air crisp. Cover the crisping lid.
5. Cook at 400 degrees F for 8 minutes, turning halfway through.
6. Season with the salt and pepper.
7. Mix the remaining ingredients and serve with the shrimp.
- **Nutrition Info:** Calories 293, Total Fat 4.4g, Saturated Fat 1.3g, Cholesterol 261mg, Sodium 306mg, Total Carbohydrate 37.8g, Dietary Fiber 1.1g, Total Sugars 18.2g, Protein 25.1g, Potassium 229mg

114.Grilled Swordfish With Tomatoes And Oregano

Servings: 4
Cooking Time:40 Min
Ingredients:
- ½ cup plus 2 Tbsp. extra-virgin olive oil, plus more for grill
- 2 - Tbsp. pine nuts
- 2 - (12-oz.) swordfish steaks, about 1" thick
- Kosher salt, freshly ground pepper
- ¼ cup red wine vinegar
- 2 - Tbsp. drained capers, finely chopped
- 1 - Tbsp. finely chopped oregano, plus 2 sprigs for serving
- ½ tsp. honey

- 2 - large ripe heirloom tomatoes, halved, thickly sliced

Directions:
1. Set up a Ninja Foodi oven broil for medium-high warmth; delicately oil grind. Toast pine nuts in a dry little skillet over medium warmth, shaking frequently, until brilliant, about 4MIN. Let cool and put in a safe spot for serving.
2. Pat swordfish dry and season did with salt and pepper. Spot on a rimmed preparing sheet and let sit at room temperature 15MIN.
3. Then, whisk vinegar, tricks, hacked oregano, nectar, and½ cup oil in a little bowl to consolidate; put the marinade in a safe spot. Mastermind tomatoes on a rimmed platter, covering somewhat; put in a safe spot.
4. Rub swordfish done with the staying 2 Tbsp. oil and Ninja Foodi oven broil, undisturbed, until barbecue marks show up, about 4MIN. cautiously turn over and cook on the second side until fish is misty entirely through, about 4MIN. Move to saved platter with tomatoes and top with oregano branches. Season with increasingly salt and pepper. Pour held marinade over and let sit in any event 15MIN and as long as 60 minutes. To serve, disperse saved pine nuts over.
- **Nutrition Info:** Calories 210, fat 10g, carbohydrate 0g, Protein 30g.

115.Salmon And Kale Meal

Servings: 4
Cooking Time: 5 Minutes
Ingredients:
- 1 lemon, juiced
- 2 salmon fillets
- ¼ cup extra virgin olive oil
- 1 teaspoon Dijon mustard
- 4 cups kale, thinly sliced, ribs removed
- 1 teaspoon salt
- 1 avocado, diced
- 1 cup pomegranate seeds
- 1 cup walnuts, toasted
- 1 cup goat parmesan cheese, shredded

Directions:
1. Season salmon with salt and keep it on the side.
2. Place a trivet in your Ninja Foodi.
3. Place salmon over the trivet.
4. Lock the lid and cook on high pressure for 15 minutes.
5. Release pressure naturally over 10 minutes.
6. Transfer salmon to a serving platter.
7. Take a bowl and add kale, season with salt.
8. Take another bowl and make the dressing by adding lemon juice, Dijon mustard, olive oil, and red wine vinegar.

9. Season kale with dressing, and add diced avocado, pomegranate seeds, walnuts, and cheese.
10. Toss and serve with the fish.
11. Enjoy!
- **Nutrition Info:** Calories: 234 Fat: 14 g Saturated Fat: 6 g Carbohydrates: 12 g Fiber: 2 g Sodium: 118 mg Protein: 16 g

116.Grilled Salmon Steaks With Cilantro-garlic Yogurt Sauce

Servings: 4
Cooking Time:30 Min
Ingredients:
- Vegetable oil (for the grill)
- 2 - Serrano chiles
- 2 - garlic cloves
- 1 - cup cilantro leaves with tender stems
- ½ - cup plain whole-milk Greek yogurt
- 1 - Tbsp. extra-virgin olive oil
- 1 - tsp. honey
- 2 - (12-oz.) bone-in salmon steaks
- Kosher salt

Directions:
1. Set up a Ninja Foodi oven broil for medium-high warmth; oil grind. Expel and dispose of seeds from 1 Chile. Purée the two chiles, garlic, cilantro, yogurt, oil, nectar, and ¼ cup water in a blender until smooth; season well with salt. Move half of sauce to a little bowl and put in a safe spot for serving.
2. Season salmon steaks daintily with salt. Barbecue, turning on more than one occasion until substance is beginning to turn misty, about 4MIN. Keep on Ninja Foodi oven broiling, turning regularly and seasoning with residual sauce, until misty completely through, about 4MIN longer. Present with held sauce nearby.
- **Nutrition Info:** Calories 282, fat 15g, carbohydrate 0g, Protein 34g.

117.Adventurous Sweet And Sour Fish

Servings: 8
Cooking Time: 6 Minutes
Ingredients:
- 2 drops liquid Stevia
- ¼ cup butter
- 1 pound fish chunks
- 1 tablespoon vinegar
- Salt and pepper to taste

Directions:
1. Set your Ninja Foodi to Sauté mode. Add butter and let it melt.
2. Add fish chunks and Sauté for 3 minutes. Add Stevia, salt, and pepper and stir.
3. Lock the crisping lid and cook on Air Crisp mode for 3 minutes at 360°F.
4. Serve once done and enjoy!
- **Nutrition Info:** Calories: 274 Fat: 15 g Carbohydrates: 2 g Protein: 33 g

118.Grilled Citrus Fish

Servings: 2
Cooking Time: 15 Minutes
Ingredients:
- 2 tablespoons oil
- 2 tablespoons honey
- 1 tablespoon orange juice
- 1 tablespoon lemon juice
- 1 teaspoon orange zest
- 1 teaspoon lemon zest
- 1 teaspoon garlic, minced
- 1 teaspoon ginger, minced
- 1 tablespoon parsley, minced
- Salt and pepper to taste
- 2 white fish fillets

Directions:
1. Add grill grate to the Ninja Foodi Grill.
2. Choose grill function.
3. Set it to high.
4. Set the time to 15 minutes and press start.
5. Mix all the ingredients except fish fillets.
6. Spread half of the mixture on both sides of the fish.
7. Add fish fillets to the grill grate.
8. Close the hood and grill for 15 minutes, brushing with the remaining mixture.

119.Swordfish With Caper Sauce

Servings: 4
Cooking Time: 8 Minutes
Ingredients:
- Pepper as needed
- Salt as needed
- 2 tablespoon capers drained
- 1 tablespoon extra virgin olive oil
- 1 tablespoon lemon juice
- 1 lemon, sliced into 8 slices
- 4 tablespoons unsalted butter
- 4 swordfish steaks, 1 inch thick

Directions:
1. Take a large shallow bowl and whisk together the lemon juice and oil
2. Season with swordfish steaks with salt and pepper on each side, place in the oil mixture
3. Turn to coat both sides and refrigerate for 15 minutes
4. Insert the grill grate and close the hood
5. Pre-heat Ninja Foodi by pressing the "GRILL" option at and setting it to "MAX" and timer to 8 minutes
6. Let it pre-heat until you hear a beep
7. Arrange the swordfish over the grill grate, lock lid and cook for 9 minutes
8. Place a medium saucepan over medium heat and melt butter
9. Add the lemon slices and capers to the pan and cook for 1 minute
10. Then turn off the heat
11. Remove the swordfish from the grill and serve with caper sauce over it
12. Enjoy!

- **Nutrition Info:** Calories: 472 Fat: 31 g Saturated Fat: 6 g Carbohydrates: 2 g Fiber: 0.5 g Sodium: 540 mg Protein: 48 g

120.Japanese Flounder With Chives

Servings: 4
Cooking Time: 12 Minutes
Ingredients:
- 4 flounder fillets
- Sea salt and freshly cracked mixed peppercorns, to taste
- 1 ½ tablespoons dark sesame oil
- 2 tablespoons sake
- 1/4 cup soy sauce
- 1 tablespoon grated lemon rind
- 2 garlic cloves, minced
- 2 tablespoons chopped chives, to serve

Directions:
1. Place all the ingredients, without the chives, in a large-sized mixing dish. Cover and allow it to marinate for about 2 hours in your fridge.
2. Remove the fish from the marinade and cook in the air fryer cooking basket at 360 degrees f for 10 to 12 minutes; flip once during cooking.
3. Pour the remaining marinade into a pan that is preheated over a medium-low heat; let it simmer, stirring continuously, until it has thickened.
4. Pour the prepared glaze over flounder and serve garnished with fresh chives.
- **Nutrition Info:** 288 calories; 18.3g fat; 5.1g carbs; 19.8g protein; 3.2g sugars; 0.4g fiber

121.Grilled Turbot With Celery Leaf Salsa Verde

Servings: 8
Cooking Time:40 Min
Ingredients:
- 2 - whole turbot, heads and fins removed, split in half along the backbone
- 1¼ cups extra-virgin olive oil, divided
- Kosher salt
- 8 - sprigs rosemary, divided
- 1½ cups finely chopped parsley
- ½ cup finely chopped celery leaves
- 1 - garlic clove, finely grated
- ½ - lemon
- ½ tsp. Aleppo-style or other mild red pepper flakes
- Freshly ground black pepper
- Aioli or store-bought mayonnaise (for serving)

Directions:
1. Set up a Ninja Foodi oven broil for medium-low backhanded warmth. Detach 4 huge sheets of foil. Rub fish with ½ cup oil (2 Tbsp. per piece) and season with salt. Working each in turn, place a filet in the focal point of a sheet of foil and top with 2 rosemary twigs. Crease in short sides of the foil over fish, at that point overlap in long sides and move edges together to seal.
2. Spot pockets on the cool side of the Ninja Foodi oven broil, spread barbecue, and cook fish, turning once, 20–25MIN. open a pocket to check fish. The substance ought to be somewhat murky and the tip of a blade should slide through without any problem. Barbecue somewhat more if necessary.
3. In the interim, consolidate parsley, celery leaves, and garlic in a medium bowl. Finely get-up-and-go the lemon into a bowl, at that point crush in the juice. Include red pepper drops and blend in remaining ¾ cup oil; season with salt and dark pepper. Let salsa Verde sits 10MIN for flavors to meet up.
4. Move fish to a platter and present with salsa Verde and aioli
- **Nutrition Info:** Calories 234, fat 10g, carbohydrate 0g, Protein 33g.

122.Crispy Cod Fish

Servings: 4
Cooking Time: 15 Minutes
Ingredients:
- 4 cod fish fillets
- Salt and sugar to taste
- 1 teaspoon sesame oil
- 250 ml water
- 5 tablespoons light soy sauce
- 1 teaspoon dark soy sauce
- 3 tablespoons oil
- 5 slices ginger

Directions:
1. Pat the cod fillets dry.
2. Season with the salt, sugar, and sesame oil. Marinate for 15 minutes.
3. Set the Ninja Foodi to Air Crisp.
4. Put the fish on top of the basket. Cook at 350°F for 3 minutes.
5. Flip and cook for 2 minutes. Take the fish out and set aside.
6. Put the rest of the ingredients in the pot.
7. Set it to Sauté. Simmer and pour over the fish before serving.
8. serving Suggestions:
9. Top with chopped green onion.
- **Nutrition Info:** Calories: 303 Total Fat: 13.1 g Saturated Fat: 1.9 g Cholesterol: 99 mg Sodium: 144 mg Total Carbohydrate: 2.9 g Dietary Fiber: 0.5 g Total Sugars: 0.1 g Protein: 41.5 g Potassium: 494 mg

123.Crumbed Flounder Fillet

Servings: 4
Cooking Time: 12 Minutes
Ingredients:
- ¼ cup vegetable oil
- 1 cup breadcrumbs
- 4 flounder fillets

- 1 egg, beaten

Directions:
1. Set Ninja Foodi Grill to Air Fry.
2. Preheat to 350°F.
3. Combine oil and breadcrumbs in a bowl.
4. Mix until crumbly.
5. Coat the fish with the egg and dredge with the breadcrumb mixture.
6. Add fish fillets to the air fryer basket.
7. Cook for 12 minutes.
8. serving Suggestionss:
9. Garnish with lemon wedges.
10. preparation/Cooking Tips:
11. You can also use olive oil in place of vegetable oil.
- **Nutrition Info:** Calories: 257 Fat: 19 g Carbohydrates: 5 g Protein: 14 g

124. Home Haddock

Servings: 3
Cooking Time: 13 Minutes
Ingredients:
- ¼ teaspoon salt
- ¾ cup breadcrumbs
- ¼ cup parmesan cheese, grated
- ¼ teaspoon ground thyme
- ¼ cup butter, melted
- 1 pound haddock fillets
- ¾ cup milk

Directions:
1. Take the fish fillets and carefully dredge them in milk
2. Season them well with salt, keep them on the side
3. Take a medium-sized bowl, add cheese, thyme, parmesan, breadcrumbs, and mix
4. Take your fillets and coat them with breadcrumbs
5. Pre-heat your Ninja Foodi Grill in Bake mode to a temperature of 325 degrees F, setting the timer to 13 minutes
6. Once you hear the beep, the appliance is ready
7. Transfer the prepared fillets to Grill Grate and cook for 8 minutes, flip and cook for 5 minutes more
8. Once you have a flaky texture, serve, and enjoy!
- **Nutrition Info:** Calories: 450 Fat: 27 g Saturated Fat: 12 g Carbohydrates: 16 g Fiber: 22 g Sodium: 1056 mg Protein: 44 g

125. Tilapia With Cheesy Caper Sauce

Servings: 4
Cooking Time: 12 Minutes
Ingredients:
- 4 tilapia fillets
- 1 tablespoon extra-virgin olive oil
- Celery salt, to taste
- Freshly cracked pink peppercorns, to taste
- For the creamy caper sauce:

- 1/2 cup crème fraîche
- 2 tablespoons mayonnaise
- 1/4 cup cottage cheese, at room temperature
- 1 tablespoon capers, finely chopped

Directions:
1. Toss the tilapia fillets with olive oil, celery salt, and cracked peppercorns until they are well coated.
2. Place the fillets in a single layer at the bottom of the air fryer cooking basket. Air-fry at 360 degrees f for about 12 minutes; turn them over once during cooking.
3. Meanwhile, prepare the sauce by mixing the remaining items.
4. Lastly, garnish air-fried tilapia fillets with the sauce and serve immediately!
- **Nutrition Info:** 253 calories; 13.1g fat; 3.5g carbs; 21.5g protein; 0.6g sugars; 0.1g fiber

126. Shrimp Fajitas

Servings: 12
Cooking Time: 20 Minutes
Ingredients:
- 1 lb. shrimp, peeled and deveined
- 1 onion, diced
- 1 red bell pepper, chopped
- 1 green bell pepper, chopped
- 2 tablespoons taco seasoning
- Cooking spray
- Tortillas

Directions:
1. Spray air fryer basket with oil.
2. Mix shrimp, onion and bell peppers in a bowl.
3. Spray with oil and season with taco seasoning.
4. Set your Ninja Foodi Grill to air fry.
5. Add shrimp mixture to the air fryer basket.
6. Air fry at 390 degrees F for 10 to 12 minutes.
7. Shake and cook for another 10 minutes.
8. Spread on top of tortillas.

127. Buttered Up Scallops

Servings: 8
Cooking Time: 5 Minutes
Ingredients:
- 4 garlic cloves, minced
- 4 tablespoons rosemary, chopped
- 2 pounds sea scallops
- ½ cup butter
- Salt and pepper to taste

Directions:
1. Set your Ninja Foodi to Sauté and add butter, rosemary, and garlic.
2. Sauté for 1 minute. Add scallops, salt, and pepper.
3. Sauté for 2 minutes. Lock the crisping lid and crisp for 3 minutes at 350°F. Serve and enjoy!

- **Nutrition Info:** Calories: 279 Fat: 16 g Carbohydrates: 5 g Protein: 25 g

128.Garlicky Grilled Squid With Marinated Peppers

Servings: 4
Cooking Time:20 Min
Ingredients:
- 1/3 - cup coarsely chopped blanched hazelnuts or almonds
- 2 - Tbsp. plus½ cup extra-virgin olive oil, divided
- Kosher salt
- 4 - large red bell peppers
- 2 - Tbsp. sherry vinegar or red wine vinegar
- 1 - tsp. hot smoked Spanish paprika
- 3 - garlic cloves, divided
- 1½ lb. cleaned squid, bodies and tentacles separated
- ½ - small red onion, very thinly sliced
- 1 - cup mint leaves, torn if large
- ½ lemon

Directions:
1. Preheat stove to 350°F. Toast hazelnuts on a rimmed preparing sheet, hurling once, until brilliant earthy colored, 7–10MIN. Let cool, at that point pulverize nuts utilizing the side of a culinary expert's blade or coarsely cleave. Move to a little bowl. Blend in 2 Tbsp. oil and season with salt. Put in a safe spot.
2. Set up a Ninja Foodi oven broil for high warmth and spot a wire rack on one side, arranging it opposite to the barbecue grind. Spot chime peppers legitimately on the mesh and Ninja Foodi oven broil, turning at times, until roasted all finished and substance is delicate, 8–10MIN.
3. Move ringer peppers to a medium bowl and spread firmly with cling wrap. Let sit 10–20MIN. Take skins out from peppers and scoop out seeds; dispose of. Tear or cut peppers into big pieces and spot them in a perfect medium bowl. Include vinegar, paprika, and ¼ cup oil and finely grind 1 garlic clove into a bowl. Season with salt and hurl well to cover peppers.
4. Return Ninja Foodi oven broil to high warmth. Finely grind the staying 2 garlic cloves into a huge bowl; mix remaining ¼ cup oil. Pat squid dry at that point add to oil blend; hurl well to cover. Working in clumps, Ninja Foodi oven broil squid on a wire rack on the barbecue until marks show up on bodies and limbs start too fresh around the edges, 45–60 seconds for each side. Move to a perfect huge bowl and season with salt.
5. Spot onion and Mint in a little bowl. Finely grind the pizzazz from lemon half-finished; at that point crush in the juice. Season with salt and hurl to join.
6. Partition marinated peppers and squid among plates. Spoon hazelnuts over and top with Mint plate of mixed greens.
- **Nutrition Info:** Calories 105, fat 1g, carbohydrate 12g, Protein 13g.

129.Grilled Lemon Pepper Shrimp

Servings: 4
Cooking Time: 10 Minutes
Ingredients:
- 1 lb. shrimp, peeled and deveined
- Cooking spray
- Pinch lemon pepper seasoning

Directions:
1. Spray the shrimp with oil.
2. Sprinkle with lemon pepper seasoning.
3. Set Ninja Foodi Grill to air fry.
4. Cook at 350 degrees F for 3 to 5 minutes per side.

130.Parmesan And Paprika Baked Tilapia

Servings: 6
Cooking Time: 15 Minutes
Ingredients:
- 1 cup parmesan cheese, grated
- 1 teaspoon paprika
- 1 teaspoon dried dill weed
- 2 pounds tilapia fillets
- 1/3 cup mayonnaise
- 1/2 tablespoon lime juice
- Salt and ground black pepper, to taste

Directions:
1. Mix the mayonnaise, parmesan, paprika, salt, black pepper, and dill weed until everything is thoroughly combined.
2. Then, drizzle tilapia fillets with the lime juice.
3. Cover each fish fillet with parmesan/mayo mixture; roll them in parmesan/paprika mixture. Bake at 335 for about 10 minutes. Serve and eat warm.
- **Nutrition Info:** 294 calories; 16.1g fat; 2.7g carbs; 35.9g protein; 0.1g sugars; 0.2g fiber

MEAT RECIPES

131.Ninja Foodi Grilled Steaks

Servings: 2 To 3
Cooking Time: 1½ Hrs, Or Up To 4 Days
Ingredients:
- 2 - large ribeye or
- Kosher salt and freshly ground black pepper

Directions:
1. Season steaks liberally with salt. Set on a plate and let relaxation for at the least 40MIN or up to four days. If resting longer than 40MIN, transfer to a twine rack set in a rimmed baking sheet and refrigerate, uncovered, until equipped to prepare dinner.
2. Light one chimney complete of charcoal. When all charcoal is lit and included with gray ash, pour out and set up coals on one facet of the charcoal grate. Set cooking grate in location, cowl grill, and permit to preheat for 5MIN. Clean and oil grilling grate. Season steak with pepper and area at the cooler side of the grill. Cover and prepare dinner, with all vents open, flipping and taking temperature every few MIN until steaks sign in 105°F (41°C) for medium-uncommon or one hundred 15°F (46°C) for medium on an immediate-read thermometer, 10 to 15MIN total.
3. Transfer steaks to the recent aspect of grill and prepare dinner, flipping often till a deep char has developed an inner temperature registers a hundred 25°F (fifty two°C) for medium-rare or 135°F (fifty seven°C) for medium, about 2MIN overall. Transfer steaks to a reducing board and allow to relaxation for at the least 5MIN and up to ten. Carve and serve straight away.
- **Nutrition Info:** Calories 212, fat 10g, carbohydrate 0g, Protein 38g.

132.Hybrid Beef Prime Roast

Servings: 4
Cooking Time: 45 Minutes
Ingredients:
- 2 pounds chuck roast
- 1 tablespoon olive oil
- 1 teaspoon salt
- 1 teaspoon ground black pepper
- 1 teaspoon onion powder
- 1 teaspoon garlic powder
- 4 cups beef stock

Directions:
1. Place roast in Ninja Food pot and season it well with salt and pepper

2. Add oil and set the pot to Sauté mode, sear each side of the roast for 3 minutes until lightly browned
3. Add beef broth, onion powder, garlic powder, and stir
4. Lock lid and cook on HIGH pressure for 40 minutes
5. Once the timer goes off, naturally release the pressure over 10 minutes
6. Open the lid and serve hot. Enjoy!

133.Ninja Foodi Barbecue Short Ribs

Servings: 6-8
Cooking Time: 5 Hrs
Ingredients:
- For the rub
- 3 Tbsp Kosher salt
- 2 - Tbsp black pepper
- 2 - Tbsp white pepper
- 1 - Tbsp paprika
- 2 - teaspoon garlic powder
- 8 - full short ribs, cut into individual ribs
- 1 - cup apple juice in a spray bottle
- 3 to 4 - chunks of medium smoking wood,

Directions:
1. In a little bowl join dark pepper, white pepper, salt, paprika, and garlic powder to make the rub. Season ribs all over generously with the rub.
2. Fire up smoker or barbecue to 225°F, including pieces of smoking wood lumps when at temperature. At the point when the wood is touched off and creating smoke, place the ribs in the smoker or Ninja Foodi oven broil, meat side up, and smoke until ribs arrive at 180 degrees on a moment read thermometer embedded into the center of the meat, around 4 to 5 HRS. Shower ribs with squeezed apple consistently during cooking.
3. Take ribs out from the smoker, let rest for 10MIN, at that point serve.
- **Nutrition Info:** Calories 249, fat 22g, carbohydrate 0g, Protein 11g.

134.Lamb Curry

Servings: 4
Cooking Time: 10minutes
Ingredients:
- 1½ lb. lamb stew meat, cubed
- 1 tablespoon lime juice
- 4 cloves garlic, minced
- ½ cup coconut milk
- 1-inch piece fresh ginger, grated
- Salt and pepper to taste
- 1 tablespoon coconut oil
- 14 oz. diced tomatoes

- ¾ teaspoon turmeric
- 1 tablespoon curry powder
- 1 onion, diced
- 3 carrots, sliced

Directions:
1. In a bowl, toss the lamb meat in lime juice, garlic, coconut milk, ginger, salt, and pepper. Marinate for 30 minutes.
2. Put the meat with its marinade and the rest of the ingredients into the Ninja Foodi.
3. Mix well. Seal the pot. Set it to Pressure. Cook at high pressure for 20 minutes.
4. Release the pressure naturally.
5. serving Suggestions:
6. Garnish with chopped cilantro.
- **Nutrition Info:** Calories: 631 Total Fat: 31.4 g Saturated Fat: 18.4 g Cholesterol: 204 mg Sodium: 230 mg Total Carbohydrate: 19.7 g Dietary Fiber: 5.7 g Total Sugars: 9.5 g Protein: 67.2 g Potassium: 1490 mg

135.Panko Chicken Breast

Servings: 2
Cooking Time: 15 Minutes
Ingredients:
- 1 large egg, beaten
- 1/4 cup flour, preferably all-purpose
- 3/4 cup panko bread crumbs
- 1/3 cup Parmesan, freshly grated
- 2 tsp lemon zest
- 1 tsp dried oregano
- 1/2 tsp cayenne pepper
- Salt
- Black pepper
- 2 chicken breasts, boneless skinless

Directions:
1. Beat eggs in one bowl and spread the flour in another shallow bowl.
2. Whisk panko with cayenne, salt, black pepper, oregano, lemon zest, and parmesan in a shallow tray.
3. Take the chicken breasts and coat them with flour, then dip in eggs.
4. Coat the chicken breasts with the panko mixture and place them in the Air Fryer.
5. Place this Air Fryer inside the Ninja Foodi Oven and Close its lid.
6. Rotate the Ninja Foodi dial to select the "Air Fry" mode.
7. Press the Time button and again use the dial to set the cooking time to 10 minutes.
8. Now press the Temp button and rotate the dial to set the temperature at 350 degrees F.
9. Flip the chicken and return to cooking for another 5 minutes on the same mode and temperature.
10. Serve warm.

- **Nutrition Info:** Calories 453 ; Fat 2.4 g ; Carbs 18 g ; Fiber 2.3 g ; Sugar 1.2 g ; Protein 23.2 g

136.Mediterranean Lamb Roast

Servings: 4
Cooking Time: 10minutes
Ingredients:
- 2 tablespoons olive oil
- 5 lb. leg of lamb
- Salt and pepper to taste
- 1 teaspoon dried marjoram
- 3 cloves garlic, minced
- 1 teaspoon dried sage
- 1 teaspoon dried thyme
- 1 teaspoon ground ginger
- 1 bay leaf, crushed
- 2 cups broth
- 3 lb. potatoes, sliced into cubes
- 2 tablespoons arrowroot powder
- 1/3 cup water

Directions:
1. Set the Ninja Foodi to Sauté. Pour in the olive oil. Add the lamb.
2. Coat with the oil. Season with the herbs and spices. Sear on both sides.
3. Pour in the broth. Add the potatoes. Close the pot. Set it to Pressure.
4. Cook at high pressure for 50 minutes. Release the pressure naturally.
5. Dissolve the arrowroot powder in water.
6. Stir in the diluted arrowroot powder into the cooking liquid.
7. Let sit for a few minutes before serving.
8. serving Suggestions:
9. Serve with cauliflower rice.
- **Nutrition Info:** Calories: 688 Total Fat: 24.8 g Saturated Fat: 8.1 g Cholesterol: 255 mg Sodium: 417 mg Total Carbohydrate: 27.7 g Dietary Fiber: 4.2 g Total Sugars: 2.2 g Protein: 83.8 g Potassium: 1705 mg

137.One Dish Chicken Bake

Servings: 4
Cooking Time: 40 Minutes
Ingredients:
- 1 can (14.5 oz.) canned tomatoes, diced
- 1 tbsp olive oil
- 2 tbsp fresh parsley, chopped
- 1 yellow onion, chopped
- 3 garlic cloves, minced
- 1 tsp dried oregano
- 4 boneless chicken breasts
- Salt and black pepper, to taste
- 3/4 cup gruyere cheese, grated
- 1 tsp Italian seasoning
- 1 tbsp parsley, for garnish

Directions:

1. Grease the Ninja baking dish with cooking spray.
2. Toss the tomatoes with olive oil, garlic, onions, Italian seasoning, oregano, and parsley in a bowl.
3. Spread this tomato mixture in the prepared baking dish.
4. Rub the chicken with salt, and black pepper then place over the tomatoes.
5. Transfer this baking dish to the Ninja oven and Close its lid.
6. Rotate the Ninja Foodi dial to select the "Bake" mode.
7. Press the Time button and again use the dial to set the cooking time to 35 minutes.
8. Now press the Temp button and rotate the dial to set the temperature at 400 degrees F.
9. Drizzle the cheese over the chicken and bake for 5 minutes.
10. Serve warm.
- **Nutrition Info:** Calories 297 ; Fat 14 g ; Carbs 8 g ; Fiber 1 g ; Sugar 3 g ; Protein 32 g

138.Chicken Quesadilla

Servings: 8
Cooking Time: 30 Minutes
Ingredients:
- 4 tortillas
- Cooking spray
- 1/2 cup sour cream
- 1/2 cup salsa
- Hot sauce
- 12 oz. chicken breast fillet, chopped and grilled
- 3 jalapeño peppers, diced
- 2 cups cheddar cheese, shredded
- Chopped scallions

Directions:
1. Add grill grate to the Ninja Foodi Grill.
2. Close the hood.
3. Choose grill setting.
4. Preheat for 5 minutes.
5. While waiting, spray tortillas with oil.
6. In a bowl, mix sour cream, salsa and hot sauce. Set aside.
7. Add tortilla to the grate.
8. Grill for 1 minute.
9. Repeat with the other tortillas.
10. Spread the toasted tortilla with the salsa mixture, chicken, jalapeño peppers, cheese and scallions.
11. Place a tortilla on top. Press.
12. Repeat these steps with the remaining 2 tortillas.
13. Take the grill out of the pot.
14. Choose roast setting.
15. Cook the quesadillas at 350 degrees F for 25 minutes.

139.Chicken Margherita

Servings: 8
Cooking Time: 15 Mins
Ingredients:
- 4 tbsp vegetable oil
- 1 1/2 cups of balsamic vinegar
- 6 minced garlic cloves
- Cilantro, rosemary, and pepper for seasoning (about ¼ tsp of each)
- ½ tsp salt
- 8 chicken breast fillets
- 8 slices of mozzarella cheese
- 2 diced tomatoes
- 1/2 cup fresh chopped basil

Directions:
1. Whisk the vinegar, cloves, oil, and seasoning to make a marinade. Soak the chicken for a half hour.
2. Place your Ninja Foodi grill grate in the unit and close the hood. Choose GRILL, set temperature to HIGH, and set time to 15 minutes. Select START/STOP to start your pre-heating.
3. When pre-heating is done, place the marinated chicken onto the grill and cook for 6 minutes.
4. Top chicken with cheese, tomatoes, and basil
5. Resume cooking for a further 5 – 10 mins or until the chicken is golden brown
6. Serve immediately
- **Nutrition Info:** Calories: 514 Fat: 26g Saturated Fat: 5g Trans Fat: 0g Carbohydrates: 30g Fiber: 2g Sodium: 24mg Protein: 37g

140.Beef Chops With English Mustard And Coriander

Servings: 3
Cooking Time: 27 Minutes
Ingredients:
- 1 ½ teaspoon english mustard
- 3 boneless beef chops
- 1/3 teaspoon garlic pepper
- 2 teaspoons oregano, dried
- 2 tablespoons vegetable oil
- 1 ½ tablespoons fresh coriander, chopped
- 1/2 teaspoon onion powder
- 1/2 teaspoon basil, dried
- Grated rind of 1/2 small-sized lime
- 1/2 teaspoon fine sea salt

Directions:
1. Firstly, make the rub for the beef chops by mixing all the ingredients, except the chops and the new potatoes.
2. Now, evenly spread the beef chops with the english mustard rub.

3. Then, arrange the new potatoes in the bottom of the air fryer cooking basket. Top them with the prepared beef chops.
4. Roast for about 27 minutes at 365 degrees f, turning halfway through. Serve on individual plates with a keto salad on the side, if desired.
- **Nutrition Info:** 402 calories; 44.5g fat; 2g carbs; 31.9g protein; 0.4g sugars; 0.6g fiber

141.Cheeseburger

Servings: 4
Cooking Time: 10 Minutes
Ingredients:
- 1 1/2 lb. ground beef
- 1 egg, beaten
- 1 tablespoon breadcrumbs
- 4 cheese slices
- 1 onion, minced
- Salt and pepper to taste
- 1 red bell pepper, chopped
- 4 burger buns

Directions:
1. Insert grill grate to your Ninja Foodi Grill.
2. Choose grill setting.
3. Set it to high. Set time to 10 minutes.
4. Preheat your unit.
5. In a bowl, mix ground beef, onion, bell pepper, breadcrumbs and egg.
6. Form patties from the mixture.
7. Season patties with salt and pepper.
8. Add patties to the grill.
9. Cook for 8 to 10 minutes.
10. Add cheese on top of the beef and cook for another 1 minute.
11. Serve patties and cheese on burger buns.
12. Serving Suggestions: Serve with desired condiments.

142.Roast Beef With Chimichurri

Servings: 6
Cooking Time: 30 Minutes
Ingredients:
- 2 lb. roast beef
- 2 tablespoons olive oil
- Salt and pepper to taste
- Chimichurri
- ¼ cup olive oil
- ½ cup cilantro
- ½ cup parsley
- 2 tablespoons fresh oregano, sliced
- ¼ red wine vinegar
- 2 cloves garlic, minced
- Salt and pepper to taste

Directions:
1. Preheat your unit by pressing air crisp.
2. Press start.
3. Preheat for 4 minutes.
4. Brush roast beef with oil.

5. Season with salt and pepper.
6. Select roast function.
7. Cook at 250 degrees F for 3 hours.
8. Add all the ingredients to a food processor.
9. Pulse until smooth.
10. Serve the roast beef with chimichurri.

143.Eggs And Sausage With Keto Rolls

Servings: 6
Cooking Time: 14 Minutes
Ingredients:
- 1 teaspoon dried dill weed
- 1 teaspoon mustard seeds
- 6 turkey sausages
- 3 bell peppers, seeded and thinly sliced
- 6 medium-sized eggs
- 1/2 teaspoon fennel seeds
- 1 teaspoon sea salt
- 1/3 teaspoon freshly cracked pink peppercorns
- Keto rolls:
- 1/2 cup ricotta cheese, crumbled
- 1 cup part skim mozzarella cheese, shredded
- 1 egg
- 1/2 cup coconut flour
- 1/2 cup almond flour
- 1 teaspoon baking soda
- 2 tablespoons plain whey protein isolate

Directions:
1. Set your air fryer to cook at 325 degrees f. Cook the sausages and bell peppers in the air fryer cooking basket for 8 minutes.
2. Crack the eggs into the ramekins; sprinkle them with salt, dill weed, mustard seeds, fennel seeds, and cracked peppercorns. Cook an additional 12 minutes at 395 degrees f.
3. To make the keto rolls, microwave the cheese for 1 minute 30 seconds, stirring twice. Add the cheese to the bowl of a food processor and blend well. Fold in the egg and mix again.
4. Add in the flour, baking soda, and plain whey protein isolate; blend again. Scrape the batter onto the center of a lightly greased cling film.
5. Form the dough into a disk and transfer to your freezer to cool; cut into 6 pieces and transfer to a parchment-lined baking pan (make sure to grease your hands.
6. Bake in the preheated oven at 400 degrees f for about 14 minutes.
7. Serve eggs and sausages on keto rolls.
- **Nutrition Info:** 494 calories; 30.1g fat; 9.2g carbs; 45.1g protein; 2.3g sugars; 2.1g fiber

144.Primavera Chicken

Servings: 4

Cooking Time: 25 Minutes
Ingredients:
- 4 boneless chicken breasts
- 2 tbsp olive oil
- Salt, to taste
- Black pepper, to taste
- 1 zucchini, sliced
- 3 medium tomatoes, sliced
- 1/2 red onion, sliced
- 1 cup mozzarella, cheese shredded
- 1 tsp Italian seasoning
- 2 yellow bell peppers, sliced
- Freshly parsley, for garnish

Directions:
1. Carve one side slit in the chicken breasts and stuff them with all the veggies.
2. Place these stuffed chicken breasts in a casserole dish, then drizzle oil, Italian seasoning, black pepper, salt, and Mozzarella over the chicken.
3. Place this casserole dish in the Ninja Foodi Oven and Close its lid.
4. Rotate the Ninja Foodi dial to select the "Bake" mode.
5. Press the Time button and again use the dial to set the cooking time to 25 minutes.
6. Now press the Temp button and rotate the dial to set the temperature at 370 degrees F.
7. Garnish with parsley and serve warm.
- **Nutrition Info:** Calories 440 ; Fat 7.9 g ; Carbs 21.8 g ; Sugar 7.1 g ; Fiber 2.6 g ; Protein 37.2 g

145.Grilled Herbed Steak

Servings: 4
Cooking Time: 10 Minutes
Ingredients:
- 4 steaks
- 4 sprigs rosemary, chopped
- 1 teaspoon dried basil
- 1 teaspoon dried tarragon
- Garlic salt to taste

Directions:
1. Add grill grate to the Ninja Foodi Grill.
2. Close the hood and choose grill setting.
3. Set it to 15 minutes.
4. Set it to high.
5. Press start to preheat.
6. Rub both sides of steak with garlic salt.
7. Sprinkle with herbs.
8. Add steaks to the grill grate.
9. Cook for 5 minutes per side.
10. Serving Suggestions: Garnish with fresh rosemary sprig.

146.Middle Eastern Lamb Stew

Servings: 4
Cooking Time: 20 Minutes
Ingredients:

- 2 tablespoons olive oil
- 1½ lb. lamb stew meat, sliced into cubes
- 1 onion, diced
- 6 garlic cloves, chopped
- 1 teaspoon cumin
- 1 teaspoon coriander
- 1 teaspoon turmeric
- 1 teaspoon cinnamon
- Salt and pepper to taste
- 2 tablespoons tomato paste
- ¼ cup red wine vinegar
- 2 tablespoons honey
- 1¼ cups chicken broth
- 15 oz. chickpeas, rinsed and drained
- ¼ cup raisins

Directions:
1. Choose Sauté on the Ninja Foodi. Add the oil. Cook the onion for 3 minutes.
2. Add the lamb and seasonings. Cook for 5 minutes, stirring frequently.
3. Stir in the rest of the ingredients. Cover the pot. Set it to Pressure.
4. Cook on high pressure for 50 minutes. Release the pressure naturally.
5. serving Suggestions:
6. Serve with quinoa.
- **Nutrition Info:** Calories: 867 Total Fat: 26.6 g Saturated Fat: 6.3 g Cholesterol: 153 mg Sodium: 406 mg Total Carbohydrate: 87.4 g Dietary Fiber: 20.4 g Total Sugars: 27.9 g Protein: 71.2 g Potassium: 1815 mg

147.Loaded Turkey Meatloaf With Cheese

Servings: 6
Cooking Time: 45 Minutes
Ingredients:
- 2 pounds turkey mince
- 1/2 cup scallions, finely chopped
- 2 garlic cloves, finely minced
- 1 teaspoon dried thyme
- 1/2 teaspoon dried basil
- 3/4 cup colby cheese, shredded
- 1 tablespoon tamari sauce
- Salt and black pepper, to your liking
- 1/4 cup roasted red pepper tomato sauce
- 3/4 tablespoons olive oil
- 1 medium-sized egg, well beaten

Directions:
1. In a nonstick skillet, that is preheated over a moderate heat, sauté the turkey mince, scallions, garlic, thyme, and basil until just tender and fragrant.
2. Then set your air fryer to cook at 360 degrees. Combine sautéed mixture with the cheese and tamari sauce; then form the mixture into a loaf shape.
3. Mix the remaining items and pour them over the meatloaf. Cook in the air fryer baking pan for 45 to 47 minutes. Eat warm.

- **Nutrition Info:** 324 calories; 19.3g fat; 2.7g carbs; 35.5g protein; 1.1g sugars; 0.6g fiber

148.Korean Beef Bulgogi Burgers

Servings: 4
Cooking Time: 18 Minutes
Ingredients:
- 1 ½ pounds ground beef
- 1 teaspoon garlic, minced
- 2 tablespoons scallions, chopped
- Sea salt and cracked black pepper, to taste
- 1 teaspoon gochugaru (korcan chili powder
- 1/2 teaspoon dried marjoram
- 1 teaspoon dried thyme
- 1 teaspoon mustard seeds
- 1/2 teaspoon shallot powder
- 1/2 teaspoon cumin powder
- 1/2 teaspoon paprika
- 1 tablespoon liquid smoke flavoring

Directions:
1. In a mixing bowl, thoroughly combine all ingredients until well combined.
2. Shape into four patties and spritz them with cooking oil on both sides. Bake at 357 degrees f for 18 minutes, flipping over halfway through the cooking time.
3. Serve warm.
- **Nutrition Info:** 377 calories; 19.3g fat; 2.4g carbs; 45.9g protein; 0.7g sugars; 0.8g fiber

149.Pork With Gravy

Servings: 4
Cooking Time: 30minutes
Ingredients:
- 5 pork chops
- 1 tablespoon olive oil
- 1 teaspoon salt
- ½ teaspoon pepper
- ½ teaspoon garlic powder
- 2 cups beef broth
- 1 packet ranch dressing mix
- 10½ oz. cream of chicken soup
- 1 packet brown gravy mix
- 2 tablespoons corn starch dissolved in 2 tablespoons water

Directions:
1. Season both sides of the pork chops with salt, pepper, and garlic powder.
2. Pour the olive oil into the Ninja Foodi. Set it to Sauté.
3. Brown the pork chops on both sides. Remove and set aside.
4. Pour the beef broth to deglaze the pot.
5. Add the rest of the ingredients except the corn starch. Seal the pot.
6. Set it to Pressure. Cook at high pressure for 8 minutes. Release the pressure naturally.
7. Remove the pork chops. Turn the pot to Sauté. Stir in the corn starch.
8. Simmer to thicken. Pour the gravy over the pork chops.
9. serving Suggestions:
10. Serve with mashed potatoes.
- **Nutrition Info:** Calories: 357 Total Fat: 26.8 g Saturated Fat: 9 g Cholesterol: 74 mg Sodium: 1308 mg Total Carbohydrate: 6 g Dietary Fiber: 0.1 g Total Sugars: 0.8 g Protein: 21.6 g Potassium: 396 mg

150.Grilled Steak & Potatoes

Servings: 4
Cooking Time: 50 Minutes
Ingredients:
- 1/4 cup avocado oil
- 4 potatoes
- 2 tablespoons steak seasoning
- 3 sirloin steaks
- Salt to taste

Directions:
1. Poke potatoes with fork.
2. Coat potatoes with half of avocado oil.
3. Season with salt.
4. Add to the air fryer basket.
5. Choose air fry function in your Ninja Foodi Grill.
6. Seal the hood and cook at 400 degrees F for 35 minutes.
7. Flip and cook for another 10 minutes.
8. Transfer to a plate.
9. Add grill grate to the Ninja Foodi Grill.
10. Add steaks to the grill grate.
11. Set it to high.
12. Cook for 7 minutes per side.
13. Serve steaks with potatoes.
14. Serving Suggestions: Serve with steak sauce and hot sauce.

151.Korean Chili Pork

Servings: 4
Cooking Time: 8 Minutes
Ingredients:
- 2 pounds pork, cut into ⅛-inch slices
- 5 minced garlic cloves
- 3 tablespoons minced green onion
- 1 yellow onion, sliced
- ½ cup soy sauce
- ½ cup brown sugar
- 3 tablespoons Korean red chili paste or regular chili paste
- 2 tablespoons sesame seeds
- 3 teaspoons black pepper
- Red pepper flakes to taste

Directions:
1. Take a zip-lock bag, add all the ingredients. Shake well and refrigerate for 6-8 hours to marinate.
2. Take Ninja Foodi Grill, orchestrate it over your kitchen stage, and open the top.

3. Mastermind the barbecue mesh [NH3]and close the top cover.
4. Click Grill and choose the Med grill function. flame broil work. [NH4]Modify the clock to 8 minutes and press Start/Stop. Ninja Foodi will begin to warm up.
5. Ninja Foodi is preheated and prepared to cook when it begins to signal. After you hear a signal, open the top.
6. Fix finely sliced pork on the barbeque mesh.
7. Cover and cook for 4 minutes. Then open the cover, switch the side of the pork.
8. Cover it and cook for another 4 minutes.
9. Serve warm with chopped lettuce (optional).
- **Nutrition Info:** Calories: 621 Fat: 31 g Saturated Fat: 12.5 g Trans Fat: 0 g Carbohydrates: 29 g Fiber: 3 g Sodium: 1428 mg Protein: 53 g

152.Country-style Nutty Turkey Breast

Servings: 2
Cooking Time: 25 Minutes
Ingredients:
- 1 ½ tablespoons coconut aminos
- 1/2 tablespoon xanthan gum
- 2 bay leaves
- 1/3 cup dry sherry
- 1 ½ tablespoons chopped walnuts
- 1 teaspoon shallot powder
- 1 pound turkey breasts, sliced
- 1 teaspoon garlic powder
- 2 teaspoons olive oil
- 1/2 teaspoon onion salt
- 1/2 teaspoon red pepper flakes, crushed
- 1 teaspoon ground black pepper

Directions:
1. Begin by preheating your air fryer to 395 degrees f. Place all ingredients, minus chopped walnuts, in a mixing bowl and let them marinate at least 1 hour.
2. After that, cook the marinated turkey breast approximately 23 minutes or until heated through.
3. Pause the machine, scatter chopped walnuts over the top and air-fry an additional 5 minutes.
- **Nutrition Info:** 395 calories; 19.5g fat; 1.1g carbs; 51.5g protein; 0.4g sugars; 0.5g fiber

153.Easy Fruitcake With Cranberries

Servings: 8
Cooking Time: 20 Minutes
Ingredients:
- 1 cup almond flour
- 1/3 teaspoon baking soda
- 1/3 teaspoon baking powder
- 3/4 cup erythritol
- 1/2 teaspoon ground cloves
- 1/3 teaspoon ground cinnamon
- 1/2 teaspoon cardamom
- 1 stick butter
- 1/2 teaspoon vanilla paste
- 2 eggs plus 1 egg yolk, beaten
- 1/2 cup cranberries, fresh or thawed
- 1 tablespoon browned butter
- For ricotta frosting:
- 1/2 stick butter
- 1/2 cup firm ricotta cheese
- 1 cup powdered erythritol
- 1/4 teaspoon salt
- Zest of 1/2 lemon

Directions:
1. Start by preheating your air fryer to 355 degrees f.
2. In a mixing bowl, combine the flour with baking soda, baking powder, erythritol, ground cloves, cinnamon, and cardamom.
3. In a separate bowl, whisk 1 stick butter with vanilla paste; mix in the eggs until light and fluffy. Add the flour/sugar mixture to the butter/egg mixture. Fold in the cranberries and browned butter.
4. Scrape the mixture into the greased cake pan. Then, bake in the preheated air fryer for about 20 minutes.
5. Meanwhile, in a food processor, whip 1/2 stick of the butter and ricotta cheese until there are no lumps.
6. Slowly add the powdered erythritol and salt until your mixture has reached a thick consistency. Stir in the lemon zest; mix to combine and chill completely before using.
7. Frost the cake and serve.
- **Nutrition Info:** 286 calories; 27g fat; 9.1g carbs; 7.8g protein; 1.1g sugars; 5g fiber

154.Roast Beef With Garlic

Servings: 4
Cooking Time: 1 Hour And 20 Minutes
Ingredients:
- 2 lb. beef roast, sliced
- 6 cloves garlic
- Salt and pepper to taste
- 2 tablespoons vegetable oil

Directions:
1. Coat beef roast with oil.
2. Season with salt and pepper.
3. Place inside the Ninja Foodi Grill pot.
4. Sprinkle garlic on top.
5. Choose bake setting.
6. Set it to 400 degrees F and cook for 30 minutes.
7. Reduce temperature to 375 degrees F and cook for another 40 minutes.
8. Serving Suggestions: Serve with mashed potato and gravy.

155.Fried Chicken

Servings: 6
Cooking Time: 45 Minutes
Ingredients:
- 2 tablespoons onion powder
- 2 tablespoons garlic powder
- 1 tablespoon mustard powder
- 2 tablespoons chili powder
- Salt and pepper to taste
- 4 cups buttermilk
- 8 chicken thighs
- 2 cups all-purpose flour
- 3/4 cup vegetable oil
- 2 tablespoons sugar
- 3 tablespoons paprika

Directions:
1. Mix the spice powders, salt and pepper in a bowl.
2. Transfer half of mixture to another bowl.
3. Pour in buttermilk to the second bowl and mix well.
4. Coat the chicken pieces with this mixture.
5. Cover and marinate in the refrigerator for 8 hours.
6. Add flour to the remaining spice blend.
7. Toss the chicken in this mixture.
8. Add to the air fryer basket.
9. Select air fryer function.
10. Cook at 360 degrees for 25 to 30 minutes.
11. Coat chicken with oil.
12. Cook for another 15 minutes.

156.Grilled Pork Chops

Servings: 4
Cooking Time: 15 Minutes
Ingredients:
- 4 pork chops
- Barbecue sauce
- Salt and pepper to taste

Directions:
1. Add grill grate to your Ninja Foodi Grill.
2. Set it to grill. Close the hood.
3. Preheat to high for 15 minutes.
4. Season pork chops with salt and pepper.
5. Add to the grill grates.
6. Grill for 8 minutes.
7. Flip and cook for another 7 minutes, brushing both sides with barbecue sauce.
8. Serving Suggestions: Let rest for 5 minutes before slicing and serving.

157.Buffalo Chicken Wings

Servings: 4
Cooking Time: 30 Minutes
Ingredients:
- 2 lb. chicken wings
- 2 tablespoons oil
- 1/2 cup Buffalo sauce

Directions:
1. Coat the chicken wings with oil.
2. Add these to an air fryer basket.
3. Choose air fry function.
4. Cook at 390 degrees F for 15 minutes.
5. Shake and then cook for another 15 minutes.
6. Dip in Buffalo sauce before serving.

158.Crying Tiger (grilled Steak With Dry Chili Dipping Sauce)

Servings: 4
Cooking Time: 30min
Ingredients:
- 4 - rib-eye or New York strip steaks, about 1½-inches thick
- 2 - Tbsp dark soy sauce
- 1 - Tbsp oyster sauce
- 1 - Tbsp light or dark brown sugar
- 1 - Tbsp plain vegetable oil
- 2 - plum tomatoes

Directions:
1. Combine the soy sauce, clam sauce, earthy colored sugar, and vegetable oil in a medium blending bowl. Coat the steaks with the soy sauce blend and let them marinate while you chip away at the plunging sauce.
2. Strip and deseed the tomatoes. Cleave the mash finely, and add it to arranged dried bean stew plunging sauce (Jaew); put in a safe spot.
3. Light one stack brimming with charcoal. At the point when all the charcoal is lit and secured with dim debris, spill out and spread the coals equally over the whole surface of coal grind. Set cooking grate set up, spread Ninja Foodi oven broil, and permit to preheat for 5MIN. On the other hand, set all the burners on a gas Ninja Foodi oven broil to high warmth. Clean and oil the barbecuing grate.
4. Ninja Foodi oven broil the steaks, turning every now and again until the ideal doneness is reached. Expel from Ninja Foodi oven broil and let rest for 5MIN.
5. Cut the steaks into ¼-inch cuts and present with the plunging sauce. Warm clingy rice as an afterthought is enthusiastically suggested
- **Nutrition Info:** Calories 288, fat 11g, carbohydrate 3g, Protein 36g.

159.Juicy Korean Chii Pork Delight

Servings: 4
Cooking Time: 8 Minutes
Ingredients:
- Red pepper flakes
- 3 teaspoons pepper
- 2 tablespoon sesame seeds
- 3 tablespoons Korean Red Chili Paste
- ½ cup brown sugar

- ½ cup of soy sauce
- 1 yellow onion, sliced
- 3 tablespoons green onion, minced
- 5 garlic cloves, minced
- 2 pounds pork, cut into 1/8 inch slices

Directions:
1. Take a re-sealable zip bag and add all of the listed ingredients
2. Zip up the bag and let it sit in your fridge for 6-8 hours
3. Pre-heat your Ninja Foodi Grill in MED heat setting timer to 8 minutes
4. Arrange the sliced-up pork over your grill grate
5. Lock lid and cook for 4 minutes, flip the meat and cook for 4 minutes more
6. Serve with chopped lettuce
7. Enjoy!
- **Nutrition Info:** Calories: 621 Fat: 31 g Saturated Fat: 12 g Carbohydrates: 29 g Fiber: 3 g Sodium: 1428 mg Protein: 53 g

160. Chicken Sausage With Nestled Eggs

Servings: 6
Cooking Time: 17 Minutes
Ingredients:
- 6 eggs
- 2 bell peppers, seeded and sliced
- 1 teaspoon dried oregano
- 1 teaspoon hot paprika
- 1 teaspoon freshly cracked black pepper
- 6 chicken sausages
- 1 teaspoon sea salt
- 1 1/2 shallots, cut into wedges
- 1 teaspoon dried basil

Directions:
1. Take four ramekins and divide chicken sausages, shallot, and bell pepper among those ramekins. Cook at 315 degrees f for about 12 minutes.
2. Now, crack an egg into each ramekin. Sprinkle the eggs with hot paprika, basil, oregano, salt, and cracked black pepper. Cook for 5 more minutes at 405 degrees f.
- **Nutrition Info:** 211 calories; 14.6g fat; 5.9g carbs; 14.7g protein; 1.4g sugars; 0.7g fiber

161. Ninja Foodi Porterhouse Steaks

Servings: 4
Cooking Time: 3 Hrs
Ingredients:
- 2 - whole porterhouse steaks, at least 1½ inches
- Kosher salt and freshly ground black pepper
- 8 chunks hickory or mesquite hardwood

Directions:
1. Season steaks softly with salt and pepper on all surfaces, including edges. Stack steaks on a wood cutting board, at that point, embed up to four metallic sticks via the two steaks to ensure about them. Turn them on their facets, and spread them out on the sticks. They must stay on their edges without falling.
2. Light 8 coals utilizing a smokestack starter. The spot right on one edge of the coal grind in a charcoal Ninja Foodi oven broil. Then again, set one lot of burners on a gasoline barbecue to low. Spot 2 wood pieces on coals encompass the cooking mesh and spot steaks on the cooking grate with tenderloins confronting upwards and bones pointing toward the coals.
3. Spread Ninja Foodi oven broil and set-top and base vents to ¾ close. Position top vents over steaks. Cook, signifying 8 additional coals and final wood lumps to maintain the temperature below the Ninja Foodi oven broil at around a hundred seventy-five to two hundred°F. Screen the inner temperature of the steaks continuously and cook until steaks register a hundred and ten to one hundred fifteen°F for medium-uncommon or a hundred and twenty°F for medium, 1½ to 2 HRS. Expel steaks from Ninja Foodi oven broil and put a part on a reducing board.
4. Light one smokestack brimming with charcoal. At the point, while all of the charcoal is lit and secured with dark debris, spill out and mastermind the coals on one facet of the charcoal mesh. Set cooking grate installation, spread Ninja Foodi oven broil, and permit to preheat for 5MIN. On the alternative hand, set a huge part of the burners on a fuel Ninja Foodi oven broil to the most noteworthy warm temperature setting, unfold, and preheat for 10MIN. Clean and oil the Ninja Foodi oven broiling grate.
5. Spot steaks straightforwardly over the recent aspect of the Ninja Foodi oven broil. Spread and cook dinner for forty-five seconds. Flip steaks, spread, and cook dinner for forty-five seconds longer. Evacuate to a reducing board, cut, and serve.

162. Coffee Rib-eye

Servings: 4
Cooking Time: 30 Minutes
Ingredients:
- 1 teaspoon onion powder
- 4 rib eye steaks
- 1 tablespoon vegetable oil
- 2 tablespoons coffee
- 1 teaspoon garlic powder
- 2 tablespoons ground chipotle pepper
- 1/2 teaspoon ground ginger

- 1/2 teaspoon mustard powder
- Salt and pepper to taste

Directions:
1. Brush both sides of steak with oil.
2. In a bowl, mix the remaining ingredients.
3. Sprinkle steak with spice mixture.
4. Add grill grate to your Ninja Foodi Grill.
5. Seal the hood and choose grill setting.
6. Set it to high. Start to preheat.
7. Add grill to the grate.
8. Once the temperate reaches 11o degrees F, flip the beef.
9. Wait until the pot beeps.
10. Let it rest for 10 minutes before slicing and serving.
11. Serving Suggestions: Serve with steamed veggies.

163.The Epic Carne Guisada

Servings: 4
Cooking Time: 30 Minutes
Ingredients:
- 3 pounds beef stew
- 3 tablespoon seasoned salt
- 1 tablespoon oregano chili powder
- 1 tablespoon organic cumin
- 1 pinch crushed red pepper
- 2 tablespoons olive oil
- 1/2 medium lime, juiced
- 1 cup beef bone broth
- 3 ounces tomato paste
- 1 large onion, sliced

Directions:
1. Trim the beef stew as needed into small bite-sized portions
2. Toss the beef stew pieces with dry seasoning
3. Set your Ninja Foodi to Sauté mode and add oil, allow the oil to heat up
4. Add seasoned beef pieces and brown them
5. Combine the browned beef pieces with the rest of the ingredients
6. Lock up the lid and cook on HIGH pressure for 30 minutes
7. Release the pressure naturally
8. Enjoy!

164.Ninja Foodi Italian Chicken Skewers

Servings: 8
Cooking Time:25 Min
Ingredients:
- 1 lb. boneless skinless chicken breasts, cut into large cubes
- kosher salt
- Freshly ground black pepper
- 2 tbsp. tomato paste
- ¼ c. extra-virgin olive oil, plus more for drizzling
- 3 - garlic cloves, Minced

- 1 - tbsp. chopped fresh Italian parsley, plus more leaves for garnish
- 8 - skewers, soaked in water for 20MIN
- 1 - baguette French bread, cut into cubes

Directions:
1. Season chicken with salt and pepper. Make the marinade: consolidate tomato glue, olive oil, garlic cloves, and slashed parsley in a huge bowl. Add chicken and hurl to completely cover. Refrigerate 30MIN.
2. Preheat Ninja Foodi oven broil to medium-high. Stick chicken and bread. Shower with olive oil and season with salt and pepper.
3. Ninja Foodi oven broil, turning every so often until chicken is cooked through and bread marginally burned, about 10MIN. Embellishment with parsley.
- **Nutrition Info:** Calories 260, fat 8g, carbohydrate 7g, Protein 38g.

165.Paprika Chicken

Servings: 6
Cooking Time: 30 Minutes
Ingredients:
- 2 lb. chicken wings
- 2 tablespoons olive oil
- 1 tablespoon smoked paprika
- 1 teaspoon garlic powder
- Salt and pepper to taste

Directions:
1. Coat chicken wings with oil.
2. Sprinkle with paprika, garlic powder, salt and pepper.
3. Add chicken wings to the air crisp tray.
4. Select air crisp.
5. Cook at 400 degrees For 15 minutes per side.

166.Beef Fajita Keto Burrito

Servings: 4
Cooking Time: 12 Minutes
Ingredients:
- 1 pound rump steak
- 1 teaspoon garlic powder
- 1/2 teaspoon onion powder
- 1/2 teaspoon cayenne pepper
- 1 teaspoon piri piri powder
- 1 teaspoon mexican oregano
- Salt and ground black pepper, to taste
- 1 cup mexican cheese blend
- 1 head romaine lettuce, separated into leaves

Directions:
1. Toss the rump steak with the garlic powder, onion powder, cayenne pepper, piri piri powder, mexican oregano, salt, and black pepper.
2. Cook in the preheated air fryer at 390 degrees f for 10 minutes. Slice against the

grain into thin strips. Add the cheese blend and cook for 2 minutes more.

3. Spoon the beef mixture onto romaine lettuce leaves; roll up burrito-style and serve.

- **Nutrition Info:** 365 calories; 20g fat; 7.8g carbs; 40.1g protein; 2.8g sugars; 3.7g fiber

167.Romantic Mustard Pork

Servings: 4
Cooking Time: 30 Minutes
Ingredients:
- 2 tablespoons butter
- 2 tablespoons Dijon mustard (Keto-Friendly)
- 4 pork chops
- Salt and pepper to taste
- 1 tablespoon fresh rosemary, coarsely chopped

Directions:
1. Take a bowl and add pork chops, cover with Dijon mustard and carefully sprinkle rosemary, salt, and pepper. Let it marinate for 2 hours
2. Add butter and marinated pork chops to your Ninja Foodi pot
3. Lock lid and cook on Low-Medium Pressure for 30 minutes
4. Release pressure naturally over 10 minutes. Take the dish out, serve, and enjoy!

168.Bratwursts

Servings: 4
Cooking Time: 12 Minutes
Ingredients:
- 1 pack bratwursts

Directions:
1. Preheat your unit to 350 degrees F for 5 minutes.
2. Add the bratwursts to the air crisp tray.
3. Set it to air crisp.
4. Cook for 10 minutes, flipping once.

169.Barbecue Beef Short Ribs

Servings: 2
Cooking Time: 3 Hours And 15 Minutes
Ingredients:
- 2 beef short ribs
- ¾ cup beef broth
- ¼ cup red wine
- ¼ cup onion, diced
- ½ cup barbecue sauce
- Spice mixture
- 1 teaspoon garlic powder
- 1 teaspoon onion powder
- 1 tablespoon cornstarch
- Salt and pepper to taste

Directions:
1. Mix spice mixture ingredients in a bowl.
2. Season beef short ribs with this mixture.

3. Add beef ribs to a small baking pan.
4. Pour in the broth and wine.
5. Sprinkle with onion.
6. Choose roast setting.
7. Roast at 250 degrees for 3 hours.
8. Stir in barbecue sauce to the cooking liquid.

170.Classic Cookies With Hazelnuts

Servings: 6
Cooking Time: 10 Minutes
Ingredients:
- 1 cup almond flour
- 1/2 cup coconut flour
- 1 teaspoon baking soda
- 1 teaspoon fine sea salt
- 1 stick butter
- 1 cup swerve
- 2 teaspoons vanilla
- 2 eggs, at room temperature
- 1 cup hazelnuts, coarsely chopped

Directions:
1. Begin by preheating your air fryer to 350 degrees f.
2. Mix the flour with the baking soda, and sea salt.
3. In the bowl of an electric mixer, beat the butter, swerve, and vanilla until creamy. Fold in the eggs, one at a time, and mix until well combined.
4. Slowly and gradually, stir in the flour mixture. Finally, fold in the coarsely chopped hazelnuts.
5. Divide the dough into small balls using a large cookie scoop; drop onto the prepared cookie sheets. Bake for 10 minutes or until golden brown, rotating the pan once or twice through the cooking time.
6. Work in batches and cool for a couple of minutes before removing to wire racks and serve.

- **Nutrition Info:** 328 calories; 32.3g fat; 5g carbs; 6.7g protein; 1.9g sugars; 2.4g fiber

171.Sausage & Peppers

Servings: 6
Cooking Time: 18 Minutes
Ingredients:
- 1 white onion, sliced into rings
- 2 bell peppers, sliced
- 2 tablespoons vegetable oil, divided
- Salt and pepper to taste
- 6 sausages
- 6 hotdog buns

Directions:
1. Preheat the unit by pressing grill.
2. Set it to low.
3. Set it to 26 minutes.
4. Press start.
5. Coat the onion and bell peppers with oil.

6. Season with salt and pepper.
7. After the unit beeps, add the onion and bell pepper to the grill grate.
8. Cook for 12 minutes.
9. Transfer to a plate.
10. Add the sausages to the grill.
11. Cook for 6 minutes.
12. Add the sausages to the hotdog buns.
13. Top with the onion and pepper mixture.

172. Birthday Chocolate Raspberry Cake

Servings: 4
Cooking Time: 25 Minutes
Ingredients:
- 1/3 cup monk fruit
- 1/4 cup unsalted butter, room temperature
- 1 egg plus 1 egg white, lightly whisked
- 3 ounces almond flour
- 2 tablespoons dutch-process cocoa powder
- 1/2 teaspoon ground cinnamon
- 1 tablespoon candied ginger
- 1/8 teaspoon table salt
- For the filling:
- 2 ounces fresh raspberries
- 1/3 cup monk fruit
- 1 teaspoon fresh lime juice

Directions:
1. Firstly, set your air fryer to cook at 315 degrees f. Then, spritz the inside of two cake pans with the butter-flavored cooking spray.
2. In a mixing bowl, beat the monk fruit and butter until creamy and uniform. Then, stir in the whisked eggs. Stir in the almond flour, cocoa powder, cinnamon, ginger and salt.
3. Press the batter into the cake pans; use a wide spatula to level the surface of the batter. Bake for 20 minutes or until a wooden stick inserted in the center of the cake comes out completely dry.
4. While your cake is baking, stir together all of the ingredients for the filling in a medium saucepan. Cook over high heat, stirring frequently and mashing with the back of a spoon; bring to a boil and decrease the temperature.
5. Continue to cook, stirring until the mixture thickens, for another 7 minutes. Let the filling cool to room temperature.
6. Spread 1/2 of raspberry filling over the first crust. Top with another crust; spread remaining filling over top. Spread frosting over top and sides of your cake.
- **Nutrition Info:** 217 calories; 18.8g fat; 8.6g carbs; 7.5g protein; 1.7g sugars; 4.6g fiber

173. Tantalizing Beef Jerky

Servings: 8
Cooking Time: 20 Minutes
Ingredients:
- ½ pound beef, sliced into 1/8-inch-thick strips
- ½ cup of soy sauce
- 2 tablespoons Worcestershire sauce
- 2 teaspoons ground black pepper
- 1 teaspoon onion powder
- ½ teaspoon garlic powder
- 1 teaspoon salt

Directions:
1. Add listed ingredient to a large-sized Ziploc bag. Seal it shut.
2. Shake well, leave it in the fridge overnight.
3. Lay strips on dehydrator trays, making sure not to overlap them.
4. Lock the air crisping lid and set the temperature to 135°F. Cook for 7 hours.
5. Store in an airtight container and enjoy!
- **Nutrition Info:** Calories: 62 Fat: 7 g Carbohydrates: 2 g Protein: 9 g

174. Parmesan Chicken Nuggets

Servings: 4
Cooking Time: 8 Minutes
Ingredients:
- 1 pound chicken breast, ground
- 1 teaspoon hot paprika
- 2 teaspoon sage, ground
- 1/3 teaspoon powdered ginger
- 1/2 teaspoon dried thyme
- 1/3 teaspoon ground black pepper, to taste
- 1 teaspoon kosher salt
- 2 tablespoons melted butter
- 3 eggs, beaten
- 1/2 cup parmesan cheese, grated

Directions:
1. In a mixing bowl, thoroughly combine ground chicken together with spices and an egg. After that, stir in the melted butter; mix to combine well.
2. Whisk the remaining eggs in a shallow bowl.
3. Form the mixture into chicken nugget shapes; now, coat them with the beaten eggs; then, dredge them in the grated parmesan cheese.
4. Cook in the preheated air fryer at 405 degrees f for 8 minutes.
- **Nutrition Info:** 347 calories; 23.6g fat; 1.5g carbs; 30.5g protein; 0.5g sugars; 0g fiber

175. Chicken & Zucchini

Servings: 6
Cooking Time: 20 Minutes
Ingredients:
- 1/4 cup olive oil
- 1 tablespoon lemon juice
- 2 tablespoons red wine vinegar
- 1 teaspoon oregano
- 1 tablespoon garlic, chopped
- 2 chicken breast fillet, sliced into cubes

- 1 zucchini, sliced
- 1 red onion, sliced
- 1 cup cherry tomatoes, sliced
- Salt and pepper to taste

Directions:
1. In a bowl, mix the olive oil, lemon juice, vinegar, oregano and garlic.
2. Pour half of mixture into another bowl.
3. Toss chicken in half of the mixture.
4. Cover and marinate for 15 minutes.
5. Toss the veggies in the remaining mixture.
6. Season both chicken and veggies with salt and pepper.
7. Add chicken to the air fryer basket.
8. Spread veggies on top.
9. Select air fry function.
10. Seal and cook at 380 degrees F for 15 to 20 minutes.

176.Baked Butter Thighs

Servings: 6
Cooking Time: 35 Minutes
Ingredients:
- Zest of 1 lemon
- 3 lb. (6) bone-in, skin-on chicken thighs
- Salt, to taste
- 1/2 cup butter
- 1 lb. baby potatoes, quartered
- 5 garlic cloves, minced
- 1 tbsp fresh thyme leaves
- 1 lemon, cut into rounds
- Black pepper, to taste
- 1 tbsp freshly chopped parsley, for garnish

Directions:
1. Pat dry all the chicken thighs and rub them with salt and black pepper.
2. Whisk butter with lemon zest, thyme, and garlic in a small bowl.
3. Rub this butter thyme mixture over the chicken thighs liberally
4. Place these chicken thighs, potatoes, and lemon rounds in a casserole dish.
5. Transfer the casserole dish to the Ninja Foodi oven and Close its lid.
6. Rotate the Ninja Foodi dial to select the "Bake" mode.
7. Press the Time button and again use the dial to set the cooking time to 35 minutes.
8. Now press the Temp button and rotate the dial to set the temperature at 420 degrees F.
9. Serve warm.
- **Nutrition Info:** Calories 231 ; Fat 20.1 g ; Carbs 30.1 g ; Fiber 0.9 g ; Sugar 1.4 g ; Protein 14.6 g

177.Chili Dogs

Servings: 16
Cooking Time: 40 Mins
Ingredients:

- If making the chili -
- 1 ½ jar of pasta sauce
- 2 tsp of butter or margarine
- 2 pounds of ground beef
- At least 2 tsp chili powder
- 2 tsp vegetable oil
- 4 minced garlic cloves
- 1 white onion, finely chopped
- 2 tsp salt
- Also requires –
- Hot dog buns
- 2 tbsp butter
- 16 beef hot dogs

Directions:
1. Prepare the chili. If it is store-bought, follow instructions. If making fresh chili, heat the olive oil and butter in a skillet then fry the ground beef, garlic, and onions.
2. Use the back of a spoon to break it up and cook until browning before adding the other ingredients. Simmer for 15 mins.
3. Place your Ninja Foodi grill grate in the unit and close the hood. Choose GRILL, set temperature to MAX, and set time to 10 minutes. Select START/STOP to start your pre-heating.
4. When the pre-heating timer goes off, place the hot dogs on the grill grate, close the hood, and cook for 3-5 mins. Flip halfway through.
5. Butter the buns. They can also be heated on the grill, oven, or microwave as you like.
6. Put the dogs in buns and top with chili and your other favorite toppings.
- **Nutrition Info:** Calories: 448 Fat: 29g Saturated Fat: 11g Trans Fat: 0g Carbohydrates: 26g Fiber: 1g Sodium: 1103mg Protein: 21g

178.Pork Sandwich

Servings: 4
Cooking Time: 21 Minutes
Ingredients:
- Marinade
- 1 teaspoon onion powder
- 1 clove garlic, minced
- 1 tablespoon fresh cilantro, chopped
- 2 tablespoons soy sauce
- 2 tablespoons lime juice
- 2 teaspoons cumin
- 1 ½ cups orange juice
- Salt and pepper to taste
- Spread
- ¼ cup mayonnaise
- ¼ cup sour cream
- 1 teaspoon cumin
- 1 tablespoon lime juice
- Sandwich
- 2 pork fillets

- 3 bell peppers, sliced into strips and roasted
- 8 slices French bread

Directions:
1. Combine marinade ingredients in a bowl.
2. Add pork fillets to the bowl.
3. Cover and refrigerate for 5 hours.
4. Strain and discard marinade.
5. Add pork to the grill grate.
6. Set the unit to grill.
7. Choose high setting.
8. Set time to 11 minutes.
9. Press start.
10. Mix the spread ingredients in a bowl.
11. Spread mixture on French bread slices.
12. Add pork to the bread along with the red bell pepper.
13. Grill sandwich for 10 minutes

179.A Keto-friendly Philly Willy Steak And Cheese

Servings: 4
Cooking Time: 40 Minutes
Ingredients:
- 2 tablespoons olive oil
- 2 large onion, sliced
- 8 ounces mushrooms, sliced
- 1-2 teaspoons Keto-friendly steak seasoning
- 1 tablespoon butter
- 2 pounds beef chuck roast
- 12 cup beef stock

Directions:
1. Set your Ninja Foodi to Sauté mode and add oil, let it heat up
2. Rub seasoning over roast and Sauté for 1-2 minutes per side
3. Remove and add butter, onion
4. Add mushrooms, pepper, stock, and roast
5. Lock lid and cook on HIGH pressure for 35 minutes
6. Naturally, release the pressure over 10 minutes
7. Shred meat and sprinkle cheese if using, enjoy!

180.Picnic Blackberry Muffins

Servings: 8
Cooking Time: 12 Minutes
Ingredients:
- 1 ½ cups almond flour
- 1/2 teaspoon baking soda
- 1 teaspoon baking powder
- 1/4 teaspoon kosher salt
- 1/2 cup swerve
- 2 eggs, whisked
- 1/2 cup milk
- 1/4 cup coconut oil, melted
- 1/2 teaspoon vanilla paste
- 1/2 cup fresh blackberries

Directions:
1. In a mixing bowl, combine the almond flour, baking soda, baking powder, swerve, and salt. Whisk to combine well.
2. In another mixing bowl, mix the eggs, milk, coconut oil, and vanilla.
3. Now, add the wet egg mixture to dry the flour mixture. Then, carefully fold in the fresh blackberries; gently stir to combine.
4. Scrape the batter mixture into the muffin cups. Bake your muffins at 350 degrees f for 12 minutes or until the tops are golden brown.
5. Sprinkle some extra icing sugar over the top of each muffin if desired.
6. Serve
- **Nutrition Info:** 192 calories; 17.3g fat; 5.5g carbs; 5.7g protein; 2g sugars; 2.7g fiber_____

181.Chocolate Almond Cookies

Servings: 10
Cooking Time: 15 Minutes
Ingredients:
- 2 cups almond flour
- 1/2 cup coconut flour
- 5 ounces swerve
- 5 ounces butter, softened
- 1 egg, beaten
- 1 teaspoon vanilla essence
- 4 ounces double cream
- 3 ounces bakers' chocolate, unsweetened
- 1 teaspoon cardamom seeds, finely crushed

Directions:
1. Start by preheating your air fryer to 350 degrees f.
2. In a mixing bowl, thoroughly combine the flour, swerve, and butter. Mix until your mixture resembles breadcrumbs.
3. Gradually, add the egg and vanilla essence. Shape your dough into small balls and place in the parchment-lined air fryer basket.
4. Bake in the preheated air fryer for 10 minutes. Rotate the pan and bake for another 5 minutes. Transfer the freshly baked cookies to a cooling rack.
5. As the biscuits are cooling, melt the double cream and bakers' chocolate in the air fryer safe bowl at 350 degrees f. Add the cardamom seeds and stir well.
6. Spread the filling over the cooled biscuits and sandwich together and serve.
- **Nutrition Info:** 303 calories; 29.6g fat; 8.5g carbs; 6.5g protein; 1.6g sugars; 4.3g fiber

182.Authentic Korean Flank Steak

Servings: 4
Cooking Time: 10minutes
Ingredients:

- 1 teaspoon red pepper flakes
- ½ cup and 1 tablespoon soy sauce
- 1½ pounds flank steak
- ¼ cup and 2 tablespoons vegetable oil
- ½ cup of rice wine vinegar
- 3 tablespoons sriracha
- 2 cucumbers, seeded and sliced
- 4 garlic cloves, minced
- 2 tablespoons ginger, minced
- 2 tablespoons honey
- 3 tablespoons sesame oil
- 1 teaspoon sugar
- Salt to taste

Directions:
1. Take a bowl and add ½ cup soy sauce, half of the rice wine, honey, ginger, garlic, 2 tablespoons sriracha, 2 tablespoons sesame oil, and vegetable oil.
2. Mix well, pour half of the mixture over steak and rub well.
3. Cover steak and let it sit for 10 minutes.
4. Prepare the salad mix by add remaining rice wine vinegar, sesame oil, sugar red pepper flakes, sriracha sauce, soy sauce, and salt in a salad bowl.
5. Preheat your Ninja Foodi Grill on High, with the timer set to 12 minutes.
6. Transfer steak to your Grill and cook for 6 minutes per side.
7. Slice and serve with the salad mix.
8. Enjoy!
- **Nutrition Info:** Calories: 327 Fat: 4 g Saturated Fat: 0.5 g Carbohydrates: 33 g Fiber: 1 g Sodium: 142 mg Protein: 24 g

183.Chicken Schnitzel

Servings: 2
Cooking Time: 12 Minutes
Ingredients:
- 1 lb. chicken thighs, skinless, boneless
- ½ cup seasoned bread crumbs
- 1 tsp salt
- ½ tsp ground black pepper
- ¼ cup flour
- 1 egg, beaten
- Avocado oil or cooking spray

Directions:
1. Place one chicken thigh in between 2 sheets of parchment sheet and use a mallet to flatten the chicken.
2. Similarly, flatten the remaining thighs using this method.
3. Now mix bread crumbs with black pepper and salt in a shallow bowl.
4. Spread flour in another bowl and whisk the egg in yet another bowl.
5. First coat the chicken with flour then dip into the egg.

6. Place the flatten chicken in the crumbs and flip to coat well, then shake off excess.
7. Keep the chicken thighs in the Air Fryer basket.
8. Transfer this Air Fryer to the Ninja Foodi oven and Close its lid.
9. Rotate the Ninja Foodi dial to select the "Air Fry" mode.
10. Press the Time button and again use the dial to set the cooking time to 6 minutes.
11. Now press the Temp button and rotate the dial to set the temperature at 375 degrees F.
12. Flip the cooked chicken and continue cooking for another 6 minutes on the same mode and temperature.
13. Serve warm.
- **Nutrition Info:** Calories 388 ; Fat 8 g ; Carbs 8 g ; Fiber 1 g ; Sugar 2 g ; Protein 13 g

184.Ninja Foodi Rotisserie Porchetta

Servings: 10
Cooking Time: 6 Hrs
Ingredients:
- For the Brine:
- 2 - quarts cold water
- 1/3 - cup salt
- ¼ - cup white sugar
- 1 - whole pork loin, trimmed of silver skin and excess fat
- For the Rub:
- 1 - Tbsp whole black peppercorns
- 1 - Tbsp fennel seed
- 2 - Tbsp finely chopped fresh sage
- 1 - Tbsp finely chopped fresh rosemary
- 1 - Tbsp freshly Minced garlic
- 2 - Tsp finely chopped fresh thyme
- 2 - Tsp crushed red pepper
- 1 - teaspoon lemon zest
- 1 - whole boneless pork belly

Directions:
1. To make the saline solution: In a huge bowl, whisk together water, salt, and sugar until solids are broken down. Lower pork midsection in saline solution. A spot in cooler and brackish water for 2 HRS.
2. To make the rub: Place peppercorns and fennel seed in a cast-iron skillet over medium-high warmth; toast flavors until fragrant, about 2MIN. Move to a zest processor and procedure until coarsely ground. Move flavor blend to a little bowl and blend in sage, rosemary, garlic, thyme, squashed red pepper, and lemon get-up-and-go. Put in a safe spot.
3. Lay pork midsection, skin side down, on an enormous cutting board. Score tissue with a sharp blade at an edge about each inch. Rehash the other way to make a precious

stone example. Season pork tummy generously with salt. Sprinkle rub equally across pork stomach, utilizing hands to pat rub into meat and cut cleft.

4. Take out pork flank from brackish water; pat dry with paper towels. A spot in the focal point of pork paunch. Move pork paunch around pork flank so it completely encases midsection. Tie move close with butcher twine about each inch.

5. Light one fireplace loaded with charcoal. At the point when all the charcoal is lit and secured with dim debris, spill out and orchestrate the coals on either side of the charcoal mesh and spot a foil skillet between the two heaps of coals. Spread barbecue and permit to preheat for 5MIN. Run spit of the rotisserie through the center of pork roll and secure closures with rotisserie forks. Spot on the rotisserie, spread, and cook at medium warmth until the skin has obscured and crisped and pork registers 155ºF when a moment read thermometer is embedded into the thickest piece of the meat, around 3 HRS, renewing coals to keep up temperature varying. Take out from the barbecue and let rest for 10MIN. Take it out spit, cut, and serve.

- **Nutrition Info:** Calories 224, fat 16g, carbohydrate 1g, Protein 19g.

185.Ninja Foodi Sticky Grilled Chicken

Servings: 4
Cooking Time:2 Hrs 35 Min
Ingredients:
- ½ c. low-sodium soy sauce
- ½ c. balsamic vinegar
- 3 tbsp. honey
- 2 - cloves garlic, Minced
- 2 - green onions, thinly sliced
- 2½ lb. chicken drumsticks
- Vegetable oil, for grill
- 2 tbsp. sesame seeds, for garnish

Directions:
1. In an enormous bowl, whisk together soy sauce, balsamic vinegar, nectar, garlic, and green onions. Put aside ¼ cup marinade.
2. Add chicken to an enormous resalable plastic pack and pour it in the outstanding marinade. Let marinate in the cooler at any rate 2 HRS or up to expedite.
3. At the point when prepared to barbecue, heat Ninja Foodi oven broils to high. Oil meshes and barbecue chicken, seasoning with the held marinade and turning each 3 to 4MIN, until sang and cooked through, 24 to 30MIN aggregate.
4. Embellishment with sesame seeds before serving.

- **Nutrition Info:** Calories 440, fat 8g, carbohydrate 51g, Protein 40g.

186.Simple/aromatic Meatballs

Servings: 4
Cooking Time: 11 Minutes
Ingredients:
- 2 cups ground beef
- 1 egg, beaten
- 1 teaspoon taco seasoning
- 1 tablespoon sugar-free marinara sauce
- 1 teaspoon garlic, minced
- 1/2 teaspoon salt

Directions:
1. Take a big mixing bowl and place all the ingredients into the bowl
2. Add all the ingredients into the bowl.
3. Mix all the ingredients by using a spoon or fingertip.
4. Then make the small size meatballs and put them in a layer in the air fryer rack
5. Lower the air fryer lid. Cook the meatballs for 11 minutes at 350 F.
6. Serve immediately and enjoy it!

187.Grilled Mayo Short Loin Steak

Servings: 4
Cooking Time: 15 Minutes
Ingredients:
- 1 cup mayonnaise
- 1 tablespoon fresh rosemary, finely chopped
- 2 tablespoons worcestershire sauce
- Sea salt, to taste
- 1/2 teaspoon ground black pepper
- 1 teaspoon smoked paprika
- 1 teaspoon garlic, minced
- 1 ½ pounds short loin steak

Directions:
1. Combine the mayonnaise, rosemary, worcestershire sauce, salt, pepper, paprika, and garlic; mix to combine well.
2. Now, brush the mayonnaise mixture over both sides of the steak. Lower the steak onto the grill pan.
3. Grill in the preheated air fryer at 390 degrees f for 8 minutes. Turn the steaks over and grill an additional 7 minutes.
4. Check for doneness with a meat thermometer. Serve warm.

- **Nutrition Info:** 620 calories; 50g fat; 2.7g carbs; 39.7g protein; 1.2g sugars; 0.3g fiber

188.Garlic Chicken And Pepper Skewers

Servings: 4
Cooking Time: 15 Mins
Ingredients:
- ½ cup of vegetable oil
- ½ cup of white wine vinegar

- 4 cloves of garlic, minced
- 1 pound of chicken cut into small chunks
- 3 bell peppers (any color) cut into chunks
- 1 onion cut into chunks
- Wooden skewers
- Salt and pepper to taste

Directions:
1. Place your Ninja Foodi grill grate in the unit and close the hood. Choose GRILL, set temperature to MAX, and set time to 10 minutes. Select START/STOP to start your pre-heating.
2. Whisk together the oil, vinegar, and garlic with the salt and pepper
3. Toss in the vegetable and chicken chunks until coated in the mix
4. Assemble chicken and vegetables on wooden skewers as preferred
5. When pre-heating is done, place the skewers into the grill. Close the hood and cook for ten minutes, flipping halfway through.
6. Remove the chicken and leave to cool for 5 mins.
7. Serve immediately
- **Nutrition Info:** Calories: 398 Fat: 36g Saturated Fat: 5g Trans Fat: 0g Carbohydrates: 20g Fiber: 1g Sodium: 1298mg Protein: 3g

189.Honey Sriracha Chicken

Servings: 4
Cooking Time: 15 Minutes
Ingredients:
- 2 lb. chicken tenders
- 2 tablespoons olive oil
- Salt and pepper to taste
- Honey sriracha sauce
- ½ cup honey
- 2 teaspoons sriracha
- 1 tablespoon garlic powder
- 2 tablespoons soy sauce
- 2 teaspoons cornstarch

Directions:
1. Brush chicken with oil.
2. Season with salt and pepper.
3. Place inside the unit, on the air crisp basket.
4. Select air crisp setting.
5. Air fry at 370 degrees F for 5 minutes per side.
6. Mix the sauce ingredients in a bowl.
7. Dip the chicken in the sauce.
8. Place the chicken back to the air crisp tray.
9. Cook at 400 degrees F for 5 minutes.

190.Cajun Chicken

Servings: 6
Cooking Time: 20 Minutes
Ingredients:

- 6 chicken drumsticks
- Olive oil
- Seasoning
- 1 teaspoon onion powder
- 1 teaspoon paprika
- ½ teaspoon dried thyme
- ½ teaspoon dried basil
- ½ teaspoon dried oregano
- ½ teaspoon garlic powder
- ½ teaspoon cayenne pepper
- Salt and pepper to taste

Directions:
1. Combine seasoning ingredients in a bowl.
2. Brush chicken with oil.
3. Sprinkle both sides with seasoning.
4. Add to the air crisp basket.
5. Select air crisp setting.
6. Set to 400 degrees F.
7. Cook for 10 minutes per side.

191.Wine Marinated Flank Steak

Servings: 4
Cooking Time: 12 Minutes
Ingredients:
- 1 ½ pounds flank steak
- 1/2 cup red wine
- 1/2 cup apple cider vinegar
- 2 tablespoons soy sauce
- Salt, to taste
- 1/2 teaspoon ground black pepper
- 1/2 teaspoon red pepper flakes, crushed
- 1/2 teaspoon dried basil
- 1 teaspoon thyme

Directions:
1. Add all ingredients to a large ceramic bowl. Cover and let it marinate for 3 hours in your refrigerator.
2. Transfer the flank steak to the air fryer basket that is previously greased with nonstick cooking oil.
3. Cook in the preheated air fryer at 400 degrees f for 12 minutes, flipping over halfway through the cooking time.
- **Nutrition Info:** 312 calories; 15.5g fat; 2.5g carbs; 36.8g protein; 1.9g sugars; 0.2g fiber

192.Generous Pesto Beef Meal

Servings: 4
Cooking Time: 14 Minutes
Ingredients:
- ½ teaspoon pepper
- ½ teaspoon salt
- ½ cup feta cheese, crumbled
- 2/3 cup pesto
- ½ cup walnuts, chopped
- 4 cups grape tomatoes, halved
- 4 cups penne pasta, uncooked
- 10 ounces baby spinach, chopped

- 4 beef (6 ounces each) tenderloin steaks

Directions:
1. Cook the pasta according to the package instructions.
2. Drain the pasta and rinse it.
3. Keep the pasta on the side.
4. Season the tenderloin steaks with pepper and salt.
5. Preheat your Ninja Foodi Grill to High, and set the timer to 7 minutes.
6. You will hear a beep once the preheating sequence is complete.
7. Transfer steak to your grill and cook for 7 minutes, flip and cook for 7 minutes more.
8. Take a bowl and add pasta, walnuts, spinach, tomatoes, and pesto.
9. Mix well.
10. Garnish your steak with cheese and serve with the prepared sauce.
11. Enjoy!
- **Nutrition Info:** Calories: 361 Fat: 5 g Saturated Fat: 1 g Carbohydrates: 16 g Fiber: 4 g Sodium: 269 mg Protein: 33 g

193.Pork Belly Marinated In Char Siu Sauce

Servings: 8
Cooking Time: 10-16 Hrs
Ingredients:
- ½ cup char siu sauce
- ½ cup pineapple juice
- 5 - cloves garlic, finely Minced
- 1 - Tbsp Kosher salt
- 1 - teaspoon freshly ground black pepper
- 4lbs pork belly, skin on
- 4 to 6 - chunks apple wood

Directions:
1. In a medium bowl, combine roast siu sauce, pineapple juice, garlic, salt, and dark pepper.
2. Score the skin of the pork askew every 2-inches; rehash the other way, making a jewel design. Spot pork in a huge resalable plastic pack and pour in the marinade. Seal and hurl to uniformly cover. Marinate in the fridge for at any rate 4 HRS to expedite.
3. Take out the pork stomach and permit it to come to room temperature while setting up the smoker or Ninja Foodi oven broil. Fire up smoker or barbecue to 225°F for aberrant warmth, including lumps of apple wood when at temperature. At the point when the wood is touched off and creating smoke, place the pork in the smoker or Ninja Foodi oven broil, skin side up, and smoke until pork registers 160 degrees on a moment read thermometer embedded into the focal point of the gut, around 4 to 5 HRS.
4. Spot pork tummy on a medium-hot Ninja Foodi oven broil, skin side down, or in a

grill, skin side up, and cook until skin is fresh. Evacuate to a cutting board, let rest for 10 to 15MIN, at that point cut and serve.
- **Nutrition Info:** Calories 234, fat 5g, carbohydrate 23g, Protein 22g.

194.Honey & Rosemary Chicken

Servings: 6
Cooking Time: 35 Minutes
Ingredients:
- 1 teaspoon paprika
- Salt to taste
- 1/2 teaspoon baking powder
- 2 lb. chicken wings
- 1/4 cup honey
- 1 tablespoon lemon juice
- 1 tablespoon garlic, minced
- 1 tablespoon rosemary, chopped

Directions:
1. Choose air fry setting in your Ninja Foodi Grill.
2. Set it to 390 degrees F.
3. Set the time to 30 minutes.
4. Press start to preheat.
5. While waiting, mix the paprika, salt and baking powder in a bowl.
6. Add the wings to the crisper basket.
7. Close and cook for 15 minutes.
8. Flip and cook for another 15 minutes.
9. In a bowl, mix the remaining ingredients.
10. Coat the wings with the sauce and cook for another 5 minutes.

195.Rib Eye Steak With Onions & Peppers

Servings: 2
Cooking Time: 20 Minutes
Ingredients:
- 1/2 teaspoon cumin
- 2 rib eye steaks
- 1 tablespoon vegetable oil
- 1 teaspoon smoked paprika
- 1/2 teaspoon onion powder
- 1 red bell pepper, sliced
- 1/2 teaspoon garlic powder
- Salt and pepper to taste
- 1 white onion, sliced into rings
- 1/4 cup fajita sauce

Directions:
1. Combine cumin, onion powder, garlic powder, paprika, salt and pepper to taste.
2. Add grill grate to your Ninja Foodi Grill.
3. Place the veggie tray on the grill grate. Seal the hood.
4. Choose grill setting.
5. Preheat it to medium for 20 minutes.
6. Coat steaks with half of oil.
7. Sprinkle with half of spice blend.
8. Toss the onions and bell pepper with remaining oil and spice blend.

9. Add steaks on the grill grate.
10. Cook for 10 minutes.
11. Brush both sides with fajita sauce.
12. Cook for another 10 minutes.
13. Add veggies to the veggie tray.
14. Cook with the steak for 10 minutes.
15. Serving Suggestions: Serve with fresh green salad or pasta.

196.Tangy And Saucy Beef Fingers

Servings: 4
Cooking Time: 14 Minutes
Ingredients:
- 1 ½ pounds sirloin steak
- 1/4 cup red wine
- 1/4 cup fresh lime juice
- 1 teaspoon garlic powder
- 1 teaspoon shallot powder
- 1 teaspoon celery seeds
- 1 teaspoon mustard seeds
- Coarse sea salt and ground black pepper, to taste
- 1 teaspoon red pepper flakes
- 2 eggs, lightly whisked
- 1 cup parmesan cheese
- 1 teaspoon paprika

Directions:
1. Place the steak, red wine, lime juice, garlic powder, shallot powder, celery seeds, mustard seeds, salt, black pepper, and red pepper in a large ceramic bowl; let it marinate for 3 hours.
2. Tenderize the cube steak by pounding with a mallet; cut into 1-inch strips.
3. In a shallow bowl, whisk the eggs. In another bowl, mix the parmesan cheese and paprika.
4. Dip the beef pieces into the whisked eggs and coat on all sides. Now, dredge the beef pieces in the parmesan mixture.
5. Cook at 400 degrees f for 14 minutes, flipping halfway through the cooking time.
6. Meanwhile, make the sauce by heating the reserved marinade in a saucepan over medium heat; let it simmer until thoroughly warmed. Serve the steak fingers with the sauce on the side.
- **Nutrition Info:** 475 calories; 26.3g fat; 7.9g carbs; 45g protein; 1.1g sugars; 0.6g fiber

197.Old-fashioned Walnut And Rum Cookies

Servings: 8
Cooking Time: 35 Minutes
Ingredients:
- 1/2 cup walnuts, ground
- 1/2 cup coconut flour
- 1 cup almond flour
- 3/4 cup swerve

- 1 stick butter, room temperature
- 2 tablespoons rum
- 1/2 teaspoon pure vanilla extract
- 1/2 teaspoon pure almond extract

Directions:
1. In a mixing dish, beat the butter with swerve, vanilla, and almond extract until light and fluffy. Then, throw in the flour and ground walnuts; add in rum.
2. Continue mixing until it forms a soft dough. Cover and place in the refrigerator for 20 minutes. In the meantime, preheat the air fryer to 330 degrees f.
3. Roll the dough into small cookies and place them on the air fryer cake pan; gently press each cookie using a spoon.
4. Bake butter cookies for 15 minutes in the preheated air fryer. Bon appétit!
- **Nutrition Info:** 228 calories; 22.3g fat; 4g carbs; 3.5g protein; 0.9g sugars; 2.3g fiber

198.Barbecue Chicken Breast

Servings: 4
Cooking Time: 50 Minutes
Ingredients:
- 4 chicken breast fillets
- 2 tablespoons vegetable oil
- Salt and pepper to taste
- 1 cup barbecue sauce

Directions:
1. Add grill grate to the Ninja Foodi Grill.
2. Close the hood.
3. Choose grill setting.
4. Preheat to medium for 25 minutes.
5. Press start.
6. Brush chicken breast with oil.
7. Sprinkle both sides with salt and pepper.
8. Add chicken and cook for 10 minutes.
9. Flip and cook for another 10 minutes.
10. Brush chicken with barbecue sauce.
11. Cook for 5 minutes.
12. Brush the other side and cook for another 5 minutes.

199.Roast Beef & Grilled Potatoes

Servings: 6
Cooking Time: 45 Minutes
Ingredients:
- 2 1/2 teaspoons onion powder
- 3 lb. top round roast
- 4 cups potatoes, grilled
- 2 1/2 teaspoons garlic powder
- Salt and pepper to taste

Directions:
1. Combine onion powder, garlic powder, salt and pepper in a bowl.
2. Rub top round roast with dry rub.
3. Set the Ninja Foodi Grill to broil.
4. Preheat it to high for 10 minutes.

5. Add the roast beef and cook for 25 minutes.
6. Turn and cook for another 20 minutes.
7. Serve with grilled potatoes.
8. Serving Suggestions: Slice against the grain and serve.

200.Spicy Ranch Fried Chicken

Servings: 4
Cooking Time: 20 Minutes
Ingredients:
- ½ cup buffalo sauce
- ½ cup ranch seasoning
- 4 cups buttermilk
- 2 chicken thighs
- 2 chicken breast fillets
- 2 cups all-purpose flour
- Cooking spray

Directions:
1. Mix buffalo sauce and ranch seasoning in a bowl.
2. Pour into a sealable plastic bag.
3. Add buttermilk to the bag.
4. Place the chicken inside the bag.
5. Marinate in the refrigerator for 1 hour.
6. Remove from marinade.
7. Coat chicken with flour.
8. Spray with oil.
9. Select air crisp in your unit.
10. Set it to 360 degrees F and preheat for 10 minutes.
11. Add chicken to the air crisp basket.
12. Cook for 20 minutes, flipping once.

201.Lovely American Grilled Burger

Servings: 4
Cooking Time: 20 Minutes
Ingredients:
- 1 tablespoon olive oil
- 1-pound ground beef
- 4 seed hamburger buns, cut in half
- ½ teaspoon salt
- 1 large egg, whisked
- ½ teaspoon pepper
- ½ cup breadcrumbs

Directions:
1. Take a medium-sized bowl and add listed ingredients, except oil and buns
2. Mix well and make about 4 patties out of the mixture
3. Brush the patties with olive oil
4. Pre-heat your Ninja Food Grill to HIGH setting, set a timer to 10 minutes
5. Once beeping sound is heard, transfer 2 patties to Grill and cook for 5 minutes per side
6. Grill remaining patties in a similar manner
7. Serve with the buns
8. Enjoy!

- **Nutrition Info:** Calories: 301 Fat: 15 g Saturated Fat: 3 g Carbohydrates: 11 g Fiber: 0.3 g Sodium: 398 mg Protein: 28 g

202.Onion Beef Roast

Servings: 6
Cooking Time: 30 Minutes
Ingredients:
- 2 sticks of celery, sliced
- 1 bulb of garlic, peeled and crushed
- A bunch of herbs of your choice
- 2 pounds topside of beef
- 2 medium onions, chopped
- Salt and ground black pepper to taste
- 1 tablespoon butter
- 3 tablespoons olive oil

Directions:
1. In a mixing bowl, add the ingredients. Combine the ingredients to mix well with each other.
2. Take Ninja Foodi Grill, arrange it over your kitchen platform, and open the top lid. Lightly grease the cooking pot with some oil or cooking spray.
3. Press "ROAST" and adjust the temperature to 380°F. Adjust the timer to 30 minutes and then press "START/STOP." Ninja Foodi will start preheating.
4. Ninja Foodi is preheated and ready to cook when it starts to beep. After you hear a beep, open the top lid.
5. Arrange the bowl mixture directly inside the pot.
6. Close the top lid and allow it to cook until the timer reads zero.
7. Serve warm.

203.Rosemary Lamb Chops

Servings: 4
Cooking Time: 10 Minutes
Ingredients:
- 3 lb. lamb chops
- 4 rosemary sprigs
- Salt to taste
- 1 tablespoon olive oil
- 2 tablespoons butter
- 1 tablespoon tomato paste
- 1 cup beef stock
- 1 green onion, sliced

Directions:
1. Season the lamb chops with rosemary, salt, and pepper.
2. Pour in the olive oil and add the butter to the Ninja Foodi. Set it to Sauté.
3. Add the lamb chops and cook for one minute per side. Add the rest of the ingredients.
4. Stir well. Cover the pot. Set it to Pressure. Cook at high pressure for 5 minutes.

5. Release the pressure naturally.
6. serving Suggestions:
7. Serve with pickled onions.
8. Tips:
9. You can also use tomato sauce in place of tomato paste.
- **Nutrition Info:** Calories: 484 Total Fat: 23 g Saturated Fat: 8.8 g Cholesterol: 214 mg Sodium: 361 mg Total Carbohydrate: 1.2 g Dietary Fiber: 0.5 g Total Sugars: 0.4 g Protein: 64.4 g Potassium: 824 mg

204.Grilled Steak With Asparagus

Servings: 5
Cooking Time: 20 Minutes
Ingredients:
- 4 strip steaks
- 3 tablespoons vegetable oil, divided
- Salt and pepper to taste
- 2 cups asparagus, trimmed and sliced

Directions:
1. Select grill setting.
2. Choose "beef".
3. Preheat the unit by pressing "start".
4. Brush steaks with half of the oil.
5. Season with salt and pepper.
6. Coat asparagus with remaining oil.
7. Sprinkle with salt and pepper.
8. Add the steak to the grill.
9. Cook for 7 to 10 minutes per side.
10. Transfer to a plate.
11. Add the asparagus to the unit.
12. Select grill. Set it to high.
13. Serve steaks with asparagus.

205.Quick Picadillo Dish

Servings: 4
Cooking Time: 16 Minutes
Ingredients:
- 1/2 pound lean ground beef
- 2 garlic cloves, minced
- 1/2 large onion, chopped
- 1 teaspoon salt
- 1 tomato, chopped
- 1/2 red bell pepper, chopped
- 1 tablespoon cilantro
- 1/2 can (4 ounces) tomato sauce
- 1 teaspoon ground cumin
- 1-2 bay leaves
- 2 tablespoons green olives, capers
- 2 tablespoons brine
- 3 tablespoons water

Directions:
1. Set your Ninja Foodi to Sauté mode and add meat, salt, and pepper, slightly brown
2. Add garlic, tomato, onion, cilantro, and Sauté for 1 minute. Add olives, brine, leaf, cumin, and mix

3. Pour in sauce, water, and stir. Lock lid and cook on HIGH pressure for 15 minutes
4. Quick-release pressure

206.Beefed Up Spaghetti Squash

Servings: 8
Cooking Time: 10-15 Minutes
Ingredients:
- 2 pounds ground beef
- 1 medium spaghetti squash
- 32 ounces marinara sauce
- 3 tablespoons olive oil

Directions:
1. Slice squash in half lengthwise and dispose of seeds.
2. Add trivet to your Ninja Foodi.
3. Add 1 cup water.
4. Arrange squash on the rack and lock the lid, cook on high pressure for 8 minutes.
5. Quick-release the pressure.
6. Remove from pot.
7. Clean the pot and set your Ninja Foodi to Sauté.
8. Add ground beef and add olive oil, and let it heat up.
9. Add ground beef and cook until slightly browned and cooked.
10. Separate strands from cooked squash and transfer to a bowl.
11. Add cooked beef, and mix with marinara sauce. Serve and enjoy!
- **Nutrition Info:** Calories: 174 Fat: 6 g Carbohydrates: 5 g Protein: 19 g

207.Competition-style Barbecue Ribs Recipe

Servings: 4
Cooking Time: 6 Hrs
Ingredients:
- 2 - racks St. Louis-cut pork ribs
- ½ - cup yellow mustard
- 1 - cup your favorite barbecue rub
- 2 - cups apple juice, divided, 1 cup placed in a squirt bottle
- 2 to 3 fist size chunks of light smoking wood, such as cherry or apple
- 1 - cup your favorite barbecue sauce
- ½ cup agave syrup (optional)
- ½ cup dark brown sugar (optional)

Directions:
1. Take the movie out from the rear of each rack, and trim the ribs of overabundance fat. Brush meat aspect of every rack with yellow mustard; at that point rub generously with grill rub on the 2 aspects.
2. Fire up smoker or barbecue to 225°F, consisting of pieces of smoking wood while at temperature. At the factor while the wood is lighted and delivering smoke,

vicinity the ribs within the smoker or Ninja Foodi oven broil, meat facet up. Smoke till ribs obscure to profound mahogany, round 3 HRS, clouding with a squeezed apple in a spurt bottle every hour.

3. Wrap every rack, meat side up, in greater-large hardcore aluminum foil, leaving an opening toward one side of the foil. Pour½ cup of squeezed apple in every foil percent through the hole, seal and notice again on smoker or Ninja Foodi oven broil for 60 minutes.

4. Take out ribs from foil and spot ribs back in the smoker and maintain on cooking until ribs have a mild twist whilst lifted from one give up, 1 to 2 HRS increasingly more, spurting with squeezed apple continually. Take ribs out from smoker or Ninja Foodi oven broil, envelope by using foil, and a gap in a vacant cooler to keep heat whilst putting in place the barbeque.

5. Light one smokestack loaded with charcoal. At the point when all charcoal is lit and secured with dim debris, spill out and unfold the coals equally over the entire surface of coal grind. Set cooking grate set up, spread Ninja Foodi oven broil, and permit to preheat for 5MIN. Clean and oil the Ninja Foodi oven broiling grate. Take the racks out from foil and brush with grill sauce. Spot ribs face down over warm fire and cook till sauce caramelizes 2 to 5MIN. Take racks out from the barbeque.

6. For extra candy and sleek ribs: Tear off two extra big sheets of aluminum foil longer than each rack. In a rectangular form, the inexact length of every rack of ribs unfold ¼ cup of agave syrup and sprinkle ¼ cup earthy colored sugar on agave on each little bit of foil. Spot ribs, meat facet down, on agave and sugar, and wrap foil shut round ribs. Spot ribs returned at the smoker for 15MIN. Take ribs out from smoker and foil, at that point reduce and serve.

- **Nutrition Info:** Calories 387, fat 25g, carbohydrate 13g, Protein 27g.

208.Lettuce Cheese Steak

Servings: 5-6
Cooking Time: 16 Minutes
Ingredients:
- 4 (8-ounce) skirt steaks
- 6 cups romaine lettuce, chopped
- ¾ cup cherry tomatoes halved
- ¼ cup blue cheese, crumbled
- Ocean salt and ground black pepper
- 2 avocados, peeled and sliced
- 1 cup croutons
- 1 cup blue cheese dressing

Directions:

1. Coat steaks with black pepper and salt.
2. Take Ninja Foodi Grill, mastermind it over your kitchen stage, and open the top[NH5]. Organize the barbecue mesh and close the top.
3. Click Grill and the High functions. Change the clock to 8 minutes and press Start/Stop. Ninja Foodi will begin pre-warming.
4. Ninja Foodi is preheated and prepared to cook when it begins to blare. After you hear a blare, open the top cover.
5. Fix finely the 2 steaks on the barbeque mesh.
6. Close the top cover and cook for 4 minutes. Presently open the top cover, flip the steaks.
7. Close the top cover and cook for 4 additional minutes. Cook until the food thermometer comes to 165°F. Cook for 3-4 more minutes if needed. Grill the remaining steaks.
8. In a mixing bowl, add the lettuce, tomatoes, blue cheese, and croutons. Combine the ingredients to mix well with each other.
9. Serve the steaks warm with the salad mixture, blue cheese dressing, and avocado slices on top.

- **Nutrition Info:** Calories: 576 Fat: 21 g Saturated Fat: 8.5 g Trans Fat: 0 g Carbohydrates: 23 g Fiber: 6.5 g Sodium: 957 mg Protein: 53.5 g

209.Grilled Ranch Chicken

Servings: 6
Cooking Time: 30 Minutes
Ingredients:
- 6 chicken thigh fillets
- 3 tablespoons ranch dressing
- Garlic salt and pepper

Directions:

1. Spread both sides of chicken with ranch dressing.
2. Sprinkle with garlic salt and pepper.
3. Set your Ninja Foodi Grill to grill.
4. Preheat it to medium.
5. Add chicken to the grill grate.
6. Cook for 15 minutes per side.

210.Thanksgiving Turkey With Mustard Gravy

Servings: 6
Cooking Time: 45 Minutes
Ingredients:
- 2 teaspoons butter, softened
- 1 teaspoon dried sage
- 2 sprigs rosemary, chopped
- 1 teaspoon salt
- 1/4 teaspoon freshly ground black pepper, or more to taste
- 1 whole turkey breast

- 2 tablespoons turkey broth
- 2 tablespoons whole-grain mustard
- 1 tablespoon butter

Directions:
1. Start by preheating your air fryer to 360 degrees f.
2. To make the rub, combine 2 tablespoons of butter, sage, rosemary, salt, and pepper; mix well to combine and spread it evenly over the surface of the turkey breast.
3. Roast for 20 minutes in an air fryer cooking basket. Flip the turkey breast over and cook for a further 15 to 16 minutes. Now, flip it back over and roast for 12 minutes more.
4. While the turkey is roasting, whisk the other ingredients in a saucepan. After that, spread the gravy all over the turkey breast.
5. Let the turkey rest for a few minutes before carving.
- **Nutrition Info:** 384 calories; 8.2g fat; 2.5g carbs; 51.5g protein; 0.2g sugars; 0.2g fiber

211.Generous Shepherd's Pie

Servings: 4
Cooking Time: 15 Minutes
Ingredients:
- 2 cups of water
- 4 tablespoons butter
- 4 ounces cream cheese
- 1 cup mozzarella
- 1 whole egg
- Salt and pepper to taste
- 1 tablespoon garlic powder
- 2-3 pounds ground beef
- 1 cup frozen carrots
- 8 ounces mushrooms, sliced
- 1 cup beef broth

Directions:
1. Add water to Ninja Foodi, arrange cauliflower on top, lock lid and cook for 5 minutes on HIGH pressure.
2. Quick-release and transfer to a blender, add cream cheese, butter, mozzarella cheese, egg, pepper, and salt. Blend well.
3. Drain water from Ninja Foodi and add beef
4. Add carrots, garlic powder, broth and pepper, and salt
5. Add in cauliflower mix and lock lid, cook for 10 minutes on HIGH pressure
6. Release pressure naturally over 10 minutes. Serve and enjoy!

212.Honey Mustard Chicken

Servings: 6
Cooking Time: 30 Minutes
Ingredients:
- 6 chicken breast fillets
- 3 tablespoons vegetable oil
- Salt and pepper to taste

- 1 cup honey mustard sauce
- 1 cup barbecue sauce

Directions:
1. Set your unit to grill.
2. Choose medium temperature.
3. Set it to 30 minutes.
4. Press start to preheat.
5. While preheating, brush both sides of chicken breast with oil.
6. Season with salt and pepper.
7. After 10 minutes, add the chicken to the grill grate.
8. Cook for 10 minutes, flipping once.
9. In a bowl, mix the honey mustard sauce and barbecue sauce.
10. Brush chicken with sauce.
11. Cook for another 10 minutes.

213.Chicken Teriyaki

Servings: 2
Cooking Time: 30 Minutes
Ingredients:
- 2 chicken breast fillets, sliced into strips
- Salt and pepper to taste
- Cooking spray
- ¼ cup teriyaki sauce

Directions:
1. Season chicken strips with salt and pepper.
2. Spray with oil.
3. Add chicken strips to the grill grate.
4. Select grill setting.
5. Choose high.
6. Cook for 5 minutes per side.
7. Brush chicken with the teriyaki sauce.
8. Cook for another 10 minutes, flipping once.

214.Asian-style Round Steak

Servings: 4
Cooking Time: 30 Minutes
Ingredients:
- 2 pounds top round steak, cut into bite-sized strips
- 2 garlic cloves, sliced
- 1 teaspoon dried marjoram
- 1/4 cup red wine
- 1 tablespoon tamari sauce
- Salt and black pepper, to taste
- 1 tablespoon olive oil
- 1 red onion, sliced
- 2 bell peppers, sliced
- 1 celery stalk, sliced

Directions:
1. Place the top round, garlic, marjoram, red wine, tamari sauce, salt and pepper in a bowl, cover and let it marinate for 1 hour.
2. Preheat your air fryer to 390 degrees f and add the oil.
3. Once hot, discard the marinade and cook the beef for 15 minutes. Add the onion,

peppers, carrot, and garlic and continue cooking until tender about 15 minutes more.

4. Open the air fryer every 5 minutes and baste the meat with the remaining marinade. Serve immediately.

- **Nutrition Info:** 418 calories; 12.2g fat; 4.8g carbs; 68.2g protein; 2.3g sugars; 0.8g fiber

215.Beef, Pearl Onions And Cauliflower

Servings: 4
Cooking Time: 12 Minutes
Ingredients:

- 1 ½ pounds new york strip, cut into strips
- 1 (1-pound head cauliflower, broken into florets
- 1 cup pearl onion, sliced
- Marinade:
- 1 tablespoon olive oil
- 2 cloves garlic, minced
- 1 teaspoon of ground ginger
- 1/4 cup tomato paste
- 1/2 cup red wine

Directions:

1. Mix all ingredients for the marinade. Add the beef to the marinade and let it sit in your refrigerator for 1 hour.
2. Preheat your air fryer to 400 degrees f. Transfer the meat to the air fryer basket. Add the cauliflower and onions.
3. Drizzle a few tablespoons of marinade all over the meat and vegetables. Cook for 12 minutes, shaking the basket halfway through the cooking time. Serve warm.

- **Nutrition Info:** 298 calories; 13.8g fat; 7.4g carbs; 37g protein; 3.1g sugars; 2g fiber

216.Braised Lamb Shanks

Servings: 4
Cooking Time: 40 Minutes
Ingredients:

- 2 tablespoons olive oil
- 4 lamb shanks
- Salt and pepper to taste
- 4 cloves garlic, minced
- ¾ cup dry red wine
- 1 teaspoon dried basil
- ¾ teaspoon dried oregano
- 28 oz. crushed tomatoes

Directions:

1. Turn the Ninja Foodi to Sauté. Add the oil. Season the lamb with salt and pepper.
2. Cook until brown. Remove and set aside. Add the garlic and cook for 15 seconds.
3. Pour in the wine. Simmer for 2 minutes. Stir in the basil, oregano, and tomatoes.
4. Put the lamb back in the pot. Seal the pot. Set it to Pressure.
5. Cook at high pressure for 45 minutes. Release the pressure naturally.

6. serving Suggestions:
7. Serve over polenta.

- **Nutrition Info:** Calories: 790 Total Fat: 31 g Saturated Fat: 9.6 g Cholesterol: 294 mg Sodium: 632 mg Total Carbohydrate: 18.3 g Dietary Fiber 6.5 g Total Sugars: 11.5 g Protein: 96.8 g Potassium: 1157 mg

217.Pork Tenderloin

Servings: 4
Cooking Time: 20 Minutes
Ingredients:

- 1 clove garlic, minced
- 1 teaspoon ginger, grated
- 1 tablespoon rice vinegar
- 2 tablespoons soy sauce
- 1 tablespoon vegetable oil
- 1 tablespoon dry sherry
- 1 tablespoon brown sugar
- Salt and pepper to taste
- 1 lb. pork tenderloin

Directions:

1. Mix all the ingredients except pork in a bowl.
2. Once fully combined, add the pork.
3. Coat evenly with the sauce.
4. Cover and marinate for 3 hours in the refrigerator.
5. Choose air crisp function.
6. Air fry at 400 degrees F for 20 minutes, stirring once or twice.

218.Chocolate Fudgy Brownies

Servings: 8
Cooking Time: 20 Minutes
Ingredients:

- 1 stick butter, melted
- 1 cup swerve
- 2 eggs
- 1 teaspoon vanilla essence
- 2 tablespoons flaxseed meal
- 1 cup coconut flour
- 1 teaspoon baking powder
- 1/2 cup cocoa powder, unsweetened
- A pinch of salt
- A pinch of ground cardamom

Directions:

1. Start by preheating your air fryer to 350 degrees f. Now, spritz the sides and bottom of a baking pan with cooking spray.
2. In a mixing dish, beat the melted butter with swerve until fluffy. Next, fold in the eggs and beat again.
3. After that, add the vanilla, flour, baking powder, cocoa, salt, and ground cardamom. Mix until everything is well combined.
4. Bake in the preheated air fryer for 20 to 22 minutes. Enjoy!

- **Nutrition Info:** 180 calories; 17.6g fat; 5.7g carbs; 3.5g protein; 0.8g sugars; 3.3g fiber

219.The Yogurt Lamb Skewers

Servings: 4
Cooking Time: 16 Minutes
Ingredients:
- 2 garlic cloves, minced
- 1 pack of 10 ounces couscous
- 1 tablespoon and 1 teaspoon cumin
- 2 lemons, juiced
- 1½ cup yogurt
- Salt to taste
- 1½ pound lamb leg, boneless, cubed
- Fresh ground black pepper
- 2 tomatoes, seeded and diced
- ½ small red onion, chopped
- 3 tablespoons olive oil
- ½ cucumber, seeded and diced
- ¼ cup finely chopped fresh parsley
- ¼ cup fresh mint, chopped
- Lemon wedges to serve

Directions:
1. Cook couscous following the package instructions, and fluff it up with a fork.
2. Whisk yogurt with garlic, cumin, lemon juice, salt, pepper in a large-sized bowl.
3. Add lamb, mix well to coat it.
4. Separate toss red onion, cucumber, tomatoes, parsley, mint, lemon juice, olive oil, salt, and couscous in a salad bowl.
5. Thread your seasoned lamb on 8 skewers and drizzle salt and pepper over them.
6. Preheat your Ninja Foodi Grill on High. Set the timer to 16 minutes.
7. Once you hear the beep, place 4 skewers on the grill.
8. Let it cook for 4 minutes per side.
9. Cook the remaining ones in a similar way.
10. Serve and enjoy!
- **Nutrition Info:** Calories: 417 Fat: 11 g Saturated Fat: 5 g Carbohydrates: 20 g Fiber: 2 g Sodium: 749 mg Protein: 13 g

220.Classic Cube Steak With Sauce

Servings: 4
Cooking Time: 14 Minutes
Ingredients:
- 1 ½ pounds cube steak
- Salt, to taste
- 1/4 teaspoon ground black pepper, or more to taste
- 4 ounces butter
- 2 garlic cloves, finely chopped
- 2 scallions, finely chopped
- 2 tablespoon fresh parsley, finely chopped
- 1 tablespoon fresh horseradish, grated
- 1 teaspoon cayenne pepper

Directions:
1. Pat dry the cube steak and season it with salt and black pepper. Spritz the air fryer basket with cooking oil. Add the meat to the basket.
2. Cook in the preheated air fryer at 400 degrees f for 14 minutes.
3. Meanwhile, melt the butter in a skillet over a moderate heat. Add the remaining ingredients and simmer until the sauce has thickened and reduced slightly.
4. Top the warm cube steaks with cowboy sauce and serve immediately.
- **Nutrition Info:** 469 calories; 30.4g fat; 0.6g carbs; 46g protein; 0g sugars; 0.4g fiber

POULTRY RECIPES

221.Turkey Burrito

Servings: 2
Cooking Time: 8 Minutes
Ingredients:
- 4 slices turkey breast already cooked
- ½ red bell pepper, sliced
- 2 eggs
- 1 small avocado, peeled, pitted, and sliced
- 2 tablespoons salsa
- Salt and black pepper to the taste
- 1/8 cup mozzarella cheese, grated
- Tortillas for serving

Directions:
1. In a bowl, whisk eggs with salt and pepper to the taste, pour them in a pan and place it in the air fryer's basket.
2. Cook at 400 degrees F for 5 minutes, take the pan out of the fryer, and transfer eggs to a plate.
3. Roll your burritos and place them in your air fryer after you've lined it with some tin foil.
4. Heat the burritos at 300 degrees F for 3 minutes, divide them among plates and serve.
5. Enjoy!

222.Classic Honey Soy Chicken

Servings: 4
Cooking Time: 18 Min
Ingredients:
- 4 boneless, skinless chicken bosoms cut into little pieces
- 4 garlic cloves, smashed
- 1 onion, diced
- ½ cup honey
- 2 tablespoon lime juice
- 2 teaspoon sesame oil
- 3 tablespoon soy sauce
- 1 tablespoon water
- 1 tablespoon cornstarch
- 1 teaspoon rice vinegar
- Black pepper and salt to taste

Directions:
1. In a mixing bowl, add the honey, sesame oil, lime juice, soy sauce, and rice vinegar. Combine well.
2. Take Ninja Foodi multi-cooker, arrange it over a cooking platform, and open the top lid.
3. In the pot, add the onion, chicken, and garlic; add the soy sauce mixture and stir gently.
4. Seal the multi-cooker by locking it with the pressure lid; ensure to keep the pressure release valve locked/sealed.

5. Select "PRESSURE" mode and select the "HI" pressure level. Then, set timer to 15 minutes and press "STOP/START"; it will start the cooking process by building up inside pressure.
6. At the point when the clock goes off, brisk discharge pressure by adjusting the pressure valve to the VENT. After pressure gets released, open the pressure lid.
7. In a bowl, mix water and cornstarch until well dissolved.
8. Select "SEAR/SAUTÉ" mode and select the "MD" pressure level; add the cornstarch mixture in the pot and combine it, stir-cook for 2 minutes.
9. Serve warm.
- **Nutrition Info:** Calories: 493, Fat: 8.5g, Saturated Fat: 1g, Trans Fat: 0g, Carbohydrates: 44.5g, Fiber: 5g, Sodium: 712mg, Protein: 41.5g

223.Grilled Orange Chicken

Servings: 5-6
Cooking Time: 10 Minutes
Ingredients:
- 1/2 teaspoon garlic salt
- 2 teaspoons ground coriander
- 12 chicken wings
- 1/4 teaspoon ground black pepper
- 1 tablespoon canola oil
- Sauce:
- 1/4 cup butter, melted
- 3 tablespoons honey
- 1/2 cup orange juice
- 1/3 cup Sriracha chili sauce
- 2 tablespoons lime juice
- 1/4 cup chopped cilantro

Directions:
1. Coat chicken with oil and season with the spices; refrigerate for 2 hours to marinate.
2. Combine all the sauce ingredients and set aside. Optionally, you can stir-cook the sauce mixture for 3-4 minutes in a saucepan.
3. Take Ninja Foodi Grill, organize it over your kitchen stage, and open the top cover.
4. Organize the barbecue mesh and close the top cover.
5. Click "GRILL" and choose the "MED" grill function. Adjust the timer to 10 minutes and afterward press "START/STOP." Ninja Foodi will begin pre-warming.
6. Ninja Foodi is preheated and prepared to cook when it begins to signal. After you hear a blare, open the top.
7. Organize chicken over the grill grate.
8. Close the top lid and cook for 5 minutes. Now open the top lid, flip the chicken.

9. Close the top lid and cook for 5 more minutes.
- **Nutrition Info:** Calories: 327, Fat: 14g, Saturated Fat: 3.5g, Trans Fat: 0g, Carbohydrates: 19g, Fiber: 1g, Sodium: 258mg, Protein: 25g

224.The Tarragon Chicken Meal

Servings: 4
Cooking Time: 5 Minutes
Ingredients:
- For Chicken
- 1 and ½ pounds chicken tenders
- Salt as needed
- 3 tablespoons tarragon leaves, chopped
- 1 teaspoon lemon zest, grated
- 2 tablespoons fresh lemon juice
- 2 tablespoons extra virgin olive oil
- For Sauce
- 2 tablespoons fresh lemon juice
- 2 tablespoons butter, salted
- ½ cup heavy whip cream

Directions:
1. Prepare your chicken by taking a baking dish and arranging the chicken over the dish in a single layer
2. Season generously with salt and pepper
3. Sprinkle chopped tarragon and lemon zest all around the tenders
4. Drizzle lemon juice and olive oil on top
5. Let them sit for 10 minutes
6. Drain them well
7. Insert Grill Grate in your Ninja Foodi Grill and set to HIGH temperature
8. Set timer to 4 minutes
9. Once you hear the beep, place chicken tenders in your grill grate
10. Let it cook for 3-4 minutes until cooked completely
11. Do in batches if needed
12. Transfer the cooked chicken tenders to a platter
13. For the sauce, take a small-sized saucepan
14. Add cream, butter and lemon juice and bring to a boil
15. Once thickened enough, pour the mix over chicken
16. Serve and enjoy!
17. Serve and enjoy once ready!
- **Nutrition Info:** Calories: 263 Fat: 18 g Saturated Fat: 4 g Carbohydrates: 7 g Fiber: 1 g Sodium: 363 mg Protein: 19 g

225.Majestic Alfredo Chicken

Servings: 4
Cooking Time: 20 Minutes
Ingredients:
- ½ cup alfredo sauce
- ¼ cup blue cheese, crumbled
- 4 slices provolone cheese
- 4 teaspoons chicken seasoning
- 4 chicken breasts, halved
- 1 tablespoon lemon juice
- 1 large apple wedged

Directions:
1. Take a medium-sized bowl and add chicken, alongside the seasoning.
2. Take another bowl and toss the apple with lemon .
3. Preheat your Ninja Foodi Grill in Med mode, set timer to 16 minutes.
4. Wait until you hear a beep sound.
5. Arrange chicken pieces to the grill grate and cook for about 8 minutes, flip and cook for 8 minutes.
6. Transfer the apple to the grill and cook for 4 minutes, giving 2 minutes to each side.
7. Serve grilled chicken with the blue cheese, apple, and alfredo sauce.
8. Enjoy!
- **Nutrition Info:** Calories: 247 Fat: 19 g Saturated Fat: 3 g Carbohydrates: 29 g Fiber: 2 g Sodium: 850 mg Protein: 14 g

226.Chicken Bean Bake

Servings: 8
Cooking Time: 20 Minutes
Ingredients:
- ½ red bell pepper, diced
- ½ red onion, diced
- 2 (8-ounce) boneless, skinless chicken breasts cut into 1-inch cubes
- 1 tablespoon extra-virgin olive oil
- 1 cup white rice
- 2 cups shredded Cheddar cheese
- 2 cups chicken broth
- 1 (15-ounce) can black beans, rinsed and drained
- 1 (1-ounce) packet taco seasoning
- 1 (15-ounce) can corn, rinsed
- 1 (10-ounce) can roasted tomatoes with chiles
- Kosher salt
- Black pepper (ground)

Directions:
1. Take Ninja Foodi multi-cooker, arrange it over a cooking platform, and open the top lid. In the pot, add the oil, select "SEAR/SAUTÉ" mode and select "MD: HI" pressure level. Press "STOP/START." After about 4-5 minutes, the oil will start simmering.
2. Put in the chicken and mix for about 2-3 minutes to brown evenly.
3. Add the onion and bell pepper, stir-cook until softened for 2 minutes. Add the rice, tomatoes, beans, corn, taco seasoning, broth, salt, and pepper, combine well.

4. Seal the multi-cooker by locking it with the pressure lid; ensure to keep the pressure release valve locked/sealed.
5. Select "PRESSURE" mode and select the "HI" pressure level. Then after, set timer to 7 minutes and press "STOP/START," it will start the cooking process by building up inside pressure.
6. When the timer goes off, quickly release pressure by adjusting the pressure valve to the VENT, after pressure gets released, open the pressure lid. Add the cheese on top.
7. Seal the multi-cooker by locking it with the Crisping Lid; ensure to keep the pressure release valve locked/sealed.
8. Select "BROIL" mode and select the "HI" pressure level. Then after, set timer to 8 minutes and press "STOP/START," it will start the cooking process by building up inside pressure.
9. When the timer goes off, quickly release pressure by adjusting the pressure valve to the VENT, after pressure gets released, open the Crisping Lid.
- **Nutrition Info:** Calories: 312, Fat: 15.5g, Saturated Fat: 6g, Trans Fat: 0g, Carbohydrates: 24.5g, Fiber: 5g, Sodium: 652mg, Protein: 24g

227.Peanut Chicken

Servings: 4
Cooking Time: 20 Minutes
Ingredients:
- 1½ lb. chicken breast, sliced into cubes
- Salt to taste
- 1 teaspoon oil
- 3 clove garlic, chopped
- 1 tablespoon ginger, chopped
- 13 oz. coconut milk
- 3 tablespoons soy sauce
- 3 tablespoons honey
- 2 tablespoons fresh lime juice
- 1 tablespoon chili garlic paste
- ½ cup peanut butter

Directions:
1. Season the chicken with salt. Set the Ninja Foodi to Sauté. Add the oil.
2. Cook the garlic and ginger for 1 minute.
3. Add the chicken and all the other ingredients except the peanut butter.
4. Mix well. Put the peanut butter on top of the chicken but do not stir.
5. Seal the pot. Set it to Pressure. Cook at high pressure for 9 minutes.
6. Release the pressure naturally.
7. serving Suggestions:
8. Serve on top of spinach leaves.
- **Nutrition Info:** Calories: 445 Total Fat: 29.1 g Saturated Fat: 15.4 g Cholesterol: 73 mg

Sodium: 645 mg Total Carbohydrate: 18 g Dietary Fiber: 2.9 g Total Sugars: 12.9 g Protein: 31.5 g Potassium: 762 mg

228.Chicken Chile Verde

Servings: 4
Cooking Time: 25 Minutes
Ingredients:
- 2 lb. chicken thighs
- 1/4 teaspoon garlic powder
- 16 ounces salsa verde
- 1/2 teaspoon ground cumin
- Salt and pepper to taste

Directions:
1. Add the chicken to the Ninja Foodi.
2. Season with the garlic powder, salsa verde, and cumin. Cover the pot.
3. Set it to pressure. Cook at high pressure for 25 minutes.
4. Release the pressure quickly. Shred the chicken using 2 forks.
5. Season with the salt and pepper.

229.Taiwanese Chicken Delight

Servings: 4
Cooking Time: 10 Minutes
Ingredients:
- 6 dried red chilis
- ¼ cup sesame oil
- 2 tablespoons ginger
- ¼ cup garlic, minced
- ¼ cup red wine vinegar
- ¼ cup coconut aminos
- Salt as needed
- 1.2 teaspoon Xanthan [NH2]gum (for the finish)
- ¼ cup Thai basil, chopped

Directions:
1. Set your Ninja Foodi to Sauté mode and add ginger, chilis, garlic. Sauté for 2 minutes.
2. Add remaining ingredients. Lock the lid and cook on high pressure for 10 minutes.
3. Quick-release the pressure. Serve and enjoy!
- **Nutrition Info:** Calories: 307 Fat: 15 g Carbohydrates: 7 g Protein: 31 g

230.Exotic Pilaf Chicken

Servings: 4
Cooking Time: 15 Minutes
Ingredients:
- 1 tablespoon unsalted butter
- 4 boneless, skin-on chicken thighs
- 1 ¾ cups water
- 1 tablespoon extra-virgin olive oil
- 1 teaspoon garlic powder
- 1 (6-ounce) box rice pilaf
- 1 teaspoon kosher salt

Directions:

1. Take Ninja Foodi multi-cooker, arrange it over a cooking platform, and open the top lid.
2. In the pot, add water, butter, and pilaf, and place a reversible rack inside the pot. Place the chicken thighs over the rack.
3. Seal the multi-cooker by locking it with the pressure lid, ensure to keep the pressure release valve locked/sealed.
4. Select "PRESSURE" mode and select the "HI" pressure level. Then after, set timer to 4 minutes and press "STOP/START," it will start the cooking process by building up inside pressure.
5. When the timer goes off, quickly release pressure by adjusting the pressure valve to the VENT. After pressure gets released, open the pressure lid.
6. In a mixing bowl, combine together the olive oil, salt, and garlic powder. Brush thickens with this mixture.
7. Seal the multi-cooker by locking it with the Crisping Lid, ensure to keep the pressure release valve locked/sealed.
8. Select "BROIL" mode and select the "HI" pressure level. Then after, set timer to 10 minutes and press "STOP/START," it will start the cooking process by building up inside pressure.
9. When the timer goes off, quickly release pressure by adjusting the pressure valve to the VENT. After pressure gets released, open the Crisping Lid. Serve warm the chicken with cooked pilaf.
- **Nutrition Info:** Calories: 425, Fat: 26g, Saturated Fat: 8.5g, Trans Fat: 0g, Carbohydrates: 12g, Fiber: 1.5g, Sodium: 524mg, Protein: 23g

231.A Genuine Hassel Back Chicken

Servings: 4
Cooking Time: 60 Minutes
Ingredients:
- 4 tablespoons butter
- Salt and pepper to taste
- 2 cups fresh mozzarella cheese, thinly sliced
- 8 large chicken breasts
- 4 large Roma tomatoes, thinly sliced

Directions:
1. Make a few deep slits in chicken breasts, and season with salt and pepper.
2. Stuff mozzarella cheese slices and tomatoes in chicken slits.
3. Grease Ninja Foodi pot with butter and arrange stuffed chicken breasts.
4. Lock the lid and Bake/Roast for 1 hour at 365°F. Serve and enjoy!
- **Nutrition Info:** Calories: 278 Fat: 15 g Carbohydrates: 3.8 g Protein: 15 g

232.Sweet And Sour Chicken Bbq

Servings: 4
Cooking Time: 40 Minutes
Ingredients:
- 6 chicken drumsticks
- 1 cup of soy sauce
- 1 cup of water
- 1 cup white vinegar
- ¾ cup of sugar
- ¾ cup onion, minced
- ¼ cup tomato paste
- ¼ cup garlic, minced
- Salt and pepper, to taste

Directions:
1. Take a Ziploc bag and add all ingredients into it
2. Marinate for at least 2 hours in your refrigerator
3. Insert the crisper basket, and close the hood
4. Pre-heat Ninja Foodi by squeezing the "AIR CRISP" alternative at 390 degrees F for 40 minutes
5. Place the grill pan accessory in the air fryer
6. Flip the chicken after every 10 minutes
7. Take a saucepan and pour the marinade into it and heat over medium flame until sauce thickens
8. Brush with the glaze
9. Serve warm and enjoy!
- **Nutrition Info:** Calories: 460, Fat: 20 g, Saturated Fat: 5 g, Carbohydrates: 26 g, Fiber: 3 g, Sodium: 126 mg, Protein: 28 g

233.Glamorous Turkey Burger

Servings: 4
Cooking Time: 40 Minutes
Ingredients:
- 1 large red onion, chopped
- ½ teaspoon pepper
- ¼ teaspoon salt
- 1 cup feta cheese, crumbled
- 2/3 cup sun-dried tomatoes, chopped
- 6 burger buns, sliced in half
- 2 pounds lean turkey, grounded
- 3 ounces plain granola

Directions:
1. Take a medium-sized mixing bowl and add listed ingredients
2. Combine them well and make 6 patties out of the mixture
3. Pre-heat your Ninja Foodi Grill in MED mode setting the timer to 14 minutes
4. Wait till you hear the beep
5. Transfer the patties to your Ninja Foodi Grill Grate
6. Cook for 7 minutes
7. Serve by placing them in your burger buns
8. Enjoy!

- **Nutrition Info:** Calories: 298 Fat: 16 g Saturated Fat: 4 g Carbohydrates: 32 g Fiber: 4 g Sodium: 168 mg Protein: 27 g

234.Excellent Chicken Tomatino

Servings: 4
Cooking Time: 12 Minutes
Ingredients:
- ½ teaspoon salt
- 1 garlic clove, minced
- 2 tablespoons olive oil
- ¾ cup vinegar
- 8 plum tomatoes
- ¼ cup fresh basil leaves
- 4 chicken breast, boneless and skinless

Directions:
1. Take your fine food processor and add olive oil, vinegar, salt, garlic, and basil. Blend the mixture well until you have a smooth texture.
2. Add tomatoes and blend once again.
3. Take a mixing bowl and add tomato mix, chicken and mix well.
4. Let the mixture chill for 1-2 hours.
5. Preheat your Ninja Foodi Grill to High and set the timer to 6 minutes.
6. Once you hear the beep, arrange your prepared chicken over the grill grate.
7. Cook for 3 minutes more.
8. Flip the chicken and cook for 3 minutes more.
9. Once properly cooked, serve and enjoy!
- **Nutrition Info:** Calories: 400 Fat: 5 g Saturated Fat: 3 g Carbohydrates: 18 g Fiber: 3 g Sodium: 230 mg Protein: 23 g

235.Chicken Chili And Beans

Servings: 4
Cooking Time: 15 Minutes
Ingredients:
- 1 and ¼ pounds chicken breast, cut into pieces
- 1 can black beans, drained and rinsed
- 1 tablespoon oil
- 1 can corn
- 1 bell pepper, chopped
- ¼ teaspoon garlic powder
- ¼ teaspoon garlic powder
- 2 tablespoons chili powder
- ¼ teaspoon salt

Directions:
1. Pre-heat Ninja Foodi by squeezing the "AIR CRISP" alternative and setting it to "360 Degrees F" and timer to 15 minutes
2. Place all the ingredients in your Ninja Foodi Grill cooking basket/alternatively, you may use a dish to mix the ingredients and then put the dish in the cooking basket
3. Stir to mix well

4. Cook for 15 minutes
5. Serve and enjoy!
- **Nutrition Info:** Calories: 220, Fat: 4 g, Saturated Fat: 1 g, Carbohydrates: 24 g, Fiber: 2 g, Sodium: 856 mg, Protein: 20 g

236.Feisty Hot Pepper Wings Delight

Servings: 4
Cooking Time: 25 Minutes
Ingredients:
- ½ cup hot pepper sauce
- 2 tablespoons butter, melted
- 1 tablespoon coconut oil
- 1-pound chicken wings
- 1 tablespoon ranch salad dressing
- ½ teaspoon paprika

Directions:
1. Take a bowl and add chicken, oil, ranch dressing, and paprika. Transfer to your fridge and let it chill for about 30-60 minutes.
2. Take another bowl and add the pepper sauce alongside butter.
3. Preheat your Ninja Foodi Grill in Med mode, with a timer set to 25 minutes.
4. Arrange the chicken wings over the grill grate.
5. Cook for 25 minutes.
6. Serve once done with the pepper sauce.
7. Enjoy!
- **Nutrition Info:** Calories: 510 Fat: 24 g Saturated Fat: 7 g Carbohydrates: 6 g Fiber: 0.5 g Sodium: 841 mg Protein: 54 g

237.Alfredo Chicken Apples

Servings: 4
Cooking Time: 20 Minutes
Ingredients:
- 1 large apple, wedged
- 4 teaspoon chicken seasoning
- 4 slices provolone cheese
- 1 tablespoon lemon juice
- ¼ cup blue cheese, crumbled
- 4 chicken breasts, halved
- ½ cup alfredo sauce

Directions:
1. Take a bowl and add chicken, season it well
2. Take another bowl and add in apple, lemon juice
3. Pre-heat Ninja Foodi by pressing the "GRILL" option and setting it to "MED" and timer to 20 minutes
4. Let it pre-heat until you hear a beep
5. Arrange chicken over Grill Grate, lock lid and cook for 8 minutes, flip and cook for 8 minutes more
6. Grill apple in the same manner for 2 minutes per side (making sure to remove chicken beforehand)

7. Serve chicken with pepper, apple, blue cheese, and alfredo sauce
8. Enjoy!
- **Nutrition Info:** Calories: 247, Fat: 19 g, Saturated Fat: 6 g, Carbohydrates: 29 g, Fiber: 6 g, Sodium: 853 mg, Protein: 14 g

238.Hearty Chicken Zucchini Kabobs

Servings: 4
Cooking Time: 15 Minutes
Ingredients:
- 1-pound chicken breast, boneless, skinless and cut into cubes of 2 inches
- ¼ cup extra-virgin olive oil
- 2 tablespoons oregano
- 2 tablespoons Greek yogurt, plain
- 4 lemons juice
- 1 red onion, quartered
- 1 zucchini, sliced
- 1 lemon zest
- ½ teaspoon ground black pepper
- 4 garlic cloves, minced
- 1 teaspoon of sea salt

Directions:
1. Take a mixing bowl, add the Greek yogurt, lemon juice, oregano, garlic, zest, salt, and pepper, combine them well
2. Add the chicken and coat well, refrigerate for 1-2 hours to marinate
3. Arrange the grill grate and close the lid
4. Pre-heat Ninja Foodi by pressing the "GRILL" option and setting it to "MED" and timer to 7 minutes
5. Take the skewers, thread the chicken, zucchini and red onion and thread alternatively
6. Let it pre-heat until you hear a beep
7. Arrange the skewers over the grill grate lock lid and cook until the timer reads zero
8. Baste the kebabs with a marinating mixture in between
9. Take out your when it reaches 165 degrees F
10. Serve warm and enjoy!
- **Nutrition Info:** Calories: 277, Fat: 15 g, Saturated Fat: 4 g, Carbohydrates: 10 g, Fiber: 2 g, Sodium: 146 mg

239.Chicken Cacciatore

Servings: 4
Cooking Time: 32 Minutes
Ingredients:
- 4 chicken thighs
- 2 tablespoons olive oil
- 1/2 onion, chopped
- 2 cloves garlic, minced
- 3 stalks celery, chopped
- 4 oz. mushrooms
- 14 oz. stewed tomatoes

- 2 teaspoons herbs de Provence
- 3/4 cup water
- 3 cubes chicken bouillon, crumbled
- 2 tablespoons tomato paste

Directions:
1. Set the Ninja Foodi to sauté. Add the oil and chicken.
2. Cook the chicken for 6 minutes per side. Remove the chicken and set aside.
3. Add the onion, garlic, celery, and mushrooms. Cook for 5 minutes, stirring frequently.
4. Put the chicken back. Pour in the tomatoes and tomato paste.
5. Add the rest of the ingredients. Seal the pot.
6. Set it to pressure. Cook at high pressure for 15 minutes. Release the pressure quickly.

240.Honey Teriyaki Chicken

Servings: 4
Cooking Time: 20 Minutes
Ingredients:
- 4 chicken breasts, sliced into strips
- 1 cup soy sauce
- ½ cup water
- 2/3 cup honey
- 2 teaspoons garlic, minced
- ½ cup rice vinegar
- ½ teaspoon ground ginger
- ¼ teaspoon crushed red pepper flakes
- 3 tablespoons corn starch dissolved in 3 tablespoons cold water

Directions:
1. Put the chicken inside the Ninja Foodi.
2. Add the rest of the ingredients except the corn starch mixture.
3. Put on the lid. Set it to Pressure. Cook at high pressure for 30 minutes.
4. Release the pressure naturally. Set it to Sauté.
5. Stir in the corn starch and simmer until the sauce has thickened.
6. serving Suggestions:
7. Garnish with sesame seeds and serve with fried rice.
- **Nutrition Info:** Calories: 495 Total Fat: 10.4 g Saturated Fat: 2.9 g Cholesterol: 125 mg Sodium: 717 mg Total Carbohydrate: 52.1 g Dietary Fiber: 0.7 g Total Sugars: 47.5 g Protein: 44.8 g Potassium: 519 mg

241.Turkey Cream Noodles

Servings: 4
Cooking Time: 35 Minutes
Ingredients:
- 8 ounces cremini mushrooms, sliced
- 1 can (10.5 ounce) cream of celery soup
- 1 (10-ounce) package egg noodles
- 4 cups chicken stock

- 16 ounces peas
- 1 cup sour cream
- 2 tablespoons butter
- 1-pound ground turkey
- ¾ cup grated Parmesan cheese
- Kosher salt
- Freshly ground black pepper

Directions:
1. Take Ninja Foodi multi-cooker, arrange it over a cooking platform, and open the top lid.
2. In the pot, add the butter; Select "SEAR/SAUTÉ" mode and select "MD: HI" pressure level. Press "STOP/START." After about 4-5 minutes, the butter will melt.
3. Add the mushrooms, turkey, and stir-cook for about 8-10 minutes to brown evenly.
4. Add the condensed soup and stock; stir and simmer for 15 minutes.
5. Add the egg noodles and peas; stir-cook for 8-10 minutes until the noodles are cooked well.
6. Add the sour cream and Parmesan cheese; stir the mixture, season with salt and pepper.

- **Nutrition Info:** Calories: 752, Fat: 19.5g, Saturated Fat: 9g, Trans Fat: 0g, Carbohydrates: 38g, Fiber: 7.5g, Sodium: 1542mg, Protein: 52g

242.Turkey Bean Chili

Servings: 6
Cooking Time: 30 Minutes
Ingredients:
- 2 garlic cloves, minced
- 3 cans (15-ounce) of cannellini beans, rinsed and drained
- 1 onion, chopped
- 1 tablespoon oregano, dried
- 1 ½ pounds turkey, ground
- 4 cups chicken broth
- 1 tablespoon extra-virgin olive oil
- 1 tablespoon ground cumin
- ⅛ teaspoon sea salt
- ⅛ teaspoon black pepper, freshly ground
- 1 pack biscuits

Directions:
1. Take Ninja Foodi multi-cooker, arrange it over a cooking platform, and open the top lid.
2. In the pot, add the oil; Select "SEAR/SAUTÉ" mode and select "MD: HI" pressure level.
3. Press "STOP/START." After about 4-5 minutes, the oil will start simmering.
4. Add the onions, garlic, and cook (while stirring) for 2-3 minutes until they become softened and translucent.

5. Add the turkey, cumin, oregano, beans, broth, salt, and black pepper; stir the mixture.
6. Seal the multi-cooker by locking it with the pressure lid; ensure to keep the pressure release valve locked/sealed.
7. Select "PRESSURE" mode and select the "HI" pressure level. Then, set timer to 10 minutes and press "STOP/START"; it will start the cooking process by building up inside pressure.
8. At the point when the clock goes off, speedy discharge pressure by adjusting the pressure valve to the VENT. After pressure gets released, open the pressure lid.
9. Arrange the biscuits in a single layer over the mixture.
10. Seal the multi-cooker by locking it with the crisping lid; ensure to keep the pressure release valve locked/sealed.
11. Select "BROIL" mode and select the "HI" pressure level. Then, set timer to 15 minutes and press "STOP/START"; it will start the cooking process by building up inside pressure.
12. At the point when the clock goes off, speedy discharge pressure by adjusting the pressure valve to the VENT.
13. After pressure gets released, open the pressure lid.

- **Nutrition Info:** Calories: 543, Fat: 18g, Saturated Fat: 6, Trans Fat: 0g, Carbohydrates: 51g, Fiber: 15g, Sodium: 1357mg, Protein: 42g

243.Mexican Chicken Soup

Servings: 6
Cooking Time: 15 Min
Ingredients:
- 1 (14.5 ounces) can black beans, rinsed and drained
- 14 ounces canned whole tomatoes, chopped
- 5 chicken thighs, boneless, skinless
- 5 cups chicken broth
- 2 cups corn kernels
- ¼ cup cheddar cheese, shredded
- 2 tablespoon tomato puree
- 1 tablespoon chili powder
- 1 tablespoon ground cumin
- ½ teaspoon dried oregano
- 2 stemmed jalapeno peppers, cored and chopped
- 3 cloves garlic, minced
- Fresh cilantro, chopped to garnish

Directions:
1. Take Ninja Foodi multi-cooker, arrange it over a cooking platform, and open the top lid.

2. In the pot, add the chicken, chicken stock, cumin, oregano, garlic, tomato puree, tomatoes, chili powder, and jalapeno peppers; stir the mixture.
3. Seal the multi-cooker by locking it with the pressure lid; ensure to keep the pressure release valve locked/sealed.
4. Select "PRESSURE" mode and select the "HI" pressure level. Then, set timer to 10 minutes and press "STOP/START"; it will start the cooking process by building up inside pressure.
5. At the point when the clock goes off, brisk discharge pressure by adjusting the pressure valve to the VENT. After pressure gets released, open the pressure lid.
6. Shred the chicken and include it back in the pot.
7. Select "SEAR/SAUTÉ" mode and select "MD: HI" pressure level; add the beans and corn and combine, stir-cook for 4 minutes.
8. Add the cilantro and cheese on top; serve warm.
- **Nutrition Info:** Calories: 408, Fat: 15g, Saturated Fat: 3g, Trans Fat: 0g, Carbohydrates: 31g, Fiber: 9g, Sodium: 548mg, Protein: 34g

244.Shredded Salsa Chicken

Servings: 4
Cooking Time: 20 Minutes
Ingredients:
- 1 pound chicken breast, skin and bones removed
- 1 cup chunky salsa Keto friendly
- ½ teaspoon salt
- Pinch of oregano
- ¾ teaspoon cumin
- Pepper to taste

Directions:
1. Season chicken with all the listed spices, then add to Ninja Foodi
2. Cover with salsa and close the lid
3. Cook on HIGH pressure for 20 minutes
4. Quick-release the pressure
5. Add chicken to a platter then shred the chicken
6. Serve and enjoy!

245.Hassel Back Chicken

Servings: 4
Cooking Time: 1 Hour
Ingredients:
- 8 large chicken breasts
- 2 cups fresh mozzarella cheese, thinly sliced
- 4 large Roma tomatoes, thinly sliced
- 4 tablespoons butter
- Salt and pepper to taste

Directions:

1. Add chicken breasts, season with salt and pepper to make deep slits
2. Stuff with mozzarella cheese slices and tomatoes in your chicken slits
3. Grease Ninja Foodi pot with butter
4. Arrange stuffed chicken breasts
5. Close the lid and BAKE/ROAST for 1 hour at 365 degrees F
6. Serve and enjoy!

246.Chicken Parmesan

Servings: 4
Cooking Time: 20 Minutes
Ingredients:
- 2 chicken breasts, sliced into cutlets
- 6 tablespoons seasoned bread crumbs
- 2 tablespoons Parmesan cheese, grated
- 1 tablespoon butter, melted
- 6 tablespoons reduced-fat mozzarella cheese
- ½ cup marinara sauce
- Cooking spray

Directions:
1. Spray the Ninja Foodi basket with oil.
2. In a bowl, mix the bread crumbs and Parmesan cheese. In another bowl, place the butter. Coat the chicken with butter and dip into the bread crumb mix.
3. Place the cutlets on the basket. Seal the crisping lid. Set it to Air Crisp.
4. Cook at 375°F for 6 minutes.
5. Flip and top with the marinara and mozzarella.
6. serving Suggestions:
7. Serve with pasta or salad.
- **Nutrition Info:** Calories: 307 Total Fat: 14.4 g Saturated Fat: 6.5 g Cholesterol: 87 mg Sodium: 599 mg Total Carbohydrate: 13.3 g Dietary Fiber: 1.4 g Total Sugars: 3.4 g Protein: 30.8 g Potassium: 303 mg

247.Baked Coconut Chicken

Servings: 4
Cooking Time: 12 Minutes
Ingredients:
- 2 large eggs
- 2 teaspoons garlic powder
- 1 teaspoon salt
- ½ teaspoon ground black pepper
- ¾ cup coconut aminos
- 1-pound chicken tenders
- Cooking spray as needed

Directions:
1. Pre-heat Ninja Foodi by squeezing the "AIR CRISP" alternative and setting it to "400 Degrees F" and timer to 12 minutes
2. Take a large-sized baking sheet and spray it with cooking spray

3. Take a wide dish and add garlic powder, eggs, pepper, and salt
4. Whisk well until everything is combined
5. Add the almond meal and coconut and mix well
6. Take your chicken tenders and dip them in the egg followed by dipping in the coconut mix
7. Shake off any excess
8. Transfer them to your Ninja Foodi Grill and spray the tenders with a bit of oil.
9. Cook for 12-14 minutes until you have a nice golden-brown texture
10. Enjoy!
- **Nutrition Info:** Calories: 180, Fat: 1 g, Saturated Fat: 0 g, Carbohydrates: 3 g, Fiber: 1 g, Sodium: 214 mg, Protein: 0 g

248. Turkey Tomato Burgers

Servings: 6
Cooking Time: 40 Minutes
Ingredients:
- 2/3 cup sun-dried tomatoes, chopped
- 1/4 teaspoon salt
- 1 cup crumbled feta cheese
- 2 pounds lean ground turkey
- 1/4 teaspoon pepper
- 1 large red onion, chopped
- 6 burger buns of your choice, sliced in half

Directions:
1. In a mixing bowl, add all the ingredients. Combine the ingredients to mix well with each other.
2. Prepare six patties from the mixture.
3. Take Ninja Foodi Grill, arrange it over your kitchen platform, and open the top lid.
4. Arrange the grill grate and close the top lid.
5. Press "GRILL" and select the "MED" grill function. Adjust the timer to 14 minutes and then press "START/STOP." Ninja Foodi will start pre-heating.
6. Ninja Foodi is preheated and ready to cook when it starts to beep. After you hear a beep, open the top lid.
7. Arrange the patties over the grill grate.
8. Close the top lid and cook for 7 minutes. Now open the top lid, flip the patties.
9. Close the top lid and cook for 7 more minutes.
10. Serve warm with ciabatta rolls. Add your choice of toppings: lettuce, tomato, cheese, ketchup, cheese, etc.
- **Nutrition Info:** Calories: 298, Fat: 16g, Saturated Fat: 2.5g, Trans Fat: 0g, Carbohydrates: 32g, Fiber: 4g, Sodium: 321mg, Protein: 27.5g

249. Cabbage And Chicken Meatballs

Servings: 4
Cooking Time: 4-6 Minutes

Ingredients:
- 1-pound ground chicken
- ¼ cup heavy whip cream
- 2 teaspoons salt
- ½ teaspoon ground caraway seeds
- 1½ teaspoons freshly ground black pepper, divided
- ¼ teaspoon ground allspice
- 4-6 cups green cabbage, thickly chopped
- ½ cup almond milk
- 2 tablespoons unsalted butter

Directions:
1. Transfer meat to a bowl and add cream, 1 teaspoon salt, caraway, ½ teaspoon pepper, allspice, and mix it well. Let the mixture chill for 30 minutes
2. Once the mixture is ready, use your hands to scoop the mixture into meatballs.
3. Add half of your balls to the Ninja Foodi pot, and cover with half of the cabbage.
4. Add remaining balls and cover with the rest of the cabbage.
5. Add milk, pats of butter, season with salt and pepper.
6. Lock the lid and cook on high pressure for 4 minutes. Quick-release the pressure.
7. Unlock the lid and serve. Enjoy!
- **Nutrition Info:** Calories: 294 Fat: 26 g Carbohydrates: 4 g Protein: 12 g

250. Honey Chicken Wings

Servings: 4
Cooking Time: 20 Minutes
Ingredients:
- 1 lb. chicken wings
- ¼ cup honey
- 2 tablespoons hot sauce
- 1½ tablespoons soy sauce
- 1 tablespoon butter
- 1 tablespoon lime juice

Directions:
1. Place the chicken wings in the Ninja Foodi basket. Add the basket to the pot.
2. Cover the crisping lid. Set it to Air Crisp. Cook at 360°F for 30 minutes.
3. Flip every 10 minutes. Remove the wings and set aside. Set the pot to Sauté.
4. Add the rest of the ingredients and mix well. Simmer for 3 minutes.
5. Toss the wings in the mixture before serving.
6. serving Suggestions:
7. Garnish with chopped chives.
- **Nutrition Info:** Calories: 619 Total Fat: 22.6 g Saturated Fat: 8.3 g Cholesterol: 217 mg Sodium: 1295 mg Total Carbohydrate: 36.1 g Dietary Fiber: 0.2 g Total Sugars: 35.2 g Protein: 66.6 g Potassium: 622 mg

251.Honey-mustard Chicken Tenders

Servings: 4
Cooking Time: 4 Minutes
Ingredients:
- ½ cup Dijon mustard
- 2 tablespoons honey
- 2 tablespoons olive oil
- 1 teaspoon freshly ground black pepper
- 2 pounds chicken tenders
- ½ cup walnuts

Directions:
1. Whisk together the mustard, honey, olive oil, and pepper in a medium bowl. Add the chicken and toss to coat.
2. Finely grind the walnuts by pulsing them in a food processor or putting them in a heavy-duty plastic bag and pounding them with a rolling pin or heavy skillet.
3. Insert the Grill Grate and close the hood. Select GRILL, set the temperature to HIGH, and set the time to 4 minutes. Select START/STOP to begin preheating.
4. Toss the chicken tenders in the ground walnuts to coat them lightly.
5. Grill the chicken tenders for about 4 minutes, until they have taken on grill marks and are cooked through. Serve hot, at room temperature, or refrigerate and serve cold.

252.Shredded Up Salsa Chicken

Servings: 4
Cooking Time: 20 Minutes
Ingredients:
- 1-pound chicken breast, skin and bones removed
- ¾ teaspoon cumin
- ½ teaspoon salt
- Pinch of oregano
- Pepper to taste
- 1 cup chunky salsa Keto friendly

Directions:
1. Season chicken with spices and add to the Ninja Foodi.
2. Cover with salsa and lock the lid, cook on high pressure for 20 minutes.
3. Quick-release the pressure. Add chicken to a platter and shred the chicken. Serve and enjoy!
- **Nutrition Info:** Calories: 125 Fat: 3 g Carbohydrates: 2 g Protein: 22 g

253.Delicious Maple Glazed Chicken

Servings: 4
Cooking Time: 15 Minutes
Ingredients:
- 2 pounds chicken wings, bone-in
- 1 teaspoon black pepper, ground
- ¼ cup teriyaki sauce

- 1 cup maple syrup
- 1/3 cup soy sauce
- 3 garlic cloves, minced
- 2 teaspoons garlic powder
- 2 teaspoons onion powder

Directions:
1. Take a mixing bowl, add garlic, soy sauce, black pepper, maple syrup, garlic powder, onion powder, and teriyaki sauce, combine well
2. Add the chicken wings and combine well to coat
3. Arrange the grill grate and close the lid
4. Pre-heat Ninja Foodi by pressing the "GRILL" option and setting it to "MED" and timer to 10 minutes
5. Let it pre-heat until you hear a beep
6. Arrange the chicken wings over the grill grate lock lid and cook for 5 minutes
7. Flip the chicken and close the lid, cook for 5 minutes more
8. Cook until it reaches 165 degrees F
9. Serve warm and enjoy!
- **Nutrition Info:** Calories: 543, Fat: 26 g, Saturated Fat: 6 g, Carbohydrates: 46 g, Fiber: 4 g, Sodium: 648 mg, Protein: 42 g

254.Lemon Chicken With Garlic

Servings: 4
Cooking Time: 14 Minutes
Ingredients:
- 6 chicken thighs
- Salt and pepper to taste
- 1/2 teaspoon red chili flakes
- 1/2 teaspoon garlic powder
- 1/2 teaspoon smoked paprika
- 2 tablespoons olive oil
- 3 tablespoons butter
- 1 onion, chopped
- 4 cloves garlic, minced
- 1 tablespoon lemon juice
- 1/4 cup low sodium broth
- 2 teaspoons Italian seasoning
- Lemon zest
- 2 tablespoons heavy cream

Directions:
1. Sprinkle the chicken thighs with salt, pepper, chili flakes, garlic powder, and paprika.
2. Set the Ninja Foodi to sauté. Add the olive oil.
3. Cook the chicken for 3 minutes per side. Remove from the pot and set aside.
4. Melt the butter in the pot. Add the onion and garlic. Deglaze the pot with the lemon juice. Cook for 1 minute. Add the chicken broth, seasoning, and lemon zest.
5. Set the pot to pressure. Seal it. Cook at high pressure for 7 minutes.

6. Release the pressure naturally. Stir in the heavy cream before serving.

255. Grilled Chicken Tacos:

Servings: 8
Cooking Time: 18 Minutes
Ingredients:
- 2 tablespoons chipotle in adobo sauce, chopped
- 2 teaspoons sugar
- 1/3 cup olive oil
- 1/3 cup lime juice
- 1/3 cup red wine vinegar
- 2 teaspoons salt 2
- teaspoons pepper
- 1 cup fresh cilantro, chopped
- 2 lbs. boneless skinless chicken thighs
- Taco wraps: 8 flour tortillas
- 4 poblano peppers 1
- tablespoon olive oil
- 2 cups shredded Jack cheese

Directions:
1. Take the first six ingredients in a blender jug and blend them.
2. Once blended, mix with chipotles and cilantro.
3. Mix chicken with this cilantro marinade and cover to refrigerate for 8 hours.
4. Grease the poblanos with cooking oil and keep them aside.
5. Prepare and preheat the Ninja Foodi Grill on a High-temperature setting.
6. Once it is preheated, open the lid and place the peppers in the grill.
7. Cover the Ninja Foodi Grill's lid and let it grill on the "Grilling Mode" for 2 minutes.
8. Flip the peppers and then continue grilling for another 2 minutes.
9. It's time to grill the chicken in the same grill.
10. Place the chicken in the grill and cover the lid.
11. Select the High-temperature setting on the Grill.
12. Ninja grill the chicken for 5 minutes per side then transfer to a plate.
13. Now peel and slice the peppers in half then also slice the chicken.
14. Spread each tortilla and add half cup chicken, half peppers, and ¼ cup cheese.
15. Fold the tortilla and carefully place in the grill and cover its lid.
16. Grill each for 2 minutes per side on the medium temperature setting.
17. Serve.

256. Rosemary Chicken

Servings: 4
Cooking Time: 6 Minutes
Ingredients:
- ½ cup balsamic vinegar
- 2 tablespoons olive oil
- 2 rosemary sprigs, coarsely chopped
- 2 pounds boneless, skinless chicken breasts, pounded to a ½-inch thickness

Directions:
1. Combine the balsamic vinegar, olive oil, and rosemary in a shallow baking dish. Add the chicken breasts and turn to coat. Cover with plastic wrap and refrigerate for at least 30 minutes or overnight.
2. Insert the Grill Grate and close the hood. Select GRILL, set the temperature to HIGH, and set the time to 6 minutes. Select START/STOP to begin preheating.
3. When the unit beeps to signify it has preheated, place the s chicken breasts on the Grill Grate. Close the hood and cook for 6 minutes until they have taken on grill marks and are cooked through.

257. Turkey Yogurt Meal

Servings: 4
Cooking Time: 20 Minutes
Ingredients:
- Black pepper (ground) and salt to taste
- 14 ounces yogurt
- 2 turkey breasts, skinless, boneless and cubed
- 2 teaspoons olive oil
- 1 yellow onion, chopped
- 1 teaspoon turmeric powder
- 1 tablespoon ginger, grated

Directions:
1. Take Ninja Foodi multi-cooker, arrange it over a cooking platform, and open the top lid.
2. In the pot, add the oil, select "SEAR/SAUTÉ" mode and select "MD: HI" pressure level. Press "STOP/START." After about 4-5 minutes, the oil will start simmering.
3. Add the onions and cook (while stirring) until they become softened and translucent for 4 minutes.
4. Add the ginger and turmeric, stir-cook for 1 more minute. Add remaining ingredients, stir gently.
5. Seal the multi-cooker by locking it with the pressure lid; ensure to keep the pressure release valve locked/sealed.
6. Select "PRESSURE" mode and select the "HI" pressure level. Then after, set timer to 20 minutes and press "STOP/START," it will start the cooking process by building up inside pressure.
7. When the timer goes off, naturally release inside pressure for about 8-10 minutes, then, quick-release pressure by adjusting the pressure valve to the VENT
8. Serve warm.

- **Nutrition Info:** Calories: 176, Fat: 4.5g, Saturated Fat: 0g, Trans Fat: 0g, Carbohydrates: 7g, Fiber: 0g, Sodium: 854mg, Protein: 21g

258.Hot And Sassy Bbq Chicken

Servings: 4
Cooking Time: 18 Minutes
Ingredients:
- 2 tablespoons honey
- 2 cups BBQ sauce
- 1 tablespoon hot sauce
- 1-pound chicken drumstick
- Juice of 1 lime
- Pepper and salt as needed

Directions:
1. Take a bowl and add BBQ sauce, lime juice, honey, pepper, salt, hot sauce, and mix well
2. Take another mixing bowl and add ½ cup sauce and chicken mix well and add remaining ingredients
3. Let it sit for 1 hour to marinate
4. Pre-heat Ninja Foodi by pressing the "GRILL" option and setting it to "MED" and timer to 18 minutes
5. Let it pre-heat until you hear a beep
6. Arrange chicken over grill grate, cook until the timer reaches zero and internal temperature reaches 165 degrees F
7. Serve and enjoy!
- **Nutrition Info:** Calories: 423, Fat: 13 g, Saturated Fat: 6 g, Carbohydrates: 47 g, Fiber: 4 g, Sodium: 698 mg, Protein: 22 g

259.Chicken Marsala

Servings: 4
Cooking Time: 25 Minutes
Ingredients:
- 4 chicken breasts, sliced into strips
- 1 teaspoon garlic powder
- Salt and pepper to taste
- 1/2 cup all-purpose flour
- 3 tablespoons butter
- 3 tablespoons olive oil
- 3 cloves garlic, minced
- 1 shallot, sliced thinly
- 8 oz. mushrooms
- 2/3 cup Marsala wine
- 2/3 cup chicken stock
- 1/2 cup heavy cream

Directions:
1. Season the chicken with garlic powder, salt, and pepper. Coat the chicken with flour.
2. Place the chicken on the Ninja Foodi basket. Put the basket inside the pot.
3. Seal the crisping lid. Set it to air crisp. Cook at 375 degrees F for 15 minutes.
4. Remove and set aside. Set the pot to sauté. Add the butter and oil.

5. Cook the garlic, shallot, and mushrooms. Pour in the wine and chicken broth.
6. Simmer for 10 minutes. Stir in the heavy cream.
7. Toss the chicken into the mixture. Serve.

260.Mexico's Favorite Chicken Soup

Servings: 4
Cooking Time: 20 Minutes
Ingredients:
- 2 cups chicken, shredded
- 4 tablespoons olive oil
- ½ cup cilantro, chopped
- 8 cups chicken broth
- 1/3 cup salsa
- 1 teaspoon onion powder
- ½ cup scallions, chopped
- 4 ounces green chilies, chopped
- ½ teaspoon habanero, minced
- 1 cup celery root, chopped
- 1 teaspoon cumin
- 1 teaspoon garlic powder
- Salt and pepper to taste

Directions:
1. Add all ingredients to Ninja Foodi. Stir and lock the lid. Cook on high pressure for 10 minutes.
2. Release pressure naturally over 10 minutes. Serve and enjoy!
- **Nutrition Info:** Calories: 204 Fat: 14 g Carbohydrates: 4 g Protein: 14 g

261.Chicken Nuggets

Servings: 4
Cooking Time: 40 Minutes
Ingredients:
- 2 teaspoons olive oil
- 6 tablespoons breadcrumbs
- 2 tablespoons grated parmesan cheese
- 2 chicken breasts, sliced into nuggets
- Salt and pepper to taste
- Cooking spray

Directions:
1. Pour the olive oil into one bowl.
2. In another bowl, mix the bread crumbs and Parmesan.
3. Season the chicken with salt and pepper.
4. Coat with the olive oil and dip in the bread crumb mixture.
5. Place the chicken on the basket. Seal the crisping lid. Select Air Crisp.
6. Cook at 375°F for 8 minutes.
7. serving Suggestions:
8. Serve with a green salad or veggie sticks.
- **Nutrition Info:** Calories: 245 Total Fat: 11.4 g Saturated Fat: 4 g Cholesterol: 75 mg Sodium: 267 mg Total Carbohydrate: 7.8 g Dietary Fiber: 0.5 g Total Sugars: 0.6 g Protein: 27 g Potassium: 198 mg

262.Popcorn Chicken

Servings: 2
Cooking Time: 10 Minutes
Ingredients:
- 2 boneless, skinless chicken breasts
- 1 cup of breadcrumbs
- 2 beaten eggs
- 1 cup of flour
- 1 teaspoon of salt
- 1 teaspoon of black pepper
- 1 teaspoon of onion powder
- 1 teaspoon of garlic powder

Directions:
1. Preheat your air fryer to 390 degrees Fahrenheit.
2. Using a food processor, add the chicken breasts and beat it until it minced properly.
3. Using two bowls, add the flour, the eggs and mix it properly into the first bowl, then in the second bowl, add the breadcrumbs, seasonings and mix it properly.
4. Mold the minced chicken into small balls.
5. Cover the minced chicken in the flour, dip it into the egg wash, and then cover it with the seasoned breadcrumbs.
6. Place it inside your air fryer and cook it for 10 minutes at 390 degrees Fahrenheit or until it is fully done.
7. Serve and enjoy!

263.Basil And Garlic Chicken Legs

Servings: 4
Cooking Time: 35 Minutes
Ingredients:
- 4 chicken legs
- 2 teaspoons garlic, minced
- 1 lemon, sliced
- 2 tablespoons olive oil
- 4 teaspoons basil, dried
- Pinch of pepper and salt

Directions:
1. Pre-heat Ninja Foodi by squeezing the "AIR CRISP" alternative and setting it to "350 Degrees F" and timer to 20 minutes
2. Coat chicken with oil using a brush and drizzle with rest of the ingredients
3. Transfer to Ninja Foodi Grill
4. Add lemon slices around the chicken legs
5. Close the oven
6. Cook for 20 minutes
7. Serve and enjoy!
- **Nutrition Info:** Calories: 240, Fat: 18 g, Saturated Fat: 4 g, Carbohydrates: 3 g, Fiber: 2 g, Sodium: 1253 mg

264.Moroccan Roast Chicken

Servings: 4
Cooking Time: 22 Minutes
Ingredients:
- 3 tablespoons plain yogurt
- 4 skinless, boneless chicken thighs
- ½ teaspoon fresh flat-leaf parsley, chopped
- 2 teaspoons ground cumin
- 4 garlic cloves, chopped
- ½ teaspoon salt
- 2 teaspoons paprika
- ¼ teaspoon crushed red pepper flakes
- 1/3 cup olive oil

Directions:
1. Take your food processor and add garlic, yogurt, salt, oil and blend well
2. Take a mixing bowl and add chicken, red pepper flakes, paprika, cumin, parsley, garlic, and mix well
3. Let it marinate for 2-4 hours
4. Pre-heat Ninja Foodi by pressing the "ROAST" option and setting it to "400 degrees F" and timer to 23 minutes
5. Let it pre-heat until you hear a beep
6. Arrange chicken directly inside your cooking pot and lock lid, cook for 15 minutes, flip and cook for the remaining time
7. Serve and enjoy with yogurt dip!
- **Nutrition Info:** Calories: 321, Fat: 24 g, Saturated Fat: 5 g, Carbohydrates: 6 g, Fiber: 2 g, Sodium: 602 mg, Protein: 21 g

265.Classic Bbq Chicken Delight

Servings: 4
Cooking Time: 12 Minutes
Ingredients:
- 1/3 cup spice seasoning
- ½ tablespoon Worcestershire sauce
- 1 teaspoon dried onion, chopped
- 1 tablespoon bourbon
- 1 tablespoon brown sugar
- ½ cup ketchup
- 1 pinch salt
- 2 teaspoons BBQ seasoning
- 6 chicken drumsticks

Directions:
1. Take your saucepan and add listed ingredients except for drumsticks, stir cook for 8-10 minutes
2. Keep it on the side and let them cool
3. Pre-heat your Ninja Foodi Grill to MED and set the timer to 12 minutes
4. Once the beep sound is heard, arrange your drumsticks over the grill grate and brush with remaining sauce
5. Cook for 6 minutes, flip with some more sauce and grill for 6 minutes more
6. Enjoy once done!
- **Nutrition Info:** Calories: 300 Fat: 8 g Saturated Fat: 1 g Carbohydrates: 10 g Fiber: 1.5 g Sodium: 319 mg Protein: 12.5 g

266.Lemon And Chicken Extravaganza

Servings: 4
Cooking Time: 24 Minutes
Ingredients:
- 4 bone-in, skin-on chicken thighs
- Salt and pepper to taste
- 2 tablespoons butter, divided
- 2 teaspoons garlic, minced
- 1/2 cup herbed chicken stock
- 1/2 cup heavy whip cream
- 1/2 a lemon, juiced

Directions:
1. Season your chicken thighs generously with salt and pepper
2. Set your Foodi to sauté mode and add oil, let it heat up
3. Add thigh, Sauté both sides for 6 minutes. Remove thigh to a platter and keep it on the side
4. Add garlic, cook for 2 minutes. Whisk in chicken stock, heavy cream, lemon juice and gently stir
5. Bring the mix to a simmer and reintroduce chicken
6. Lock lid and cook for 10 minutes on HIGH pressure
7. Release pressure over 10 minutes. Serve and enjoy!

267.Daisy Fresh Maple Chicken

Servings: 4
Cooking Time: 15 Minutes
Ingredients:
- 2 teaspoons onion powder
- 2 teaspoons garlic powder
- 3 garlic cloves, minced
- 1/3 cup soy sauce
- 1 cup maple syrup
- ¼ cup teriyaki sauce
- 1 teaspoon black pepper
- 2 pounds chicken wings, bone-in

Directions:
1. Take a medium-sized bowl and add soy sauce, garlic, pepper, maple syrup, garlic powder, onion powder, teriyaki sauce and mix well
2. Add the chicken wings to the mixture and coat it gently
3. Preheat your Ninja Foodi Grill in MED mode, setting the timer to 10 minutes
4. Once you hear a beep, arrange your prepared wings in the grill grate

5. Cook for 5 minutes, flip and cook for 5 minutes more until the internal temperature reaches 165 degrees F
6. Serve!
- **Nutrition Info:** Calories: 543 Fat: 26 g Saturated Fat: 6 g Carbohydrates: 46 g Fiber: 4 g Sodium: 648 mg Protein: 42 g

268.Chicken Zucchini Kebabs

Servings: 4
Cooking Time: 15 Minutes
Ingredients:
- Juice of 4 lemons
- Grated zest of 1 lemon
- 1-pound boneless, skinless chicken breasts, cut into cubes of 2 inches
- 1 teaspoon sea salt
- ½ teaspoon ground black pepper
- 2 tablespoons plain Greek yogurt
- ¼ cup extra-virgin olive oil
- 1 red onion, quartered
- 1 zucchini, sliced
- 4 garlic cloves, minced
- 2 tablespoons dried oregano

Directions:
1. In a mixing bowl, add the Greek yogurt, oil, lemon juice, zest, garlic, oregano, salt, and pepper. Combine the ingredients to mix well with each other.
2. Add the chicken and coat well. Refrigerate for 1-2 hours to marinate.
3. Take Ninja Foodi Grill, arrange it over your kitchen platform, and open the top lid.
4. Arrange the grill grate and close the top lid.
5. Press "GRILL" and select the "MED" grill function. Adjust the timer to 14 minutes and then press "START/STOP." Ninja Foodi will start pre-heating.
6. Take the skewers, thread the chicken, red onion, and zucchini. Thread alternatively.
7. Ninja Foodi is preheated and ready to cook when it starts to beep. After you hear a beep, open the top lid.
8. Arrange the skewers over the grill grate.
9. Close the top lid and allow it to cook until the timer reads zero. Baste the kebabs with a marinating mixture in between. Cook until the food thermometer reaches 165°F.
10. Serve warm.
- **Nutrition Info:** Calories: 277, Fat: 15.5g, Saturated Fat: 2g, Trans Fat: 0g, Carbohydrates: 9.5g, Fiber: 2g, Sodium: 523mg, Protein: 25g

VEGETARIAN AND VEGAN RECIPES

269.Honey And Lime Salad

Servings: 4
Cooking Time: 4 Minutes
Ingredients:
- ½ pound strawberries washed, hulled and halved
- 1 can (9 ounces) pineapple chunks, drained
- 1 tablespoon lime juice, squeezed
- 6 tablespoons honey, divided
- 2 peaches, pitted and sliced

Directions:
1. Take a bowl and add pineapple, strawberries, peach, and 3 tablespoons, honey
2. Toss well
3. Pre-heat your Ninja Foodi Grill to MAX mode and set the timer to 4 minutes
4. Once you heart beeping sound, transfer fruits to the grill grate
5. Cook for 4 minutes
6. Take a small bowl and add remaining honey, lime juice, 1 tablespoon reserved pineapple juice
7. Once the fruits are cooked, transfer fruits to this mixture
8. Toss and serve
9. Enjoy!
- **Nutrition Info:** Calories: 178 Fat: 1 g Saturated Fat: 0 g Carbohydrates:47 g Fiber: 3 g Sodium: 3 mg Protein: 2 g

270.Coconut Cabbage

Servings: 4
Cooking Time: 7.5 Minutes
Ingredients:
- 1/2 cup cabbage, shredded
- 1-ounce dry coconut
- 3 large whole eggs
- 3 large egg yolks
- 1/3 medium carrot, sliced
- ½ ounces, yellow onion, sliced
- 1 teaspoon turmeric powder
- 2 tablespoons lemon juice
- 1/3 cup water
- 3 tablespoons olive oil
- ½ tablespoon mustard powder
- ½ teaspoon mild curry powder
- 1 large garlic cloves, diced
- 1 and ½ teaspoons salt

Directions:
1. Set your Ninja Foodi to "Sauté" mode
2. Add oil, stir in onions, salt
3. Cook for 4 minutes
4. Stir in spices, garlic, and Sauté for 30 seconds

5. Stir in the rest of the ingredients and close the lid
6. Cook on HIGH pressure for 3 minutes
7. Naturally, release the pressure over 10 minutes
8. Serve and enjoy!

271.Air Grilled Brussels

Servings: 4
Cooking Time: 12 Minutes
Ingredients:
- 6 slices bacon, chopped
- 1-pound brussels sprouts, halved
- 2 tablespoons olive oil, extra virgin
- 1 teaspoon salt
- ½ teaspoon black pepper, ground

Directions:
1. Add Brussels, olive oil, salt, pepper, and bacon into a mixing bowl.
2. Preheat the Ninja Foodi by pressing the Air Crisp option and setting it to 390°F.
3. Set the timer to 12 minutes.
4. Allow it to preheat until it beeps.
5. Arrange Brussels over basket and lock the lid.
6. Cook for 6 minutes.
7. Shake it and cook for 6 minutes more.
8. Serve and enjoy!
- **Nutrition Info:** Calories: 279 Fat: 18 g Saturated Fat: 4 g Carbohydrates: 12 g Fiber: 4 g Sodium: 874 mg

272.Spicy Ricotta Stuffed Mushrooms

Servings: 4
Cooking Time: 18 Minutes
Ingredients:
- 1 pound small white mushrooms
- Sea salt and ground black pepper, to taste
- 4 tablespoons ricotta cheese
- 1/2 teaspoon ancho chili powder
- 1 teaspoon paprika
- 1 egg
- 1/2 cup parmesan cheese, grated

Directions:
1. Remove the stems from the mushroom caps and chop them; mix the chopped mushrooms steams with the salt, black pepper, cheese, chili powder, and paprika.
2. Add in eggs and mix to combine well. Stuff the mushroom caps with the egg/cheese filling.
3. To with parmesan cheese. Spritz the stuffed mushrooms with cooking spray.
4. Cook in the preheated air fryer at 360 degrees f for 18 minutes.
- **Nutrition Info:** 144 calories; 8.4g fat; 7.7g carbs; 11.4g protein; 3.1g sugars; 1.6g fiber

273. Supreme Cauliflower Soup

Servings: 4
Cooking Time: 5 Minutes
Ingredients:

- ½ a small onion, chopped
- 2 tablespoons butter
- 1 large head of cauliflower, leaves and stems removed, coarsely chopped
- 2 cups chicken stock
- 1 teaspoon garlic powder
- 1 teaspoon salt
- 4 ounces cream cheese, cut into cubes
- 1 cup sharp cheddar cheese, cut
- 1/2 cup cream
- Extra cheddar, sour cream bacon strips, green onion for topping

Directions:

1. Peel the onion and chop up into small pieces.
2. Cut the leaves of the cauliflower and steam, making sure to keep the core intact.
3. Coarsely chop the cauliflower into pieces.
4. Set your Ninja Foodi to Sauté mode and add onion, cook for 2-3 minutes.
5. Add chopped cauliflower, stock, salt, and garlic powder.
6. Lock up the lid and cook on high pressure for 5 minutes. Perform a quick release.
7. Prepare the toppings. Use an immersion blender to puree your soup in the Ninja Foodi.
8. Serve your soup with a topping of sliced green onions, cheddar, crumbled bacon. Enjoy!

- **Nutrition Info:** Calories: 438 Fat: 36 g Carbohydrates: 8 g Protein: 22 g

274. Crispy Green Beans With Pecorino Romano

Servings: 3
Cooking Time: 7 Minutes
Ingredients:

- 2 tablespoons buttermilk
- 1 egg
- 4 tablespoons almond meal
- 4 tablespoons golden flaxseed meal
- 4 tablespoons pecorino romano cheese, finely grated
- Coarse salt and crushed black pepper, to taste
- 1 teaspoon smoked paprika
- 6 ounces green beans, trimmed

Directions:

1. In a shallow bowl, whisk together the buttermilk and egg.
2. In a separate bowl, combine the almond meal, golden flaxseed meal, pecorino romano cheese, salt, black pepper, and paprika.

3. Dip the green beans in the egg mixture, then, in the cheese mixture. Place the green beans in the lightly greased cooking basket.
4. Cook in the preheated air fryer at 390 degrees f for 4 minutes. Shake the basket and cook for a further 3 minutes.
5. Taste, adjust the seasonings, and serve with the dipping sauce if desired.

- **Nutrition Info:** 191 calories; 12.8g fat; 9.5g carbs; 11.4g protein; 2.8g sugars; 5g fiber

275. Grilled Veggies

Servings: 4
Cooking Time: 10 Minutes
Ingredients:

- 1 onion, sliced
- 1 red bell pepper, sliced
- 1 cup button mushrooms, sliced
- 1 zucchini, sliced
- 1 eggplant, sliced
- 1 cup asparagus, trimmed and sliced
- 1 squash, sliced
- 2 tablespoons olive oil
- Salt and pepper to taste

Directions:

1. Install grill grate to your Ninja Foodi Grill.
2. Select grill setting.
3. Preheat it to medium for 10 minutes.
4. Toss the veggies in olive oil and season with salt and pepper.
5. Add to the grill grate.
6. Grill for 10 minutes.

276. Crispy Asparagus

Servings: 4
Cooking Time: 10 Minutes
Ingredients:

- 1 lb. asparagus, trimmed
- 2 teaspoons olive oil
- Salt and pepper to taste

Directions:

1. Coat asparagus with oil.
2. Sprinkle with salt and pepper.
3. Choose air fry setting in your Ninja Foodi Grill.
4. Set it to 390 degrees F.
5. Cook asparagus in the air fryer basket for 7 to 10 minutes, shaking halfway through.

277. Colorful Vegetable Croquettes

Servings: 4
Cooking Time: 35 Minutes
Ingredients:

- 1/2 pound broccoli
- 4 tablespoons milk
- 2 tablespoons butter
- Salt and black pepper, to taste
- 1/2 teaspoon cayenne pepper
- 1/2 cup mushrooms, chopped

- 1 bell pepper, chopped
- 1 clove garlic, minced
- 3 tablespoons scallions, minced
- 2 tablespoons olive oil
- 1/2 cup almond flour
- 1/4 cup coconut flour
- 2 eggs
- 1/2 cup parmesan cheese, grated

Directions:
1. In a large saucepan, boil the broccoli for 17 to 20 minutes. Drain the broccoli and mash with the milk, butter, salt, black pepper, and cayenne pepper.
2. Add the mushrooms, bell pepper, garlic, scallions, and olive oil; stir to combine well. Shape the mixture into patties.
3. In a shallow bowl, place the flour; beat the eggs in another bowl; in a third bowl, place the parmesan cheese.
4. Dip each patty into the flour, followed by the eggs, and then the parmesan cheese; press to adhere.
5. Cook in the preheated air fryer at 375 degrees f for 16 minutes, shaking halfway through the cooking time.
- **Nutrition Info:** 280 calories; 22.5g fat; 9.8g carbs; 9.6g protein; 4g sugars; 3.2g fiber

278.Vegetable Fritters

Servings: 4
Cooking Time: 40 Minutes
Ingredients:
- 3 tablespoons ground flaxseed mixed with 1/2 cup water
- 2 potatoes, shredded
- 2 cups frozen mixed vegetables
- 1 cup frozen peas, thawed
- ½ cup onion, chopped
- ¼ cup fresh cilantro, chopped
- ½ cup almond flour
- Salt to taste
- Cooking spray

Directions:
1. Combine all the ingredients in a bowl. Form patties. Spray each patty with oil.
2. Transfer to the Ninja Foodi basket. Set it to Air Crisp. Close the crisping lid.
3. Cook at 360°F for 15 minutes, flipping halfway through.
- **Nutrition Info:** Calories: 171 Total Fat: 0.5 g Saturated Fat: 0.1 g Cholesterol: 0 mg Sodium: 107 mg Total Carbohydrate: 35.7 g Dietary Fiber: 9.1 g Total Sugars: 6.5 g Iron: 2 mg

279.Grilled Greens And Cheese On Toast

Servings: 2
Cooking Time:25min
Ingredients:

- 2 - Tbsp. extra-virgin olive oil
- 1 - large bunches Tuscan kale, stems removed
- ½ tsp. kosher salt, plus more
- ½ tsp. freshly ground black pepper
- 6 - oz. cherry tomatoes
- ½ lb. Halloumi cheese, sliced into½" planks
- 1 - lemon, halved crosswise
- 4 - thick slices country-style bread
- 1 - large garlic clove, peeled, halved

Directions:
1. Set up a Ninja Foodi oven broil for medium-high warmth. Oil grind. Hurl kale with 2 Tbsp. oil, ½ tsp. salt, and½ tsp. pepper in a huge bowl; put in a safe spot.
2. String tomatoes onto sticks, at that point shower with oil; season daintily with salt.
3. Ninja Foodi oven broil tomato sticks, Halloumi, and lemon parts turning sticks and cheddar partially through, until scorched and mellowed, 6–8MIN. Move to a platter.
4. In the interim, shower bread with oil; season delicately with salt. Ninja Foodi oven broil until brilliant earthy colored and fresh, about 2MIN per side. Move to a platter. Rub one side of each cut with the divided garlic clove.
5. Barbecue kale, setting it transversely across grind so it doesn't fall through the holes and turning sporadically, until scorched in places and mellowed all through, 2 to 3MIN. Move to platter close by Halloumi, tomatoes, and bread.
6. Push tomatoes off sticks. Crush singed lemon parts over Halloumi, tomatoes, kale, and bread. Sprinkle with oil.
- **Nutrition Info:** Calories 320, fat 9g, carbohydrate 39g, Protein 17g.

280.Asian Bok Choy

Servings: 4
Cooking Time: 10 Minutes
Ingredients:
- 4 cups bok choy
- 2 tablespoons peanut oil
- 1 tablespoon oyster sauce
- 2 teaspoons garlic, minced
- Salt to taste

Directions:
1. Coat bok choy with oil and oyster sauce.
2. Sprinkle with minced garlic and salt.
3. Add grill grate to your Ninja Foodi Grill.
4. Add bok choy on top of the grill.
5. Select grill setting. Set it to medium.
6. Grill for 10 minutes.

281.Maple Glazed Squash

Servings: 8

Cooking Time: 40 Minutes

Ingredients:
- 2 butternut squash, sliced
- 1 tablespoon vegetable oil
- Salt and pepper to taste
- 2 tablespoons butter
- 4 tablespoons maple syrup
- 4 tablespoons brown sugar

Directions:
1. Coat butternut squash with oil.
2. Season with salt and pepper.
3. Select roast setting.
4. Set it to 375 degrees F for 45 minutes.
5. Press start to preheat.
6. After the unit beeps, add the butternut squash to the grill grate.
7. Cook the squash for 20 minutes.
8. While waiting, combine the remaining ingredients.
9. Dip the squash in the sauce and return to the grill.
10. Cook for another 15 minutes.
11. Flip and cook for 5 more minutes.

282.Crispy Crunchy Broccoli Delight

Servings: 3
Cooking Time: 15 Minutes

Ingredients:
- Lemon wedges
- 2 tablespoons parmesan, grated
- Salt and pepper to taste
- 2 tablespoons extra virgin olive oil
- 1 large broccoli head, cut into florets
- ¼ cup toasted almonds, sliced
- ½ teaspoon red pepper flakes

Directions:
1. Take a medium bowl and add broccoli, toss with olive oil
2. Season well with salt and pepper
3. Add pepper flakes for heat
4. Pre-heat your Ninja Foodi Grill in AIR CRISP mode to 390 degrees F, and set the timer to 15 minutes
5. Once you hear the beep, arrange a reversible trivet in Grill Pan
6. Arrange broccoli and roast until the timer is out
7. Serve with some cheese on top and the lemon wedges on the side
8. Enjoy!
- **Nutrition Info:** Calories: 181 Fat: 11 g Saturated Fat: 3 g Carbohydrates: 9 g Fiber: 4 g Sodium: 421 mg Protein: 8 g

283.Keto Cauliflower Hash Browns

Servings: 6
Cooking Time: 17 Minutes

Ingredients:
- 1/2 cup cheddar cheese, shredded

- 1 tablespoon soft cheese, at room temperature
- 1/3 cup almond meal
- 1 ½ yellow or white medium-sized onion, chopped
- 5 ounces condensed cream of celery soup
- 1 tablespoon fresh cilantro, finely minced
- 1/3 cup sour cream
- 3 cloves garlic, peeled and finely minced
- 2 cups cauliflower, grated
- 1 1/2 tablespoons margarine, melted
- Sea salt and freshly ground black pepper, to your liking
- Crushed red pepper flakes, to your liking

Directions:
1. Grab a large-sized bowl and whisk the celery soup, sour cream, soft cheese, red pepper, salt, and black pepper. Stir in the cauliflower, onion, garlic, cilantro, and cheddar cheese. Mix until everything is thoroughly combined.
2. Scrape the mixture into a baking dish that is previously lightly greased.
3. In another mixing bowl, combine together the almond meal and melted margarine. Spread the mixture evenly over the top of the hash brown mixture.
4. Bake for 17 minutes at 290 degrees f. Eat warm, garnished with some extra sour cream if desired.
- **Nutrition Info:** 155 calories; 11.2g fat; 8.7g carbs; 5.6g protein; 2.7g sugars; 2.1g fiber

284.A Prosciutto And Thyme Eggs

Servings:5
Cooking Time: 5 Minutes

Ingredients:
- 4 kale leaves
- 4 prosciutto slices
- 3 tablespoons heavy cream
- 4 hardboiled eggs
- ¼ teaspoon pepper
- ¼ teaspoon salt
- 1½ cups of water

Directions:
1. Peel eggs and wrap in kale. Wrap in prosciutto and sprinkle salt and pepper.
2. Add water to your Ninja Foodi and lower trivet. Place eggs inside and lock the lid.
3. Cook on HIGH pressure for 5 minutes. Quick-release pressure. Serve and enjoy!
- **Nutrition Info:** Calories: 290 Fat: 23 g Carbohydrates: 4 g Protein: 16 g

285.Squash With Thyme & Sage

Servings: 4
Cooking Time: 15 Minutes

Ingredients:
- 2 lb. butternut squash, sliced into cubes

- 1 tablespoon olive oil
- Salt to taste
- 1 teaspoon fresh thyme, chopped
- 1 tablespoon fresh sage, chopped

Directions:
1. Preheat your air fryer to 390 degrees F.
2. Coat the squash cubes with oil.
3. Season with salt, pepper, thyme and sage.
4. Add to the air crisp tray.
5. Cook for 10 minutes.
6. Flip and cook for another 5 minutes.

286.Pepper Jack Cauliflower Meal

Servings: 3
Cooking Time: 3 Hours 35 Minutes
Ingredients:
- 1 head cauliflower
- ¼ cup whipping cream
- 4 ounces cream cheese
- ½ teaspoon pepper
- 1 teaspoon salt
- 2 tablespoons butter
- 4 ounces pepper jack cheese
- 6 bacon slices, crumbled

Directions:
1. Grease the Ninja Foodi and add listed ingredients (except cheese and bacon).
2. Stir and Lock the lid, cook Slow Cook Mode (low) for 3 hours.
3. Remove lid and add cheese, stir. Lock the lid again and cook for 1 hour more.
4. Garnish with bacon crumbles and enjoy!
- **Nutrition Info:** Calories: 272 Fat: 21 g Carbohydrates: 5 g Protein: 10 g

287.Mediterranean Vegetable Gratin

Servings: 4
Cooking Time: 25 Minutes
Ingredients:
- 1 eggplant, peeled and sliced
- 2 bell peppers, seeded and sliced
- 1 red onion, sliced
- 1 teaspoon fresh garlic, minced
- 4 tablespoons olive oil
- 1 teaspoon mustard
- 1 teaspoon dried oregano
- 1 teaspoon smoked paprika
- Salt and ground black pepper, to taste
- 1 tomato, sliced
- 6 ounces halloumi cheese, sliced lengthways

Directions:
1. Start by preheating your air fryer to 370 degrees f. Spritz a baking pan with nonstick cooking spray.
2. Place the eggplant, peppers, onion, and garlic on the bottom of the baking pan. Add the olive oil, mustard, and spices. Transfer

to the cooking basket and cook for 14 minutes.
3. Top with the tomatoes and cheese; increase the temperature to 390 degrees f and cook for 5 minutes more until bubbling. Let it sit on a cooling rack for 10 minutes before serving.
- **Nutrition Info:** 266 calories; 22.8g fat; 8.3g carbs; 7.4g protein; 5.1g sugars; 1.9g fiber

288.Ranch Flavored Cauliflower Steak

Servings: 4
Cooking Time: 15 Minutes
Ingredients:
- 1 head cauliflower, stemmed and leaves removed
- ¼ cup canola oil
- ½ teaspoon garlic powder
- ½ teaspoon paprika
- Salt and pepper to taste
- 1 cup cheddar cheese, shredded
- Ranch dressing, garnish
- 4 slices bacon, cooked and crumbled
- 2 tablespoons chopped fresh chives

Directions:
1. Cut cauliflower from top to bottom into 2-inch steaks, reserve the remaining cauliflower to cook
2. Take a small-sized bowl and whisk in oil, garlic powder, paprika, season with salt and pepper
3. Brush each steak with oil mixture on both sides
4. Pre-heat Ninja Foodi by pressing the "GRILL" option and setting it to "MAX" and timer to 15 minutes
5. let it pre-heat until you hear a beep
6. Transfer steaks to Grill Grate, lock lid and grill for 10 minutes
7. After 10 minutes, flip steaks and top with ½ cup cheese
8. Lock lid and cook for 5 minutes more
9. Once done, drizzle with ranch dressing, top with bacon and chives
10. Enjoy!
- **Nutrition Info:** Calories: 720 Fat: 19 g Saturated Fat: 19 g Carbohydrates: 11 g Fiber: 4 g Sodium: 1555 mg Protein: 32 g

289.Very Rich And Creamy Asparagus Soup

Servings: 3
Cooking Time: 5-10 Minutes
Ingredients:
- 1 tablespoon olive oil
- 3 green onions, sliced crosswise into ¼ inch pieces
- 1 lb. asparagus, tough ends removed, cut into 1-inch pieces

- 4 cups vegetable stock
- 1 tablespoon unsalted butter
- 1 tablespoon almond flour
- 2 teaspoon salt
- 1 teaspoon white pepper
- ½ cup heavy cream

Directions:
1. Set your Ninja Foodi to Sauté mode and add oil, let it heat up.
2. Add green onions and Sauté for a few minutes, add asparagus and stock.
3. Lock the lid and cook on high pressure for 5 minutes.
4. Take a small saucepan and place it over low heat, add butter, flour and stir until the mixture foams and turns into a golden beige, this is your blond roux.
5. Remove from heat. Release pressure naturally over 10 minutes.
6. Open the lid and add roux, salt, and pepper to the soup.
7. Use an immersion blender to puree the soup.
8. Taste and season accordingly, swirl in cream, and enjoy!
- **Nutrition Info:** Calories: 192 Fat: 14 g Carbohydrates: 8 g Protein: 6 g

290.Well Dressed Brussels

Servings: 4
Cooking Time: 4-5 Hours
Ingredients:
- 2 pounds Brussels, halved
- 2 red onions, sliced
- 2 tablespoons apple cider vinegar
- 1 tablespoon extra-virgin olive oil
- 1 teaspoon ground cinnamon
- ½ cup pecans, chopped

Directions:
1. Add Brussels and onions to the Ninja Foodi. Take a small bowl and add cinnamon, vinegar, olive oil.
2. Pour mixture over sprouts and toss.
3. Place lid and cook on Slow Cook mode (low) for 4-5 hours. Enjoy!
- **Nutrition Info:** Calories: 176 Fat: 10 g Carbohydrates: 14 g Protein: 4 g

291.Vegetarian Curry With Pumpkin And Chickpeas

Servings: Up To 8 People
Cooking Time: 15 - 30
Ingredients:
- clean pumpkin: 800 gr
- chickpeas already cooked: 400 gr
- sunflower oil: liv 5
- spicy paprika: 1 teaspoon
- curry: 1 teaspoon
- onion: 1

- garlic: 2 cloves
- tomato paste: 2 teaspoons
- broth: 250 ml
- turmeric: 1 teaspoon
- basmati rice: 640 gr

Directions:
1. Remove the peel and seeds from the pumpkin; cut it into cubes the same size as the chickpeas so that you have the same cooking time.
2. Insert the mixing shovel into the bowl.
3. Pour the chopped onion and garlic, oil, pumpkin and spices (paprika - curry - turmeric) into the tub.
4. Close the lid, set 25min and press the start/stop button.
5. Brown everything for about 8min.
6. Finally, pour the chickpeas, tomato paste, broth and finish cooking for the set time.
7. In the meantime boil the basmati rice in plenty of salted water, drain it al dente and accompany it with the vegetarian curry.

292.Cauliflowers Au Gratin

Servings: Up To 6 People
Cooking Time: 15 - 30
Ingredients:
- previously boiled cauliflowers: 800 gr
- stringy sliced cheese: 4 slices
- béchamel: 1/2 liter
- Grana cheese: q.b.

Directions:
1. Boil the cauliflowers separately, in the meantime prepare 1/2 liter of béchamel sauce (doses: 500ml of milk, 50gr of flour, 50gr of butter, salt and nutmeg).
2. Remove the mixing shovel from the tank.
3. Pour some béchamel in the bottom of the tank, then distribute the cauliflower florets, lay the slices of cheese on them and cover everything with béchamel; sprinkle with grana cheese.
4. Close the lid, select the AIRGRILL program, the power level 2, set 20min and press the the start/stop button; the cooking time may vary according to the desired gratin level.

293.Perfect Baked Potato For Any Topping

Servings: 3
Cooking Time: 1hr
Ingredients:
- 6 medium potatoes
- ¼ cup of vegetable oil
- 1 tsp salt
- ¼ tsp black pepper

Directions:
1. Set your Ninja Foodi appliance to BAKE. Pre-heat to 350 degrees. Select START/STOP to start your pre-heating.

2. Rub each cleaned potato all over with ½ of the oil
3. Pierce the center of each potato with a fork
4. Bake for 45 mins or until tender
5. Adjust temp to 400 degrees after removing potatoes
6. Brush potatoes with remaining oil and season with salt and pepper
7. Bake until crispy
8. Add the topping of your choice and serve
- **Nutrition Info:** Calories: 242 Fat: 9g Saturated Fat: 1g Trans Fat: 0g Carbohydrates: 38g Fiber: 2g Sodium: 342g Protein: 4g

294.Grilled Whole Eggplant With Harissa Vinaigrette

Servings: 4
Cooking Time:45min
Ingredients:
- 1 - Large eggplant (about 1½ lb.)
- 1 - tsp. kosher salt, divided
- ¼ cup extra-virgin olive oil
- 1 - Tbsp. fresh lemon juice
- 1 - Tbsp. harissa paste
- 1 - Tbsp. honey
- ¼ cup chopped parsley
- 4 to 6 (1"-thick) slices crusty bread, toasted on grill if desired

Directions:
1. Set up a charcoal fire in a fish fry. Let coals cool to medium warm temperature.
2. Ninja Foodi oven broil eggplant straightforwardly on coals, turning at instances, until the skin is darkened and substance has crumpled, 15 to 20MIN. Transfer to a wire rack set interior a rimmed heating sheet and allow cool truly.
3. Cautiously expel skin from the eggplant, leaving stem unblemished. Season on all aspects with½ tsp. Salt. Let sit at the rack until overabundance water is depleted, 20 to 30MIN.
4. Whisk oil, lemon juice, harissa, nectar, and ultimate ½ tsp. Salt in a touch bowl to sign up for.
5. Utilizing a paring blade, make a few cuts down the length of eggplant on each side. Move to a plate and pour dressing over. Top with parsley and gift with bread close by.
6. Do Ahead: Eggplant may be dressed eight HRS ahead. Let sit at room temperature up to four HRS. Chill, if status by longer and permit take a seat at room temperature 60MIN before serving.
- **Nutrition Info:** Calories 270, fat 17g, carbohydrate 21g, Protein 10g.

295.Zucchini Fritters

Servings: 2
Cooking Time: 7 Minutes
Ingredients:
- 2 cups zucchini, grated
- 1 clove garlic, minced
- 1 egg, beaten
- ¼ cup Parmesan cheese, grated
- ½ cup breadcrumbs
- Salt and pepper to taste
- Cooking spray

Directions:
1. Combine the ingredients in a bowl.
2. Form patties from the mixture.
3. Add these to the air crisp tray.
4. Spray with oil.
5. Select air crisp.
6. Cook at 390 degrees F for 7 minutes.

296.Mexican Corn

Servings: 6
Cooking Time: 12 Minutes
Ingredients:
- 6 ears corn
- 3 tablespoons canola oil
- Salt and pepper to taste
- 1 ¼ cups Cotija cheese, crumbled
- 2 teaspoons onion powder
- 2 teaspoons garlic powder
- ½ cup sour cream
- ½ cup mayonnaise
- 2 tablespoons lime juice

Directions:
1. Select grill function.
2. Set temperature to max.
3. Set it to 12 minutes.
4. Press start to preheat.
5. Brush the corn ears with oil.
6. Sprinkle all sides with salt and pepper.
7. Place on the grill grate and cook for 6 minutes per side.
8. Mix the remaining ingredients in a bowl.
9. Cover the corn with the mixture and serve.

297.Cheesy Asparagus

Servings: 2
Cooking Time: 10 Mins
Ingredients:
- 4 spears of fresh asparagus
- 1 tbsp vegetable oil
- 1 cup grated cheese
- 1 tsp honey
- Salt and pepper to taste

Directions:
1. Place your Ninja Foodi grill grate in the unit and close the hood. Choose GRILL, set temperature to MAX, and set time to 7 minutes. Select START/STOP to start your pre-heating.

2. Trim the asparagus and sprinkle with salt and pepper before tossing in the vegetable oil.
3. Mix the grated cheese and honey with some more salt and pepper, then baste the spears with this mix.
4. Place on the grill grate, close the hood and cook for 5-7 mins until tender.
5. Serve immediately
- **Nutrition Info:** Calories: 90 Fat: 7g Saturated Fat: 1g Trans Fat: 0g Carbohydrates: 1.5g Fiber: 0g Sodium: 57mg Protein: 1g

298.Zucchini Parmesan Chips

Servings: 10
Cooking Time: 8 Minutes
Ingredients:
- ½ tsp. paprika
- ½ C. grated parmesan cheese
- ½ C. Italian breadcrumbs
- 1 lightly beaten egg
- 2 thinly sliced zucchinis

Directions:
1. Use a very sharp knife or mandolin slicer to slice zucchini as thinly as you can—Pat off extra moisture.
2. Beat egg with a pinch of pepper and salt and a bit of water.
3. Combine paprika, cheese, and breadcrumbs in a bowl.
4. Dip slices of zucchini into the egg mixture and then into breadcrumb mixture. Press gently to coat.
5. Insert the Crisper Basket, and close the hood. Select AIR CRISP, set the temperature to 350°F, and set the time to 8 minutes. Select START/STOP to begin preheating.
6. Air Frying.
7. With olive oil cooking spray, mist coated zucchini slices. Place into your air fryer in a single layer. Set temperature to 350°F, and set time to 8 minutes.
8. Sprinkle with salt and serve with salsa.

299.Lemon Pepper Brussels Sprouts

Servings: 4
Cooking Time: 10 Minutes
Ingredients:
- 1 lb. Brussels sprouts, sliced
- tablespoons olive oil
- 2 teaspoons lemon pepper seasoning
- Salt to taste

Directions:
1. Coat the Brussels sprouts with oil.
2. Season with lemon pepper seasoning and salt.
3. Spread these on the air crisp tray.
4. Select broil setting.
5. Cook at 350 degrees F for 5 minutes.

300.Tangy Asparagus And Broccoli

Servings: 4
Cooking Time: 20 Minutes
Ingredients:
- 1/2 pound asparagus, cut into 1 1/2-inch pieces
- 1/2 pound broccoli, cut into 1 1/2-inch pieces
- 2 tablespoons peanut oil
- Some salt and white pepper, to taste
- 1/2 cup chicken broth
- 2 tablespoons apple cider vinegar

Directions:
1. Place the vegetables in a single layer in the lightly greased cooking basket. Drizzle the peanut oil over the vegetables.
2. Sprinkle with salt and white pepper.
3. Cook at 380 degrees f for 15 minutes, shaking the basket halfway through the cooking time.
4. Add 1/2 cup of chicken broth to a saucepan; bring to a rapid boil and add the vinegar. Cook for 5 to 7 minutes or until the sauce has reduced by half.
5. Spoon the sauce over the warm vegetables and serve immediately.
- **Nutrition Info:** 144 calories; 9.1g fat; 7.3g carbs; 9.6g protein; 2.6g sugars; 2.8g fiber

301.Vegetable Casserole With Swiss Cheese

Servings: 6
Cooking Time: 35 Minutes
Ingredients:
- 1 tablespoon olive oil
- 1 shallot, sliced
- 2 cloves garlic, minced
- 1 red bell pepper, seeded and sliced
- 1 yellow bell pepper, seeded and sliced
- 1 ½ cups kale
- 1 pound broccoli florets, steamed
- 6 eggs
- 1/2 cup milk
- Sea salt and ground black pepper, to your liking
- 1 cup swiss cheese, shredded
- 4 tablespoons romano cheese, grated

Directions:
1. Heat the olive oil in a saucepan over medium-high heat. Sauté the shallot, garlic, and peppers for 2 to 3 minutes. Add the kale and cook until wilted.
2. Arrange the broccoli florets evenly over the bottom of a lightly greased casserole dish. Spread the sautéed mixture over the top.
3. In a mixing bowl, thoroughly combine the eggs, milk, salt, pepper, and shredded cheese. Pour the mixture into the casserole dish.

4. Lastly, top with romano cheese. Bake at 330 degrees f for 30 minutes or until top is golden brown.
- **Nutrition Info:** 212 calories; 13.4g fat; 9.8g carbs; 14.1g protein; 3.3g sugars; 2.9g fiber

302.Delicious Cajun Eggplant

Servings: 4
Cooking Time: 12 Minutes
Ingredients:
- ¼ cup olive oil
- 2 small eggplants, cut into slices
- 3 teaspoons Cajun seasoning
- 2 tablespoons lime juice

Directions:
1. Coat eggplant slices with oil, lemon juice, and Cajun seasoning.
2. Take your Ninja Foodi Grill and press Grill and set to Med mode, set the timer to 10 minutes.
3. Let it preheat.
4. Arrange eggplants over grill grate, lock the lid, and cook for 5 minutes.
5. Flip and cook for 5 minutes more.
6. Serve and enjoy!
- **Nutrition Info:** Calories: 362 Fat: 11 g Saturated Fat: 3 g Carbohydrates: 16 g Fiber: 1 g Sodium: 694 mg Protein: 8 g

303.Elegant Zero Crust Kale And Mushroom Quiche

Servings: 3
Cooking Time: 9 Hours
Ingredients:
- 6 large eggs
- 2 tablespoons unsweetened almond milk
- 2 ounces low –fat feta cheese, crumbled
- ¼ cup parmesan cheese, grated
- 1½ teaspoons Italian seasoning
- 4 ounces mushrooms, sliced
- 2 cups kale, chopped

Directions:
1. Grease the inner pot of your Ninja Foodi.
2. Take a large bowl and whisk in eggs, cheese, almond milk, seasoning and mix it well.
3. Stir in kale and mushrooms. Pour the mix into Ninja Foodi. Gently stir.
4. Place lid and cook on Slow Cook Mode (low) for 8-9 hours. Serve and enjoy!
- **Nutrition Info:** Calories: 112 Fat: 7 g Carbohydrates: 4 g Protein: 10 g

304.Eggplants Skipped

Servings: Up To 4 People
Cooking Time: 15 - 30
Ingredients:
- Eggplants: 600 gr
- Zucchinis: 250 gr
- Peppers: 350 gr
- Onions: 200 gr
- Dried herbs (thyme, oregano): 200 gr
- Garlic: 2 cloves
- Olive oil: level 5
- Salt: q.b.
- Dried herbs (thyme, oregano): 1 teaspoon

Directions:
1. Clean the eggplants and peppers, remove the seeds from them and remove the skin from the tomatoes.
2. Cut all vegetables into cubes of about 1.5 cmx1.5 cm. Finely chop garlic and onion.
3. Insert the mixing shovel into the tub.
4. Pour the oil into the tub and arrange the vegetables. Add salt and oregano. Close the lid, select the program ROAST, set 30 minutes and press the the start/stop button.
5. If they dry too much, we recommend lowering the power and adding water.

305.Mashed Cauliflower Delight

Servings: 4
Cooking Time: 5 Minutes
Ingredients:
- 1 large head cauliflower, chopped into large pieces
- 1 garlic cloves, minced
- 1 tablespoon ghee
- ½ cup cashew cream
- 2 teaspoons fresh chives, minced
- Salt and pepper to taste

Directions:
1. Add the pot to your Ninja Foodi and add water
2. Add steamer basket on top and add cauliflower pieces
3. Close the lid
4. Cook for 5 minutes on High
5. Quick-release the pressure
6. Now add the remaining ingredients
7. Open the lid and use your blender to mash the cauliflower
8. Blend until you get a smooth mixture
9. Serve and enjoy!

306.Italian Squash Meal

Servings: 4
Cooking Time: 16 Minutes
Ingredients:
- 1 medium butternut squash, peeled, seeded, and cut into ½-inch slices
- 1½ teaspoons oregano, dried
- 1 teaspoon dried thyme
- 1 tablespoon olive oil
- ½ teaspoon salt
- ¼ teaspoon black pepper

Directions:
1. Add slices alongside other ingredients into a mixing bowl.

2. Mix them well.
3. Preheat your Ninja Foodi by pressing the Grill option and setting it to MED.
4. Set the timer to 16 minutes.
5. Allow it to preheat until it beeps.
6. Arrange squash slices over the grill grate.
7. Cook for 8 minutes.
8. Flip and cook for 8 minutes more.
9. Serve and enjoy!
- **Nutrition Info:** Calories: 238 Fat: 12 g Saturated Fat: 2 g Carbohydrates: 36 g Fiber: 3 g Sodium: 128 mg Protein: 15 g

307. Sauteed Cauliflower Delight

Servings:4
Cooking Time: 15 Minutes
Ingredients:
- 1 red onion, to be chopped
- 1 cup of cherry tomatoes
- 1 teaspoon of white sugar
- ¼ cup of olive oil
- 1 head of cauliflower, to be cut into florets
- 2 tablespoons of raisins
- 1 clove of garlic, to be minced
- ¼ teaspoon of red pepper flakes
- 1 teaspoon of dried parsley
- 1 tablespoon of fresh lemon juice

Directions:
1. Put the olive oil in a large skillet and heat over medium heat. Cook and stir the onion until it becomes tender in about 5 to 10 minutes. Add cherry tomatoes, cauliflower, raisins, onion, and white sugar, cover the skillet and cook while frequently stirring until the cauliflower becomes tender in about 4 to 5 minutes.
2. Mix the parsley, garlic, and red pepper flakes inside the cauliflower mixture. Increase the heat to high and sauté until the cauliflower becomes brown in about 1-2 minutes—drizzle lemon juice over the cauliflower.
- **Nutrition Info:** 196.5 calories, Carbohydrates 17.8 grams 6% DV, Protein 3.7 grams 8% DV, Fat 13.9 grams 21% DV, Sodium 49.2mg 2% DV.

308. Mushrooms With Tahini Sauce

Servings: 5
Cooking Time: 19 Minutes
Ingredients:
- 1/2 cup tahini
- 1/2 teaspoon turmeric powder
- 1/3 teaspoon cayenne pepper
- 2 tablespoons lemon juice, freshly squeezed
- 1 teaspoon kosher salt
- 1/3 teaspoon freshly cracked black pepper
- 1 1/2 tablespoons vermouth
- 1 ½ tablespoons olive oil
- 1 ½ pounds cremini mushrooms

Directions:
1. Grab a mixing dish and toss the mushrooms with the olive oil, turmeric powder, salt, black pepper, and cayenne pepper.
2. Cook them in your air fryer for 9 minutes at 355 degrees f.
3. Pause your air fryer, give it a good stir and cook for 10 minutes longer.
4. Meanwhile, thoroughly combine lemon juice, vermouth, and tahini. Serve warm mushrooms with tahini sauce.
- **Nutrition Info:** 211 calories; 17.2g fat; 9.5g carbs; 8.2g protein; 3.2g sugars; 3.5g fiber

309. Cous Cous With Vegetables

Servings: Up To 8 People
Cooking Time: 30 - 45
Ingredients:
- carrot: 100 gr
- eggplant: 350 gr
- cherry tomatoes: 100 gr
- shallot: 1
- broth: 250 gr
- zucchini: 350 gr
- salt: q.b.
- garlic: 1 clove
- chili pepper: q.b.
- couscous: 500 gr
- water: 540 ml
- butter: q.b.
- olive oil: liv 4

Directions:
1. Insert the mixer blade into the tank.
2. Peel the garlic, cut the chilli pepper into small pieces, chop the shallot and put it all in the tank distributing it well in the bottom; add the oil.
3. Before starting to cook, wash and dice the eggplant, zucchini, carrots and cherry tomatoes (the latter must be set aside because they are added to the couscous when cold).
4. Close the lid, select the Roast program, set 45min and press the start/stop program key.
5. Fry for 3/4 minutes, add carrots, broth and cook for another 6 min.
6. Finally, pour in the eggplant and zucchini, season with salt and pepper and finish cooking by lowering the cooking power level if necessary.
7. At the end pour the vegetables into a bowl, clean the bowl (remove the shovel), pour the water inside, a teaspoon of salt, set the Roast program and bring to the boil. Turn off the machine and add the couscous in the rain, oil and stir well; leave the couscous to swell for about 3 min.

8. Add a knob of butter and cook again for another 3 min always working Roast, the power level 1 stirring regularly with a wooden ladle to shell well.
9. As soon as the vegetables have cooled down, add the cherry tomatoes and pour everything into a container together with the couscous.

310.Buffalo Cauliflower

Servings: 4
Cooking Time: 15 Minutes
Ingredients:
- 4 cups cauliflower florets
- ½ cup buffalo sauce
- 2 tablespoons olive oil
- Salt to taste
- 1 teaspoon garlic powder

Directions:
1. Coat the cauliflower with buffalo sauce and olive oil.
2. Season with salt and garlic powder.
3. Spread in the air crisp tray.
4. Choose air crisp setting.
5. Cook at 375 degrees F for 15 minutes, stirring twice.

311.Grilled Sumac Mango Salad

Servings: 6
Cooking Time: 10 Mins
Ingredients:
- 2 fresh mangoes
- 1 tbsp sumac
- ½ cup red wine vinegar
- 1 cucumber
- Salt and pepper to taste
- 1 whole red onion

Directions:
1. Chop the cucumber and onion and place in a bowl
2. Place your Ninja Foodi grill grate in the unit and close the hood. Choose GRILL, set temperature to MAX, and set time to 12 minutes. Select START/STOP to start your pre-heating.
3. Slice mangoes in half and grill for 4 to 6 mins, flipping halfway through.
4. Chop the cooked fruit into large chunks and add to the onion and cucumber
5. Mix vinegar and sumac then coat ingredients
6. Leave in the fridge to marinate overnight.
7. Serve
- **Nutrition Info:** Calories: 294 Fat: 18g Saturated Fat: 4g Trans Fat: 0g Carbohydrates: 42g Fiber: 4g Sodium: 202mg Protein: 2g

312.Celeriac With Greek Yogurt Dip

Servings: 2
Cooking Time: 20 Minutes
Ingredients:
- 1/2 pound celeriac, cut into 1 1/2-inch pieces
- 1 red onion, cut into 1 1/2-inch pieces
- 1 tablespoon sesame oil
- 1/2 teaspoon ground black pepper, to taste
- 1/2 teaspoon sea salt
- Spiced yogurt:
- 1/4 cup greek yogurt
- 2 tablespoons mayonnaise
- 1/2 teaspoon mustard seeds
- 1/2 teaspoon chili powder

Directions:
1. Place the vegetables in a single layer in the lightly greased cooking basket. Drizzle the sesame oil over vegetables.
2. Sprinkle with black pepper and sea salt.
3. Cook at 390 degrees f for 20 minutes, shaking the basket halfway through the cooking time.
4. Meanwhile, make the sauce by whisking all ingredients. Spoon the sauce over the roasted vegetables.
- **Nutrition Info:** 207 calories; 17.4g fat; 9.3g carbs; 3.6g protein; 4.1g sugars; 2.6g fiber

313.Slowly Cooked Lemon Artichokes

Servings: 4
Cooking Time: 5 Hours
Ingredients:
- 5 large artichokes
- 1 teaspoon of sea salt
- 2 stalks celery, sliced
- 2 large carrots, cut into matchsticks
- Juice from 1/2 a lemon
- ¼ teaspoon black pepper
- 1 teaspoon dried thyme
- 1 tablespoon dried rosemary
- Lemon wedges for garnish

Directions:
1. Remove the stalk from your artichokes and remove the tough outer shell.
2. Transfer the chokes to your Ninja Foodi and add 2 cups of boiling water.
3. Add celery, lemon juice, salt, carrots, black pepper, thyme, rosemary.
4. Cook on Slow Cook mode (high) for 4-5 hours.
5. Serve the artichokes with lemon wedges. Serve and enjoy!
- **Nutrition Info:** Calories: 205 Fat: 2 g Carbohydrates: 12 g Protein: 34 g

314.Peas With Bacon

Servings: Up To 8 People
Cooking Time: 30 - 45

Ingredients:
- frozen peas: 1000 gr
- smoked bacon: 150 gr
- shallots: 2
- sunflower oil: liv 5
- salt and pepper: q.b.
- stock: 250 ml

Directions:
1. Insert the mixer blade into the tank.
2. Spread the chopped onion, diced bacon, oil, close the lid, select the ROASTprogram, set 35min and press the the start/stop button.
3. After 5min add the peas, broth, salt, pepper: lower the cooking power level if necessary.

315.Fresh Cooked Corn

Servings: 2
Cooking Time: 15 Mins
Ingredients:
- 2 ears of fresh corn
- ½ tsp paprika
- 1 diced red onion
- 1 cup Greek yogurt
- 1 tsp chopped mint
- Salt and pepper to taste
- Juice of one lime

Directions:
1. Place your Ninja Foodi grill grate in the unit and close the hood. Choose GRILL, set temperature to MAX, and set time to 12 minutes. Select START/STOP to start your pre-heating.
2. Mix all ingredients in a bowl and leave to settle for 10 mins
3. When the pre-heating timer goes off, place the sweetcorn on the grill, close the lid, and allow to cook for 5 mins, flipping to ensure even grilling.
4. Coat the grilled corn in the sauce and continue to cook for another 10 mins.
5. Serve
- **Nutrition Info:** Calories: 452 Fat: 42g Saturated Fat: 15g Trans Fat: 0g Carbohydrates: 4.5g Fiber: 2g Sodium: 701mg Protein: 12g

316.Barbeque Veggie Kebabs

Servings: 2
Cooking Time: 5 Mins
Ingredients:
- 1 cup barbeque sauce
- ½ cup honey
- Chunked vegetables of your choice: corn, bell peppers, and mushrooms recommended
- ½ tsp vegetable oil
- Salt and pepper to taste

Directions:

1. Mix the oil, barbeque sauce, honey, and salt and pepper
2. Mix your chunky vegetables in this sauce and leave for 30 mins in the fridge.
3. Pour marinade over vegetables and mix well. Leave to soak for 10 mins.
4. Place your Ninja Foodi grill grate in the unit and close the hood. Choose GRILL, set temperature to MAX, and set time to 6 minutes. Select START/STOP to start your pre-heating.
5. Skewer the vegetables and place them on the grill. Close the lid cook with for 5 mins, flipping once.
6. Brush with the remaining sauce.
7. Serve immediately
- **Nutrition Info:** Calories: 182 Fat: 12g Saturated Fat: 4g Trans Fat: 0g Carbohydrates: 14g Fiber: 2g Sodium: 642mg Protein: 4g

317.Honeyed Grilled Artichokes

Servings: 4
Cooking Time: 30 Mins
Ingredients:
- 2 artichokes
- 6 cups of water
- ½ tsp salt and ½ tsp pepper
- 1 cup honey
- 4 cloves of crushed garlic
- ½ a lemon
- ½ tbsp vegetable oil

Directions:
1. Prepare the artichokes by removing the tops and the center.
2. Boil the water on a stove and add the lemon and the salt and pepper.
3. Boil the artichokes in this pot for 20 mins until tender, then leave them to dry.
4. Place your Ninja Foodi grill grate in the unit and close the hood. Choose GRILL, set temperature to MAX, and set time to 8 minutes. Select START/STOP to start your pre-heating.
5. Mix the oil, honey, and crushed garlic in a bowl. When a nice consistency, slather the artichokes with this mixture all over.
6. When the pre-heating timer goes off, place artichokes cut side up on the grill grate. Grill for 10 minutes, flipping once.
7. Serve with dipping sauce immediately.
- **Nutrition Info:** Calories: 57 Fat: 3g Saturated Fat: 1.5g Trans Fat: 0g Carbohydrates: 5g Fiber: 1g Sodium: 157mg Protein: 1.5g

318.Broccoli And Cheese Calzone

Servings:4
Cooking Time: 15 Minutes
Ingredients:

- 8 ounces of shredded part-skim mozzarella cheese
- Black pepper
- Salt
- 1 (15-ounce) container of part-skim ricotta cheese
- 1 (10-ounce) package broccoli florets, to be thawed and drained
- 2 tablespoons of grated parmesan
- 1 pound of bread or pizza dough, to be thawed

Directions:
1. Get a medium bowl, then combine mozzarella, ricotta, and broccoli. Mix very well. Then season with black pepper and salt
2. Roll dough to a 12-inch circle. Spread the cheese to fill 1 side of the circle to about 1-inch edge. Lift 1 side of the dough and fold over in other to meet the other side and form a half-moon and pinch the edges together to create a seal.
3. Preheat the oven to about 400 ºF.
4. Transfer the calzone to a large baking sheet and sprinkle it with cheese. Bake for 15 minutes until it becomes golden brown. Allow it to stand for 15 minutes before you slice.

319.Crispy Leek Strips

Servings: 6
Cooking Time: 43 Minutes
Ingredients:
- 1/2 teaspoon porcini powder
- 1 cup almond flour
- 1/2 cup coconut flour
- 1 tablespoon vegetable oil
- 2 medium-sized leeks, slice into julienne strips
- 2 large-sized dishes with ice water
- 2 teaspoons onion powder
- Fine sea salt and cayenne pepper, to taste

Directions:
1. Allow the leeks to soak in ice water for about 25 minutes; drain well.
2. Place the flour, salt, cayenne pepper, onions powder, and porcini powder into a resealable bag. Add the leeks and shake to coat well.
3. Drizzle vegetable oil over the seasoned leeks. Air fry at 390 degrees f for about 18 minutes; turn them halfway through the cooking time.
4. Serve with homemade mayonnaise or any other sauce for dipping.
- **Nutrition Info:** 114 calories; 8.7g fat; 8.4g carbs; 2.7g protein; 2.3g sugars; 2.4g fiber

320.Roasted Cauliflower

Servings: 4
Cooking Time: 20 Minutes
Ingredients:
- 2 heads cauliflower, sliced into florets
- 3 tablespoons olive oil
- Salt and pepper to taste
- Sauce
- 1 tablespoon soy sauce
- 1/4 cup olive oil
- 1 tablespoon chili paste
- 3 tablespoons honey
- 2 tablespoons rice wine vinegar
- 1/4 cup roasted peanuts, chopped
- 1 tablespoon cilantro, chopped

Directions:
1. Add air fry basket to your Ninja Foodi Grill.
2. Choose air fry function.
3. Set it to 390 degrees F for 20 minutes.
4. Press "start" to preheat.
5. In a bowl, toss cauliflower in oil.
6. Season with salt and pepper.
7. Add cauliflower to the air fry basket.
8. Seal the hood.
9. Cook for 10 minutes.
10. Stir and cook for another 8 minutes.
11. While waiting, combine all ingredients for sauce.
12. Toss the roasted cauliflower in sauce before serving.

321.Spicy Celery Sticks

Servings: 4
Cooking Time: 15 Minutes
Ingredients:
- 1 pound celery, cut into matchsticks
- 2 tablespoons peanut oil
- 1 jalapeño, seeded and minced
- 1/4 teaspoon dill
- 1/2 teaspoon basil
- Salt and white pepper to taste

Directions:
1. Start by preheating your air fryer to 380 degrees f.
2. Toss all ingredients together and place them in the air fryer basket.
3. Cook for 15 minutes, shaking the basket halfway through the cooking time. Transfer to a serving platter and enjoy!
- **Nutrition Info:** 82 calories; 6.9g fat; 4.4g carbs; 1.1g protein; 2g sugars; 2g fiber

322.Vegetarian Pizza

Servings: 2
Cooking Time: 15 Minutes
Ingredients:
- 1 pizza dough
- 1 tablespoon olive oil, divided
- 1/2 cup pizza sauce

- 1 cup mozzarella cheese, shredded
- 1/2 cup ricotta cheese
- 2 tomatoes, sliced
- 5 basil leaves, sliced

Directions:
1. Add grill grate to the Ninja Foodi Grill.
2. Press grill setting.
3. Set it to max for 6 minutes.
4. Press start to preheat.
5. Roll out the dough on your kitchen table.
6. Brush top with oil.
7. Add dough to the grill.
8. Cook for 5 minutes.
9. Flip and cook for another 5 minutes.
10. Spread pizza sauce on top of the dough.
11. Sprinkle it with mozzarella cheese and then with ricotta.
12. Add tomatoes and basil on top.
13. Grill pizza for 3 to 5 minutes or until cheese has melted.

323.Cauliflower With Cholula Sauce

Servings: 4
Cooking Time: 13 Minutes
Ingredients:
- 1/2 cup almond flour
- 2 tablespoons flaxseed meal
- 1/2 cup water
- Salt, to taste
- 1/2 teaspoon ground black pepper
- 1/2 teaspoon shallot powder
- 1/2 teaspoon garlic powder
- 1/2 teaspoon cayenne pepper
- 2 tablespoons olive oil
- 1 pound cauliflower, broken into small florets
- 1/4 cup cholula sauce

Directions:
1. Start by preheating your air fryer to 400 degrees f. Lightly grease a baking pan with cooking spray.
2. In a mixing bowl, combine the almond flour, flaxseed meal, water, spices, and olive oil. Coat the cauliflower with the prepared batter; arrange the cauliflower on the baking pan.
3. Then, bake in the preheated air fryer for 8 minutes or until golden brown.
4. Brush the cholula sauce all over the cauliflower florets and bake an additional 4 to 5 minutes.
- **Nutrition Info:** 184 calories; 15.1g fat; 9g carbs; 5.4g protein; 2.8g sugars; 5g fiber

324.Roasted Mixed Veggies

Servings: 4
Cooking Time: 15 Minutes
Ingredients:
- 1 zucchini, sliced

- 8 oz. mushrooms, sliced
- 2 tablespoons olive oil
- 1 tablespoon garlic, minced
- 1 teaspoon onion powder
- 1 teaspoon garlic powder
- Salt and pepper to taste

Directions:
1. Choose the Air Fry setting on your Ninja Foodi Grill.
2. Insert air fryer basket.
3. Preheat it to 390°F.
4. Toss zucchini and mushrooms in oil.
5. Sprinkle with garlic.
6. Season with onion powder, garlic powder, salt, and pepper.
7. Place in the basket.
8. Cook for 10 minutes.
9. Stir and cook for another 5 minutes.
10. serving Suggestionss:
11. Serve as a side dish to the main course.
12. preparation/Cooking Tips:
13. Do not overcrowd the basket with veggies.
- **Nutrition Info:** Calories: 345 Fat: 30 g Carbohydrates: 5 g Protein: 20 g

325.Garlic Pepper Potato Chips

Servings: 10
Cooking Time: 10 Minutes
Ingredients:
- 1 large potato, sliced into thin chips
- Cooking spray
- Salt and garlic powder to taste
- 1 teaspoon black pepper

Directions:
1. Spray oil on the Ninja Foodi basket.
2. Season the potato with the salt, garlic powder, and black pepper.
3. Place potato chips on the basket. Seal the crisping lid. Set it to air crisp.
4. Cook at 450 degrees F for 10 minutes or until golden and crispy.

326.Provencal Tomatoes

Servings: Up To 4 People
Cooking Time: 15 - 30
Ingredients:
- tomatoes: 4
- breadcrumbs: 80 gr
- garlic: 1 clove
- marjoram: 2 twigs
- rosemary: 1 sprig
- chopped parsley: q.b.
- salt: q.b.
- olive oil: q.b.
- butter: q.b.

Directions:
1. As a first operation cut the top of the tomatoes and remove the seeds. Apart in a bowl put all the other ingredients (except

butter) and mix them together; the mixture must be quite sandy.
2. Remove the mixing shovel from the bowl.
3. Place the tomatoes inside the bowl, season with salt and fill them with the previously prepared mixture; add on top of each of the butter flakes.
4. Close the lid, select GRILL program, power level LOW, set 20min and press the start/stop button.
5. Once cooked you can eat them hot or warm.

327.Portobello Mushroom Burgers

Servings: 2
Cooking Time: 10 Mins
Ingredients:
- 1 tbsp honey
- 3 cloves crushed garlic
- Salt and pepper to taste
- ½ tbsp olive oil
- ½ tsp soy sauce
- 2 large portobello mushrooms
- 2 hamburger buns
- Lettuce, tomato, chopped onion, and sauce to garnish as preferred

Directions:
1. Place your Ninja Foodi grill grate in the unit and close the hood. Choose GRILL, set temperature to HIGH, and set time to 10 minutes. Select START/STOP to start your pre-heating.
2. Mix all ingredients except mushrooms to make a sauce
3. Soak your prepared mushrooms in the sauce for 10 mins
4. When the pre-heating timer goes off, place the mushrooms on the grill for 5-6 minutes, flip, then cook for another 5 mins.
5. Place on buns with favorite toppings and sauces.
- **Nutrition Info:** Calories: 250 Fat: 7g Saturated Fat: 2.5g Trans Fat: 0g Carbohydrates: 32g Fiber: 1.5g Sodium: 542mg Protein: 4g

328.Buttery Spinach Meal

Servings: 4
Cooking Time: 15 Minutes
Ingredients:
- 2/3 cup Kalamata olives, halved and pitted
- 1 and ½ cups feta cheese, grated
- 4 tablespoons butter
- 2 pounds spinach, chopped and boiled
- Pepper and salt to taste
- 4 teaspoons lemon zest, grated

Directions:
1. Take a mixing bowl and add spinach, butter, salt, pepper and mix well

2. Preheat Ninja Foodi by pressing the "AIR CRISP" option and setting it to "340 Degrees F" and timer to 15 minutes
3. Let it preheat until you hear a beep
4. Arrange a reversible trivet in the Grill Pan, arrange spinach mixture in a basket, and place the basket in the trivet
5. Let them roast until the timer runs out
6. Serve and enjoy!

329.Chinese Cabbage Bake

Servings: 4
Cooking Time: 30 Minutes
Ingredients:
- 1/2 pound chinese cabbage, roughly chopped
- 2 bell peppers, seeded and sliced
- 1 jalapeno pepper, seeded and sliced
- 1 onion, thickly sliced
- 2 garlic cloves, sliced
- 1/2 stick butter
- 4 tablespoons flaxseed meal
- 1/2 cup milk
- 1 cup cream cheese
- Sea salt and freshly ground black pepper, to taste
- 1/2 teaspoon cayenne pepper
- 1 cup monterey jack cheese, shredded

Directions:
1. Heat a pan of salted water and bring to a boil. Boil the chinese cabbage for 2 to 3 minutes. Transfer the chinese cabbage to cold water to stop the cooking process.
2. Place the chinese cabbage in a lightly greased casserole dish. Add the peppers, onion, and garlic.
3. Next, melt the butter in a saucepan over a moderate heat. Gradually add the flaxseed meal and cook for 2 minutes to form a paste.
4. Slowly pour in the milk, stirring continuously until a thick sauce forms. Add the cream cheese. Season with the salt, black pepper, and cayenne pepper. Add the mixture to the casserole dish.
5. Top with the shredded monterey jack cheese and bake in the preheated air fryer at 390 degrees f for 25 minutes. Serve hot.
- **Nutrition Info:** 489 calories; 45.1g fat; 8.9g carbs; 14.2g protein; 4.4g sugars; 3.4g fiber

330.Veggie Lasagna

Servings: 8
Cooking Time: 45 Minutes
Ingredients:
- 6 cups tomato sauce
- 2 tablespoons olive oil
- 2 cloves garlic, minced
- 1 teaspoon dried basil
- 1 teaspoon dried oregano

- Salt and pepper to taste
- 1 red bell pepper, chopped
- 1 green bell pepper, chopped
- 1 cup mushrooms, diced
- 1 cup broccoli, diced
- 1 eggplant, diced
- 4 cups mozzarella cheese
- 4 cups cream
- 1 pack lasagna pasta sheets

Directions:
1. Combine all ingredients except cheese, cream and pasta sheets.
2. In another bowl, mix cheese and cream.
3. Spread some of the tomato sauce and veggie mixture on the bottom of the pot.
4. Top with the pasta sheets.
5. Spread another layer of the tomato sauce mixture, and then the cheese mixture.
6. Top with another layer of pasta sheets.
7. Repeat layers until all ingredients have been used.
8. Cover the top layer with foil.
9. Choose bake setting.
10. Cook at 350 degrees F for 45 minutes.

331.Slow-cooked Brussels

Servings: 3
Cooking Time: 4 Hours
Ingredients:
- 1 lb. brussel sprouts, bottom trimmed and cut
- 1 tablespoon olive oil
- 1½ tablespoon Dijon mustard
- ¼ cup of water
- Salt and pepper as needed
- ½ teaspoon dried tarragon

Directions:
1. Add brussel sprouts, salt, water, pepper, mustard to the Ninja Foodi.
2. Add dried tarragon and stir.
3. Lock the lid and cook on Slow Cook Mode (low) for 5 hours until the sprouts are tender.
4. Stir well and add Dijon mustard over sprouts. Stir and enjoy!
- **Nutrition Info:** Calories: 83 Fat: 4 g Carbohydrates: 11 g Protein: 4 g

332.Eggplant Parmesan Ii

Servings: 10
Cooking Time: 35 Minutes
Ingredients:
- ½ cup of grated parmesan cheese. It needs to be divided
- 1 (16 ounces) package of mozzarella cheese. You will need to shred it and also divide.
- 4 cups of Italian-seasoned bread crumbs
- 3 eggplants, to be peeled and should give about 1.25 pounds of eggplant.
- 2 large eggs, to be beaten
- 6 cups of spaghetti sauce, divided
- ½ teaspoon of dried basil

Directions:
1. Preheat the oven to 350 ºF (175 ºC)
2. After you have preheated the oven as required, you will need to open the egg and put the already sliced eggplant and after that you do the same for the bread crumbs. Then, put it in the baking sheet (single layer). Then, use about 5 minutes for each of the side to bake inside oven (remember it must have been preheated).
3. For this step, you will need a 9x13 inch baking dish, inside it, you will put the spaghetti sauce. Then, you will put a single piece of the eggplant slices inside the prepared sauce. Next is to add parmesan cheese and mozzarella. You will need to follow this procedure for all other ingredient but do for the cheeses last. Then sprinkle basil at the top.
4. Next is to bake in the preheated oven, this should last for about 35 minutes or when you observe that it has become golden brown.
- **Nutrition Info:** 487.4 calories, Carbohydrates 62.1 grams 20% DV, Protein 24.2 grams 48% DV, Fat 16 grams 25% DV, Cholesterol 72.8 mg 24%, Sodium 1663.1mg 67% DV.

333.Garlic And Swiss Chard Garlic

Servings: 4
Cooking Time: 7 Minutes
Ingredients:
- 4 bacon slices, chopped
- 1 bunch Swiss chard, chopped
- 2 tablespoons ghee
- ½ teaspoon garlic paste
- 3 tablespoons lemon juice
- ½ cup chicken stock
- Salt and pepper to taste

Directions:
1. Set your Ninja Foodi to "Sauté" mode
2. Then add bacon, stir well
3. Cook for a few minutes
4. Add ghee, lemon juice, garlic paste
5. Then give a gentle stir
6. Add Swiss chard, salt, pepper, and stock
7. Close the lid
8. Cook on HIGH pressure for 3 minutes
9. Quick-release the pressure
10. Serve and enjoy!

334.Honey Carrots

Servings: 4
Cooking Time: 10 Minutes
Ingredients:

- 2 tablespoons butter, melted
- 1 tablespoon honey
- Salt to taste
- 6 carrots, sliced
- 1 tablespoon parsley, chopped

Directions:
1. Add grill grate to your Ninja Foodi Grill.
2. Set it to grill.
3. Press max temperature and set it to 10 minutes.
4. Choose start to preheat.
5. While preheating, combine butter, honey and salt.
6. Coat the carrots with the honey mixture.
7. Add carrots to the grill.
8. Seal the hood. Cook for 4 to 5 minutes.
9. Flip and cook for another 5 minutes.
10. Sprinkle with parsley and serve.

335.Cottage And Mayonnaise Stuffed Peppers

Servings: 2
Cooking Time: 15 Minutes
Ingredients:
- 1 red bell pepper, top and seeds removed
- 1 yellow bell pepper, top and seeds removed
- Salt and pepper, to taste
- 1 cup cottage cheese
- 4 tablespoons mayonnaise
- 2 pickles, chopped

Directions:
1. Arrange the peppers in the lightly greased cooking basket. Cook in the preheated air fryer at 400 degrees f for 15 minutes, turning them over halfway through the cooking time.
2. Season with salt and pepper.
3. Then, in a mixing bowl, combine the cream cheese with the mayonnaise and chopped pickles. Stuff the pepper with the cream cheese mixture and serve.
- **Nutrition Info:** 312 calories; 25g fat; 8.7g carbs; 12.9g protein; 5.1g sugars; 1.1g fiber

336.Ratatouille

Servings: Up To 8 People
Cooking Time: 45 -60
Ingredients:
- eggplant: 350 gr
- zucchini: 350 gr
- red bell pepper: 450 gr
- onion: 200 gr
- coppered tomatoes: 400 gr
- garlic: 1
- thyme: q.b.
- laurel: q.b.
- olive oil: liv 5
- broth: 150ml

Directions:
1. Wash and cut into squares all vegetables (except onion and tomatoes) about 2 cm thick. Put the tomatoes in boiling water for a few seconds, then peel them and cut them into pieces. Cut the onion into slices.
2. Insert the stirrer blade into the tub.
3. Spread the sliced onion all over the bottom and add the oil.
4. Close the lid, set 60min and press the start/stop button.
5. Fry the onion for 4/5 minutes, add the peppers and part of the broth and cook for another 6/8 min.
6. Finally add the remaining vegetables, stock, salt and bell pepper and finish cooking.

337.Brussels Sprouts

Servings: 10
Cooking Time: 6 Minutes
Ingredients:
- 1 lb. Brussels sprouts
- 2 teaspoons olive oil
- 1/4 teaspoon garlic powder
- 1/4 teaspoon salt

Directions:
1. Put the Brussels sprouts in a bowl. Pour the olive oil into the bowl.
2. Season the sprouts with garlic powder and salt. Put the sprouts on the basket.
3. Seal the crisping lid. Set it to air crisp function.
4. Cook at 370 degrees F for 6 minutes, flipping halfway through.

338.Simple Asparagus

Servings: 3
Cooking Time: 10 Minutes
Ingredients:
- 1 pound fresh thick asparagus, trimmed
- 1 tablespoon olive oil
- Salt and ground black pepper, as required

Directions:
1. In a bowl, add all the ingredients and toss to coat well.
2. Arrange the asparagus onto a cooking tray.
3. Arrange the drip pan at the bottom of the Instant Ninja Foodi Plus Air Fryer Oven cooking chamber.
4. Select "Air Fry" and then adjust the temperature to 350 degrees F.
5. Set the timer for 10 minutes and press the "Start."
6. When the display shows "Add Food" insert the cooking tray in the center position.
7. When the display shows "Turn Food," turn the asparagus.
8. When cooking time is complete, remove the tray from Ninja Foodi and serve hot.

339.Roast Carrot And Cumin

Servings: 4
Cooking Time: 12 Minutes
Ingredients:
- 21 ounces carrots, peeled
- 1 tablespoon olive oil
- 1 teaspoon cumin seeds
- Handful fresh coriander

Directions:
1. Preheat Ninja Foodi by pressing the "AIR CRISP" option and setting it to "350 Degrees F" and timer to 12 minutes
2. let it preheat until you hear a beep
3. Take a mixing bowl and add oil, honey, and carrots
4. Give it a nice stir and make sure that they are coated well
5. Season with some dill, pepper, and salt
6. Transfer the mix to your Ninja Foodi Grill and cook for 12 minutes and enjoy it!

340.Grilled Ratatouille Pasta Salad

Servings: 4
Cooking Time:40min
Ingredients:
- 2 - medium zucchini (about 1½ lb.), halved lengthwise
- 1 - medium or 2 small eggplants (about 1 lb.), cut into 1" wedges
- ¾ cup extra-virgin olive oil, divided
- 2½ tsp. kosher salt, divided
- 1 tsp. freshly ground black pepper, divided
- 10 oz. penne or casarecce pasta
- 1 - large or 2 medium heirloom or beefsteak tomato (about 1 lb.), cut into 1" pieces
- 8 oz. Ciliegini (MIN fresh mozzarella balls), drained, halved
- 2 - Tbsp. white balsamic or white wine vinegar
- 1 - Tbsp. thyme leaves
- 1 - cup basil leaves

Directions:
1. Set up a Ninja Foodi oven broil for medium warmth. Hurl zucchini, eggplant, and ¼ cup oil on a rimmed preparing sheet; season with 1 tsp. salt and½ tsp. pepper. Barbecue, turning frequently, until hot, delicate, and singed all more than, 8 to 12MIN. come back to the heating sheet and let cool.
2. Cook pasta as per bundle directions:
3. Cut Ninja Foodi oven-broiled vegetables into scaled-down pieces and move to an enormous bowl. Include tomato, cheddar, vinegar, thyme, and 1½ tsp. salt, ½ tsp. pepper, and½ cup oil and blend to consolidate. Channel pasta and promptly add to bowl with vegetables. Blend well to join, at that point top with basil.

4. Do Ahead: Vegetables can be Ninja Foodi oven-broiled 3 days ahead. Move (entire) to an impermeable holder and chill.
- **Nutrition Info:** Calories 90, fat 3g, carbohydrate 16g, Protein 3g.

341.Garlic Carrots

Servings: 4
Cooking Time: 10 Minutes
Ingredients:
- 1 lb. carrots, diced
- 2 tablespoons olive oil
- 2 teaspoons garlic powder
- Salt and pepper to taste

Directions:
1. Toss the carrot cubes in olive oil.
2. Season with garlic powder, salt and pepper.
3. Coat evenly.
4. Spread carrots in the air crisp tray.
5. Cook at 390 degrees F for 10 minutes, stirring once.

342.Balsamic Roasted Tomatoes With Herbs

Servings: 4
Cooking Time: 5 Minutes
Ingredients:
- 1 lb. tomatoes, sliced into quarters
- ½ cup balsamic vinegar
- 1 teaspoon Italian seasoning

Directions:
1. Toss tomatoes in balsamic vinegar.
2. Sprinkle with Italian seasoning.
3. Add to the air crisp tray.
4. Select air crisp.
5. Cook at 350 degrees F for 5 minutes.

343.Stewed Beans

Servings: Up To 8 People
Cooking Time: 15 - 30
Ingredients:
- beans in jar: 750 gr
- tomato puree: 450 gr
- carrot: 1
- shallot: 2
- rosemary sprig: 1
- salt and pepper: q.b.
- olive oil: liv.4

Directions:
1. Insert the mixer blade into the tank.
2. Prepare a chopped carrot and onion and put it inside the tank together with the rosemary; add the oil, close the lid, set 25min and press the the start/stop button.
3. After 4min add the beans drained from their vegetation water and rinse them well; cook for another 3 min.

4. Add tomato, 1/2 glass of water, salt, pepper and continue cooking for the set time by lowering the power level if necessary.

344.Cheesy Barbeque Stuffed Peppers

Servings: 4
Cooking Time: 15 Mins
Ingredients:
- 2 large bell peppers of any color
- ½ a diced red onion
- 1 cup barbeque sauce
- 1 pound of tofu or other ground meat substitute
- Salt and pepper to taste
- 2 cups shredded cheddar
- 1 cup honey

Directions:
1. Clean out the peppers before slicing in half
2. Place your Ninja Foodi grill grate in the unit and close the hood. Choose GRILL, set temperature to MAX, and set time to 10 minutes. Select START/STOP to start your pre-heating.
3. Briefly brown the meat substitute with red onion and garlic until tender.
4. Add all other ingredients except cheese and mix well. Add 1 cup of cheddar.
5. Scoop the mixture into each pepper half and top with remaining cheese
6. When the pre-heating timer goes off, place the peppers on the grill for 10-15 mins.
7. Serve
- **Nutrition Info:** Calories: 334 Fat: 8g Saturated Fat: 1.5g Trans Fat: 0g Carbohydrates: 42g Fiber: 10g Sodium: 335mg Protein: 32g

345.Grilled Whole Cauliflower With Miso Mayo

Servings: 4–6
Cooking Time:40min
Ingredients:
- 1 - large head of cauliflower, leaves removed, stem trimmed
- ½ tsp. (or more) kosher salt
- 4 - Tbsp. unsalted butter
- ¼ cup vinegar-based hot sauce
- 1 - Tbsp. ketchup
- 1 - Tbsp. soy sauce
- ½ cup mayonnaise
- 2 - Tbsp. white miso
- 1 - Tbsp. fresh lemon juice
- ½ tsp. freshly ground black pepper
- 2 - scallions, thinly sliced

Directions:
1. Set up a Ninja Foodi oven broil for medium-high warmth. Sprinkle cauliflower done with salt in a huge microwave-safe bowl. Spread with cling wrap, puncture plastic a couple of times with a blade to vent, and microwave on high until a paring blade effectively slides into the stem, about 5MIN. Let cool somewhat.
2. Warmth spread, hot sauce, ketchup, and soy sauce in a little pot on the Ninja Foodi oven broil, mixing at times until margarine is liquefied, about 2MIN. Brush cauliflower is done with sauce and barbecue, secured, 10MIN. Turn cauliflower over, brush with sauce, and Ninja Foodi oven broil, secured, 10MIN. Keep on barbecuing, brushing and turning each 10MIN and warming sauce varying until cauliflower is softly singed on all sides and fork-delicate, 25 to 30MIN. The sauce ought to be spent at this point, yet in the event that not, brushes any residual sauce over. Move cauliflower to a plate and let cool somewhat.
3. Whisk mayonnaise, miso, lemon squeeze, and pepper in a medium bowl until smooth. Spread on a plate. Set cauliflower on top and disperse scallions over.
- **Nutrition Info:** Calories 130, fat 3g, carbohydrate 2g, Protein 3g.

346.Honey Dressed Asparagus

Servings: 4
Cooking Time: 15 Minutes
Ingredients:
- 2 pounds asparagus, trimmed
- 4 tablespoons tarragon, minced
- ¼ cup honey
- 2 tablespoons olive oil
- 1 teaspoon salt
- ½ teaspoon pepper

Directions:
1. Add asparagus, oil, salt, honey, pepper, tarragon into your bow. Toss them well.
2. Preheat your Ninja Foodi by pressing the Grill option and setting it to MED.
3. Set the timer to 8 minutes.
4. Allow it preheat until it makes a beep sound.
5. Arrange asparagus over grill grate and lock the lid.
6. Cook for 4 minutes.
7. Then flip asparagus and cook for 4 minutes more.
8. Serve and enjoy!
- **Nutrition Info:** Calories: 240 Fat: 15 g Saturated Fat: 3 g Carbohydrates: 31 g Fiber: 1 g Sodium: 103 mg Protein: 7 g

347.Cheddar Cauliflower Bowl

Servings: 4
Cooking Time: 5 Minutes
Ingredients:
- ¼ cup butter
- ½ sweet onion, chopped

- 1 head cauliflower, chopped
- 4 cups herbed vegetable stock
- ½ teaspoon ground nutmeg
- 1 cup heavy whip cream
- Salt and pepper as needed
- 1 cup cheddar cheese, shredded

Directions:
1. Set your Ninja Foodi to sauté mode and add butter, let it heat up, and melt.
2. Add onion and cauliflower. Sauté for 10 minutes until tender and lightly browned.
3. Add vegetable stock and nutmeg, bring to a boil.
4. Lock the lid and cook on high pressure for 5 minutes, quick release pressure once done.
5. Remove the pot from the Foodi and stir in heavy cream. Puree using an immersion blender.
6. Season with more salt and pepper and serve with a topping of cheddar. Enjoy!
- **Nutrition Info:** Calories: 227 Fat: 21 g Carbohydrates: 4 g Protein: 8 g

348.French Fries

Servings: Up To 8 People
Cooking Time: 30 - 45
Ingredients:
- fresh potatoes (to peel): 1750 gr
- fine salt: q.b.
- peanut seed oil: liv 5

Directions:
1. Insert the mixer blade into the tank.
2. Peel the potatoes and cut them into sticks about 1 cm on each side.
3. Put the sliced potatoes in running water for a few minutes and rinse them well.
4. Drain and dry them with absorbent paper.
5. Pour the potatoes and the right amount of oil into the tub.
6. Close the lid, select the AIR CRISP program, power level 3, set 40min and press the program start/stop button.
7. At the end of cooking salt and serve.

349.Garlic Brussels Sprouts

Servings: 4
Cooking Time: 35 Minutes
Ingredients:
- 1 lb. Brussels sprouts, sliced in half
- 1 tablespoon olive oil
- Salt and pepper to taste
- 2 teaspoons garlic powder

Directions:
1. Toss Brussels sprouts in oil.
2. Season with salt, pepper and garlic powder.
3. Add crisper plate in the air fryer basket.
4. Add the basket to the Ninja Foodi Grill.
5. Select air fry. Set it to 390 degrees F for 3 minutes.

6. Press start to preheat.
7. Add Brussels sprouts to the crisper plate.
8. Cook for 20 minutes.
9. Stir and cook for another 15 minutes.

350.Italian Spiced Squash

Servings: 4
Cooking Time: 16 Minutes
Ingredients:
- ¼ teaspoon black pepper
- 1 and ½ teaspoon dried oregano
- 1 tablespoon olive oil
- ½ teaspoon salt
- 1 teaspoon dried thyme
- 1 medium butternut squash, peeled and seeded, cut into ½ inch slices

Directions:
1. Take a mixing bowl and add listed ingredients alongside the slices, mix
2. Pre-heat your Ninja Foodi Grill to MED, setting the timer to 16 minutes
3. Once you hear the beep, arrange squash over the griller
4. Cook for 8 minutes, flip them over and cook for 8 minutes more
5. Serve and enjoy once done!
- **Nutrition Info:** Calories: 238 Fat: 12 g Saturated Fat: 2 g Carbohydrates: 36 g Fiber: 3 g Sodium: 128 mg Protein: 15 g

351.Mixed Air Fried Veggies

Servings: 4
Cooking Time: 20 Minutes
Ingredients:
- 1 white onion, sliced into wedges
- 1 red bell pepper, sliced
- 4 oz. mushroom buttons, sliced in half
- 1 zucchini, sliced
- 1 squash, sliced into cubes
- 1 tablespoon olive oil
- Salt and pepper to taste

Directions:
1. Select air fry setting in your Ninja Foodi Grill.
2. Add air fryer basket.
3. Toss veggies in oil and season with salt and pepper.
4. Add veggies to the basket.
5. Cook for 10 minutes.
6. Shake and cook for another 10 minutes.

352.Cheddar Cauliflower Meal

Servings: 2
Cooking Time: 15 Minutes
Ingredients:
- ½ teaspoon garlic powder
- ½ teaspoon paprika
- Ocean salt and ground dark pepper to taste

- 1 head cauliflower, stemmed and leaves removed
- 1 cup Cheddar cheese, shredded
- Ranch dressing, for garnish
- ¼ cup canola oil or vegetable oil
- 2 tablespoons chopped chives
- 4 slices bacon, cooked and crumbled

Directions:
1. Cut the cauliflower into 2-inch pieces.
2. In a blending bowl, including the oil, garlic powder, and paprika. Season with salt and ground dark pepper; join well. Coat the florets with the blend.
3. Take Ninja Foodi Grill, mastermind it over your kitchen stage, and open the top cover.
4. Mastermind the flame broil mesh and close the top cover.
5. Press "Flame broil" and select the "Maximum" barbecue work. Change the clock to 15 minutes and afterward press "START/STOP." Ninja Foodi will begin preheating.
6. Ninja Foodi is preheated and prepared to cook when it begins to signal. After you hear a blare, open the top.
7. Organize the pieces over the flame broil grind.
8. Close the top lid and cook for 10 minutes. Now open the top lid, flip the pieces and top with the cheese.
9. Close the top lid and cook for 5 more minutes. Serve warm with the chives and ranch dressing on top.

353.Mediterranean Veggies

Servings: 6
Cooking Time: 20 Minutes
Ingredients:
- 1 zucchini, sliced
- 2 tomatoes, sliced in half
- 1 red bell pepper, sliced
- 1 orange bell pepper, sliced
- 1 yellow bell pepper, sliced
- 3 oz. black olives
- 1 tablespoon olive oil
- 1 teaspoon dried parsley
- 1 teaspoon dried oregano
- 1 teaspoon dried basil leaves
- Salt and pepper to taste
- 6 cloves garlic, minced

Directions:
1. Combine all the ingredients in a large bowl.
2. Transfer to the air fryer basket.
3. Insert air fryer basket to your Ninja Foodi Grill.
4. Select the Air Fry setting.
5. Cook at 390°F for 10 minutes.
6. Stir and cook for another 10 minutes.
7. serving Suggestionss:

8. Serve with crumbled feta cheese.
9. preparation/Cooking Tips:
10. Add other colorful veggies to this recipe.
- **Nutrition Info:** Calories: 390 Fat: 30 g Carbohydrates: 10 g Protein: 19 g

354.Fried Pickles With Dijon Sauce

Servings: 2
Cooking Time: 10 Minutes
Ingredients:
- 1 egg, whisked
- 2 tablespoons buttermilk
- 1/2 cup romano cheese, grated
- 1/2 teaspoon onion powder
- 1/2 teaspoon garlic powder
- 1 ½ cups dill pickle chips, pressed dry with kitchen towels
- Mayo sauce:
- 1/3 cup mayonnaise
- 1 tablespoon dijon mustard
- 1 tablespoon ketchup
- 1/4 teaspoon ground black pepper

Directions:
1. In a shallow bowl, whisk the egg with buttermilk.
2. In another bowl, mix romano cheese, onion powder, and garlic powder.
3. Dredge the pickle chips in the egg mixture, then, in the cheese mixture.
4. Cook in the preheated air fryer at 400 degrees f for 5 minutes; shake the basket and cook for 5 minutes more.
5. Meanwhile, mix all the sauce ingredients until well combined. Serve the fried pickles with the mayo sauce for dipping.
- **Nutrition Info:** 351 calories; 28g fat; 7.6g carbs; 16.1g protein; 4.8g sugars; 1.1g fiber

355.Veggie Flatbread

Servings: 6
Cooking Time: 10 Minutes
Ingredients:
- 1 teaspoon olive oil
- 1 lb. pizza dough
- 1 tablespoon olive oil
- ¼ cup zucchini, sliced thinly
- ¼ cup squash, sliced thinly
- 1 teaspoon garlic, minced
- ½ cup Parmesan cheese, grated
- ½ teaspoon red pepper flakes

Directions:
1. Coat the dough with 1 teaspoon olive oil.
2. Let sit at room temperature for 15 minutes.
3. Select grill setting.
4. Set it to high for 10 minutes.
5. Press start to preheat.
6. Add pizza dough to the grill grate.
7. Cook for 3 minutes.
8. Flip and cook for another 1 minute.

9. Take the flatbread out of the unit.
10. Brush the top with the remaining olive oil.
11. Add the remaining ingredients on top.
12. Place inside the unit.
13. Cook for 5 minutes.
14. Let cool, slice and serve.

356.Carrot Sticks With Paprika

Servings: Up To 8 People
Cooking Time: 15 - 30
Ingredients:
- carrots: 1000gr
- sweet paprika: 1 1/2 tablespoon
- oil: liv 3

Directions:
1. Peel the carrots and cut them into sticks.
2. Insert the mixing shovel into the tank.
3. Add the carrots, oil and paprika, close the lid, select OVEN program, power level 3, set 25min and press on/off key.
4. The time may vary depending on the size of the carrots. Excellent accompanied with tzatziki sauce.

357.Delicious Beet Borscht

Servings: 3
Cooking Time: 45 Minutes
Ingredients:
- 8 cups beets
- ½ cup celery, diced
- ½ cup carrots, diced
- 2 garlic cloves, diced
- 1 medium onion, diced
- 3 cups cabbage, shredded
- 6 cups beef stock
- 1 bay leaf
- 1 tablespoon salt
- ½ tablespoon thyme
- ¼ cup fresh dill, chopped
- ½ cup of coconut yogurt

Directions:
1. Add the washed beets to a steamer in the Ninja Foodi.
2. Add 1 cup of water. Steam for 7 minutes.
3. Perform a quick release and drop into an ice bath.

4. Carefully peel off the skin and dice the beets.
5. Transfer the diced beets, celery, carrots, onion, garlic, cabbage, stock, bay leaf, thyme, and salt to your Instant Pot. Lock up the lid and set the pot to Soup mode, cook for 45 minutes.
6. Release the pressure naturally. Transfer to bowls and top with a dollop of dairy-free yogurt.
7. Enjoy with a garnish of fresh dill!
- **Nutrition Info:** Calories: 625 Fats: 46 g Carbs: 19 g Protein: 90 g

358.The Authentic Zucchini Pesto Meal

Servings: 8
Cooking Time: 10 Minutes
Ingredients:
- 1 tablespoon olive oil
- 1 onion, chopped
- 2½ pound roughly chopped zucchini
- ½ cup of water
- 1½ teaspoon salt
- 1 bunch basil leaves
- 2 garlic cloves, minced
- 1 tablespoon extra-virgin olive oil
- Zucchini for making zoodles

Directions:
1. Set the Ninja Foodi to Sauté mode and add olive oil.
2. Once the oil is hot, add onion and sauté for 4 minutes.
3. Add zucchini, water, and salt. Lock up the lid and cook on high pressure for 3 minutes.
4. Release the pressure naturally. Add basil, garlic, and leaves.
5. Use an immersion blender to blend everything well until you have a sauce-like consistency.
6. Take the extra zucchini and pass them through a Spiralizer to get noodle-like shapes.
7. Toss the zoodles with sauce and enjoy!
- **Nutrition Info:** Calories: 71 Fat: 4 g Carbohydrates: 6 g Protein: 3 g

SNACK & APPETIZER RECIPES

359.Slow Cooker Bacon Cheesy Bbq Chicken

Servings: 12
Cooking Time:2 Hrs
Ingredients:
- 12 - Schwan's Fully Cooked Bacon Slices chopped, divided
- 1 c. - Schwan's Diced Chicken Breast Meat
- 1 c. - milk
- 1/3 c. - shredded Mozzarella cheese
- 2 8 - oz packages cream cheese, room temperature
- 2 c. - shredded cheddar cheese
- 1 - Oz pig Ranch Dip Mix
- 1/3 c. - BBQ Sauce
- 2 - Tbsp chopped green onion

Directions:
1. Combine all ingredients besides 2 slices of bacon and green onions in Slow Cooker.
2. Cook on low for two-3 HRS; stirring some instances to mix elements collectively.
3. Top with ultimate bacon and inexperienced onions.
4. Serve with chips.

360.Naan Pizza

Servings: 1
Cooking Time: 5 Minutes
Ingredients:
- Cooking spray
- 1 naan bread
- ¼ cup pesto
- ½ cup baby spinach, cooked
- ½ cup cherry tomatoes, sliced in half
- 1 cup mozzarella cheese

Directions:
1. Spray your air crisp tray with oil.
2. Spread pesto on top of the naan bread.
3. Top with spinach and tomatoes.
4. Sprinkle cheese on top.
5. Add naan pizza to the air crisp tray.
6. Choose air crisp setting.
7. Cook at 350 degrees F for 7 minutes.

361.Ranch Chicken Fingers

Servings: 4
Cooking Time: 20 Minutes
Ingredients:
- 2 lb. chicken breast fillet, sliced into strips
- 1 tablespoon olive oil
- 1 oz. ranch dressing seasoning mix
- 4 cups breadcrumbs
- Salt to taste

Directions:
1. Coat chicken strips with olive oil.
2. Sprinkle all sides with ranch seasoning.
3. Cover with foil and refrigerate for 1 to 2 hours.
4. In a bowl, mix breadcrumbs and salt.
5. Dredge the chicken strips with seasoned breadcrumbs.
6. Add crisper plate to the air fryer basket inside the Ninja Foodi Grill.
7. Choose air fry setting.
8. Set it to 390 degrees F.
9. Preheat for 3 minutes.
10. Add chicken strips to the crisper plate.
11. Cook for 15 to 20 minutes, flipping halfway through.

362.Chili Cheesy Fries

Servings: 6
Cooking Time: 14 Minutes
Ingredients:
- 1 package frozen French fry
- Salt and pepper to taste
- 15 oz. chili
- ½ cup cheese, shredded

Directions:
1. Add French fries to the air crisp tray.
2. Select air crisp setting.
3. Set temperature to 400 degrees.
4. Set time to 15 minutes.
5. Flip French fries halfway through cooking.
6. In a pan over medium heat, add the chili and cheese.
7. Spread mixture over the fries.

363.Spicy Chickpeas

Servings: 4
Cooking Time: 10 Minutes
Ingredients:
- 15 oz. canned chickpeas, rinsed and drained
- 1 tablespoon olive oil
- 1 teaspoon chili powder
- 1 teaspoon ground cumin
- ½ teaspoon cayenne pepper
- Salt to taste

Directions:
1. Coat the chickpeas with oil.
2. Season with chili powder, cumin, cayenne pepper and salt.
3. Add to the air crisp tray.
4. Press air crisp function.
5. Cook at 390 degrees F for 10 minutes, stirring once or twice.

364.Pepperoni Pizza

Servings: 6
Cooking Time: 7 Minutes
Ingredients:
- 1 lb. pizza dough
- Cooking spray
- 1 cup pizza sauce

- ½ cup mozzarella cheese
- ¼ cup pepperoni slices

Directions:
1. Spray the dough with oil.
2. Knead for 5 to 10 minutes.
3. Roll onto a small pizza pan.
4. Spread pizza sauce on top.
5. Sprinkle cheese and top with pepperoni slices.
6. Add the pizza pan to the unit.
7. Select air crisp setting.
8. Air fry at 375 degrees F for 7 minutes.

365.Air Fried Churros

Servings: 6
Cooking Time: 12 Minutes
Ingredients:
- 1 cup of water
- 1/3 cup butter, cut into cubes
- 2 tbsp granulated sugar
- 1/4 tsp salt
- 1 cup flour, preferably all-purpose
- 2 large eggs
- 1 tsp vanilla extract
- oil spray
- Cinnamon Coating:
- 1/2 cup granulated sugar
- 3/4 tsp ground cinnamon

Directions:
1. Grease the Ninja baking pan with cooking spray.
2. Warm water with butter, salt, and sugar in a saucepan until it boils.
3. Now reduce its heat then slowly stir in flour and mix well until smooth.
4. Remove the mixture from the heat and leave it for 4 minutes to cool.
5. Add vanilla extract and eggs, then beat the mixture until it comes together as a batter.
6. Transfer this churro mixture to a piping bag with star-shaped tips and pipe the batter on the prepared pan to get 4-inch churros using this batter.
7. Refrigerate these churros for 1 hour then transfer them to the Air fry sheet.
8. Place the churros to the Ninja oven and Close its lid.
9. Rotate the Ninja Foodi dial to select the "Air Fry" mode.
10. Press the Time button and again use the dial to set the cooking time to 12 minutes.
11. Now press the Temp button and rotate the dial to set the temperature at 375 degrees F.
12. Meanwhile, mix granulated sugar with cinnamon in a bowl.
13. Drizzle this mixture over the air fried churros.
14. Serve.

- **Nutrition Info:** Calories 319 ; Fat 19.7 g ; Carbs 23.7 g ; Fiber 0.9 g ; Sugar 19.3 g ; Protein 5.2 g

366.Grilled Butternut Squash

Servings: 4
Cooking Time: 16 Minutes
Ingredients:
- 1 teaspoon dried thyme
- 1 medium butternut squash
- 1 tablespoon olive oil
- 1/2 teaspoon salt
- 1 ½ teaspoons dried oregano
- 1/4 teaspoon pepper

Directions:
1. Peel and slice the squash into ½ inch thick slices.
2. Remove the center of the slices to discard the seeds.
3. Toss the squash slices with remaining ingredients in a bowl.
4. Prepare and preheat the Ninja Foodi Grill on the medium temperature setting.
5. Once it is preheated, open the lid and place the squash in the grill.
6. Cover the Ninja Foodi Grill's lid and grill on the "Grilling Mode" for 8 minutes per side.
7. Serve warm.
- **Nutrition Info:** Calories 249, Total Fat 11.9 g, Saturated Fat 1.7 g, Cholesterol 78 mg, Sodium 79 mg, Total Carbs 41.8 g, Fiber 1.1 g, Sugar 20.3 g, Protein 15 g

367.Ninja Foodi Reuben Dip

Servings: 10
Cooking Time: 2 Hrs 30min
Ingredients:
- 1 - (8-ounce) package cream cheese, softened
- 1/3 - cup mayonnaise
- 1/3 - cup Thousand Island Dressing
- 1 - Tbsp milk
- ½ - pound thinly sliced deli corned beef, cut into thin strips and then chopped
- 1 - (14.5-ounce) can sauerkraut, squeezed dry in paper towels
- ½ - teaspoon Worcestershire sauce
- 1½ cups shredded Swiss cheese

Directions:
1. In a medium bowl, combine cream cheddar, mayonnaise, Thousand Island dressing, and milk. You needn't bother with it totally blended or smooth; however, get the cream cheddar separated a few.
2. Mix in outstanding fixings.
3. Move to a delicately lubed stewing pot or a simmering pot fixed with a slow cooker liner.

4. Spread stewing pot and cook on LOW for 2½ HRS, mixing part of the way through.
- **Nutrition Info:** Calories 298, fat 23g, carbohydrate 6g, Protein 18g.

368.Mediterranean Spinach

Servings: 4
Cooking Time: 15 Minutes
Ingredients:
- 2 pounds spinach, chopped and boiled
- 4 tablespoons butter
- 2/3 cup Kalamata olives, halved and pitted
- 4 teaspoons fresh lemon zest, grated
- 1 and ½ cups feta cheese, grated
- Salt and pepper to taste

Directions:
1. Add spinach, butter, salt, pepper into a bowl
2. Mix them well
3. Transfer to Ninja Foodi the seasoned spinach
4. Seal your Air Crisper
5. Air Crisp for 15 minutes at 350 degrees F
6. Serve and enjoy!

369.Fried Carrots, Zucchini And Squash

Servings: 4
Cooking Time: 35 Minutes
Ingredients:
- 1/2 lb. carrots, cubed
- 6 teaspoons olive oil, divided
- 1 lb. zucchini, sliced into rounds
- 1 lb. squash, sliced into half-moons
- Salt and pepper to taste
- 1 teaspoon dried tarragon

Directions:
1. Toss the carrots in 2 teaspoons of olive oil.
2. Place these in the Ninja Foodi basket.
3. Seal the crisping lid.
4. Choose the air crisp function.
5. Cook at 400 degrees F for 5 minutes.
6. While waiting, drizzle the zucchini and squash in the remaining olive oil.
7. Season with the salt and pepper.
8. Add the zucchini and squash in the basket.
9. Cook at 400 degrees for 30 minutes.
10. Season with the tarragon.

370.Chicken Salad With Blueberry Vinaigrette

Servings: 4
Cooking Time: 14 Minutes
Ingredients:
- 2 boneless skinless chicken breasts, halves
- 1 tablespoon olive oil
- 1 garlic clove, minced
- 1/4 teaspoon salt
- 1/4 teaspoon pepper
- Vinaigrette:
- 1/4 cup olive oil
- 1/4 cup blueberry preserves
- 2 tablespoons balsamic vinegar
- 2 tablespoons maple syrup
- 1/4 teaspoon ground mustard
- 1/8 teaspoon salt
- Dash pepper
- Salads:
- 1 package (10 oz. salad greens
- 1 cup fresh blueberries
- 1/2 cup canned oranges
- 1 cup crumbled goat cheese

Directions:
1. First season the chicken liberally with garlic, salt, pepper and oil in a bowl.
2. Cover to refrigerate for 30 minutes margination.
3. Prepare and preheat the Ninja Foodi Grill on the medium temperature setting.
4. Once it is preheated, open the lid and place the chicken in the grill.
5. Cover the Ninja Foodi Grill's lid and grill on the "Grilling Mode" for 5-7 minutes per side until the internal temperature reaches 330 degrees F.
6. Toss the remaining ingredients for salad and vinaigrette in a bowl.
7. Slice the grilled chicken and serve with salad.
- **Nutrition Info:** Calories 379, Total Fat 29.7 g, Saturated Fat 18.6 g, Cholesterol 141 mg, Sodium 193 mg, Total Carbs 23.7g, Fiber 0.9 g, Sugar 19.3 g, Protein 5.2 g

371.Air Fried Doughnuts

Servings: 6
Cooking Time: 14 Minutes
Ingredients:
- Cooking spray
- 1/2 cup milk
- 1/4 cup 1 tsp granulated sugar
- 2 1/4 tsp active dry yeast
- 2 cup flour, preferably all-purpose
- 1/2 tsp Salt
- 4 tbsp melted butter
- 1 large egg
- 1 tsp pure vanilla extract

Directions:
1. Warm up the milk in a saucepan then add yeast and 1 tsp sugar.
2. Mix well and leave this milk for 8 minutes.
3. Add flour, salt, butter, egg, vanilla, and ¼ cup sugar to the warm milk.
4. Mix well and knead over a floured surface until smooth.
5. Place this doughnut dough in a lightly greased bowl and brush it with cooking oil.
6. Cover the dough and leave it at a warm place for 1 hour.

7. Punch the raised dough then roll into ½ inch thick rectangle.
8. Cut 3" circles out of this dough sheet using a biscuit cutter.
9. Now cut the rounds from the center to make a hole.
10. Place these doughnuts on the Air Fryer.
11. Transfer these doughnuts to the Ninja oven and Close its lid.
12. Rotate the Ninja Foodi dial to select the "Air Fry" mode.
13. Press the Time button and again use the dial to set the cooking time to 6 minutes.
14. Now press the Temp button and rotate the dial to set the temperature at 375 degrees F.
15. Cook the doughnuts in batches to avoid overcrowding.
16. Serve fresh.
- **Nutrition Info:** Calories 248 ; Fat 15.7 g ; Carbs 38.4 g ;Fiber 0.3 g ; Sugar 10.1 g ; Protein 14.1 g

372.Garlic Mushrooms

Servings: 4
Cooking Time: 20 Minutes
Ingredients:
- 1 lb. mushrooms, rinsed and drained
- 1 teaspoon onion powder
- Black pepper to taste
- 1 tablespoon minced garlic
- 2 teaspoons soy sauce

Directions:
1. Mix all the ingredients in a bowl.
2. Put in the Ninja Foodi basket.
3. Seal the crisping lid.
4. Set it to air crisp.
5. Cook at 360 degrees F for 20 minutes.
6. Coat the beef cubes with the salt and pickling spice.
7. In a skillet over medium heat, pour in the olive oil.

373.Crispy Pickles

Servings: 4
Cooking Time: 30 Minutes
Ingredients:
- 1 cup all-purpose flour
- 3 eggs
- 1 cup breadcrumbs
- Garlic salt to taste
- 12 dill pickle spears
- Cooking spray

Directions:
1. Dip pickles in flour, eggs and then in a mixture of breadcrumbs and garlic salt.
2. Arrange on a plate.
3. Place inside the freezer for 30 minutes.
4. Add crisper basket to the Ninja Foodi Grill.
5. Choose air fry function.

6. Add pickles to the basket.
7. Spray with oil.
8. Cook at 375 degrees F for 18 to 20 minutes.
9. Flip and cook for another 10 minutes.

374.Cherry Jam Tarts

Servings: 12
Cooking Time: 40 Minutes
Ingredients:
- 2 sheets shortcrust pastry
- For the frangipane
- 4 oz. butter softened
- 4 oz. golden caster sugar
- 1 egg
- 1 tbsp plain flour
- 4 oz. ground almonds
- 3 oz. cherry jam
- For the icing
- 1 cup icing sugar
- 12 glacé cherries

Directions:
1. Grease the 12 cups of the muffin tray with butter.
2. Roll the puff pastry into a 10 cm sheet then cut 12 rounds out of it.
3. Place these rounds into each muffin cups and press them into these cups.
4. Transfer the muffin tray to the refrigerator and leave it for 20 minutes.
5. Add dried beans or pulses into each tart crust to add weight.
6. Transfer the muffin tray to the Ninja oven and Close its lid.
7. Rotate the Ninja Foodi dial to select the "Bake" mode.
8. Press the Time button and again use the dial to set the cooking time to 10 minutes.
9. Now press the Temp button and rotate the dial to set the temperature at 350 degrees F.
10. Now remove the dried beans from the crust and bake again for 10 minutes in the Ninja oven.
11. Meanwhile, prepare the filling beat beating butter with sugar and egg until fluffy.
12. Stir in flour and almonds ground then mix well.
13. Divide this filling in the baked crusts and top them with a tbsp cherry jam.
14. Now again, place the muffin tray in the Ninja oven.
15. Continue cooking on the "Bake" mode for 20 minutes at 350 degrees F.
16. Whisk the icing sugar with 2 tbsp water and top the baked tarts with sugar mixture.
17. Serve.
- **Nutrition Info:** Calories 398 ; Fat 13.8 g ;Carbs 33.6 g ; Fiber 1 g ; Sugar 9.3 g ;Protein 1.8 g

375.Greek Potatoes

Servings: 4
Cooking Time: 30 Minutes
Ingredients:
- 1 lb. potatoes, sliced into wedges
- 2 tablespoons olive oil
- 1 teaspoon paprika
- 2 teaspoons dried oregano
- Salt and pepper to taste
- 1/4 cup onion, diced
- 2 tablespoons lemon juice
- 1 tomato, diced
- 1/4 cup black olives, sliced
- 1/2 cup feta cheese, crumbled

Directions:
1. Add crisper plate to the air fryer basket inside the Ninja Foodi Grill.
2. Choose air fry setting.
3. Set it to 390 degrees F.
4. Preheat for 3 minutes.
5. While preheating, toss potatoes in oil.
6. Sprinkle with paprika, oregano, salt and pepper.
7. Add potatoes to the crisper plate.
8. Air fry for 18 minutes.
9. Toss and cook for another 5 minutes.
10. Add onion and cook for 5 minutes.
11. Transfer to a bowl.
12. Stir in the rest of the ingredients.

376.Crockpot Chicken Taco Dip

Servings: 9-10 Cups
Cooking Time: 5 Hrs
Ingredients:
- 1 - pound chicken breast
- 1 x 16 ounce can refried beans
- 3 - cups salsa
- 8 - ounces reduced-fat cream cheese, softened and cut into 1" cubes
- 2-3 Tbsp McCormick Gluten-Free Taco Seasoning
- ½ - cup nonfat plain Greek yogurt
- 1 - cup shredded pepper jack cheese
- 1 - jalapeno, sliced
- corn tortilla chips for serving

Directions:
1. Spot chicken bosoms at the base of your moderate cooker. Spread with beans, salsa, cream cheddar, and taco flavoring. Cook on low for 4-5 HRS, blending once in the middle of if conceivable.
2. Evacuate chicken and shred. Take about a Tbsp of warm dunk and blend into Greek yogurt to temper, at that point add Greek yogurt and mix to consolidate. Mix in destroyed chicken. Move to a stove safe serving dish and top with destroyed cheddar. Cook on sear until cheddar begins to brown and air pocket, around 3-4MIN.

Watch cautiously to abstain from consuming.
3. Top with cut jalapeno and serve quickly with chips. Extras might be refrigerated in an impermeable compartment for 5-7 days.
- **Nutrition Info:** Calories 249, fat 5g, carbohydrate 29g, Protein 23g.

377.Crispy Potato Cubes

Servings: 4
Cooking Time: 15 Minutes
Ingredients:
- 1-pound potato, peeled
- 1 tablespoon olive oil
- 1 teaspoon dried dill
- 1 teaspoon dried oregano
- 1/4 teaspoon chili flakes

Directions:
1. Preheat Ninja Foodi by squeezing the "AIR CRISP" alternative and setting it to "400 Degrees F" and timer to 15 minutes
2. Let it preheat until you hear a beep
3. Cut potatoes into cubes
4. Sprinkle potato cubes with dill, oregano, and chili flakes
5. Transfer to Foodi Grill and cook for 15 minutes
6. Stir while cooking, once they are crunchy
7. Serve and enjoy!

378.Mediterranean Vegetables

Servings: 4
Cooking Time: 15 Minutes
Ingredients:
- 1 cup cherry tomatoes
- 1 eggplant, sliced into rounds
- 1 green bell pepper, sliced into strips
- 1 carrot, sliced into rounds
- 1 teaspoon mixed herbs
- 6 tablespoons olive oil
- 2 tablespoons honey
- 1 teaspoon mustard
- 2 teaspoons garlic puree
- Salt and pepper to taste

Directions:
1. Drizzle the vegetables with the olive oil.
2. Add to the Ninja Foodi basket.
3. Seal the crisping lid.
4. Set it to air crisp.
5. Cook at 360 degrees F for 15 minutes.
6. Mix the rest of the ingredients.
7. Pour the sauce over the vegetables before serving.

379.Ninja Grill Hot Dogs

Servings: 4
Cooking Time: 12 Minutes
Ingredients:
- 1 cup cabbage slaw

- 4 bacon slices, crispy
- 4 hot dogs
- 1/8 cup onion, chopped
- 4 hot dog buns, cut in half

Directions:
1. Sear the bacon in a skillet until crispy from both the sides.
2. Wrap a bacon strip around each hot dog and secure it by inserting a toothpick.
3. Prepare and preheat the Ninja Foodi Grill in a High-temperature setting.
4. Once it is preheated, open the lid and place 2 hot dogs in the grill.
5. Cover the Ninja Foodi Grill's lid and grill on the "Grilling Mode" for 6 minutes while rotating after every 2 minutes.
6. Cook all the hot dogs in batches then remove the toothpick.
7. Serve warm in a hotdog bun with cabbage slaw and onion.
8. Enjoy.
- **Nutrition Info:** Calories 301, Total Fat 32.2 g, Saturated Fat 2.4 g, Cholesterol 110 mg, Sodium 276 mg, Total Carbs 25 g, Fiber 0.9 g, Sugar 31.4 g, Protein 28.8 g

380.Baked Potato Rounds

Servings: 8
Cooking Time: 18 Minutes
Ingredients:
- 2 large potatoes, sliced into thick rounds
- Cooking spray
- Salt and pepper to taste
- 1 cup cheese, shredded
- 4 bacon slices, cooked crisp and crumbled

Directions:
1. Add the potatoes to the air crisp tray.
2. Spray the top part with oil.
3. Sprinkle with salt and pepper.
4. Select air crisp setting.
5. Air fry the potatoes at 370 degrees F for 7 to 8 minutes per side.
6. Remove from the unit.
7. Top each potato with cheese and bacon bits.
8. Air fry for another 2 minutes or until cheese has melted.

381.Goat Cheese Tarts With Tomatoes

Servings: 8
Cooking Time: 8 Minutes
Ingredients:
- Cooking spray
- 1 tablespoon honey
- 1 teaspoon dried Italian seasoning
- ½ cup goat cheese, crumbled
- 1 pack crescent rounds
- 2 tomatoes, chopped
- 2 tablespoons olive oil

Directions:

1. Spray your muffin pan with oil.
2. In a bowl, mix the honey, Italian seasoning and goat cheese.
3. Slice the dough into 8 portions.
4. Press the dough onto the cups of your muffin pan.
5. Coat the tomatoes with oil.
6. Place tomatoes on top of the dough.
7. Top with the goat cheese mixture.
8. Place inside the unit.
9. Set it to bake.
10. Cook at 330 degrees F for 8 minutes.

382.Seared Tuna Salad

Servings: 4
Cooking Time: 6 Minutes
Ingredients:
- 1/2-pounds ahi tuna, cut into four strips
- 2 tablespoons sesame oil
- 1(10 ounces) bag baby greens
- 2 tablespoons of rice wine vinegar
- 6 tablespoons extra-virgin olive oil
- 1/2 English cucumber, sliced
- 1/4 teaspoon of sea salt
- 1/2 teaspoon ground black pepper

Directions:
1. Supplement the flame broil mesh and close the hood
2. Preheat Ninja Foodi by pressing the "GRILL" option at and setting it to "MAX" and timer to 6 minutes
3. Take a small bowl, whisk together the rice vinegar, salt, and pepper
4. Slowly pour in the oil while whisking until vinaigrette is fully combined
5. Season the fish with salt and pepper, sprinkle with the sesame oil
6. Once it preheats until you hear a beep
7. Arrange the shrimp over the grill grate lock lid and cook for 6 minutes
8. Do not flip during cooking
9. Once cooked completely, top salad with tuna strip
10. Drizzle the vinaigrette over the top
11. Serve immediately and enjoy!

383.Pineapple With Cream Cheese Dip

Servings: 4
Cooking Time: 8 Minutes
Ingredients:
- DIP:
- 2 tablespoons honey
- 1 tablespoon brown sugar
- 3 oz. cream cheese, softened
- 1 tablespoon lime juice
- 1/4 cup yogurt
- 1 teaspoon grated lime zest
- Pineapple:
- 1 fresh pineapple

- 3 tablespoons honey
- 2 tablespoons lime juice
- 1/4 cup packed brown sugar

Directions:
1. First, slice the peeled pineapple into 8 wedges then cut each wedge into 2 spears.
2. Toss the pineapple with sugar, lime juice, and honey in a bowl then refrigerate for 1 hour.
3. Meanwhile, prepare the lime dip by whisking all its ingredients together in a bowl.
4. Remove the pineapple from its marinade.
5. Prepare and preheat the Ninja Foodi Grill on the medium temperature setting.
6. Once it is preheated, open the lid and place the pineapple on the grill.
7. Cover the Ninja Foodi Grill's lid and grill on the "Grilling Mode" for 4 minutes per side.
8. Serve with lime dip.
- **Nutrition Info:** Calories 368, Total Fat 6 g, Saturated Fat 1.2 g, Cholesterol 351 mg, Sodium 103 mg, Total Carbs 72.8 g, Fiber 9.2 g, Sugar 32.9 g, Protein 7.2 g

384.Cheesy Dumplings

Servings: 8
Cooking Time: 10 Mins
Ingredients:
- Vegetable oil for coating
- ½ tsp of salt
- Wonton wraps
- 1 bag of your favorite grated cheese (cheddar is suggested)
- 2 finely chopped green onions
- 1 tsp garlic powder

Directions:
1. Place your Ninja Foodi crisper basket in the unit and close the hood. Choose AIR FRY. Select START/STOP to start your pre-heating.
2. Very gently so as not to burn, melt your cheese, stirring often.
3. Mix all of your ingredients in a bowl with the melted cheese.
4. Carefully stuff your wonton wrappers.
5. Place a few of the dumplings in the crisper basket and allow to cook for 2-3 mins until golden brown. Keep shaking the basket to enjoy an even crisp.
6. Serve immediately.
- **Nutrition Info:** Calories: 192 Fat: 17g Saturated Fat: 13g Trans Fat: 0g Carbohydrates: 4g Fiber: 2g Sodium: 342mg Protein: 4g

385.Roasted Corn

Servings: 4
Cooking Time: 10 Minutes

Ingredients:
- 4 ears of corn, husks removed and sliced into 2
- 2 teaspoons olive oil
- Salt and pepper to taste

Directions:
1. Coat the corn with oil and season with salt and pepper.
2. Put in the Ninja Foodi basket.
3. Seal with the crisping lid.
4. Set it to air crisp.
5. Cook at 400 degrees F for 10 minutes.

386.Parmesan French Fries

Servings: 6
Cooking Time: 15 Minutes
Ingredients:
- 1 lb. French fries
- 1/2 cup mayonnaise
- 2 cloves garlic, minced
- 1 tablespoon oil
- Salt and pepper to taste
- 1 teaspoon garlic powder
- 1/2 cup Parmesan cheese, grated
- 1 teaspoon lemon juice

Directions:
1. Add crisper basket to your Ninja Foodi Grill.
2. Select air fry function.
3. Set it to 375 degrees F for 22 minutes.
4. Press start to preheat.
5. Add fries to the basket.
6. Cook for 10 minutes.
7. Shake and cook for another 5 minutes.
8. Toss in oil and sprinkle with Parmesan cheese.
9. Mix the remaining ingredients in a bowl.
10. Serve fries with this sauce.

387.Mayo Zucchini Mix

Servings: 4
Cooking Time: 10 Minutes
Ingredients:
- 1 tablespoon avocado oil
- 1 pound zucchinis, roughly cubed
- 1 yellow onion, chopped
- 1 teaspoon turmeric powder
- 1 cup baby kale
- 2 tablespoons mayonnaise
- 2 tablespoons mustard
- 1 cup parmesan cheese, grated

Directions:
1. Heat up the air fryer with the oil at 360 degrees f, add the onion, zucchinis and turmeric and cook for 2 minutes.
2. Add the other ingredients, toss, cook for 8 minutes more, divide between plates and serve for breakfast right away.
- **Nutrition Info:** calories 212, fat 8, fiber 8, carbs 9, protein 4

388.Avocado Bruschetta With Balsamic Reduction

Servings: 4
Cooking Time: 20min
Ingredients:

- 1 - baguette, thinly sliced
- ¼ cup olive oil, divided
- ½ cup balsamic vinegar
- 2 - Tbsp brown sugar, packed
- 2 - cups cherry tomatoes, halved
- 1 - avocado, halved, seeded, peeled and diced
- Kosher salt and freshly ground black pepper
- ¼ cup basil leaves, chiffonier

Directions:

1. Set the heat level to 350 F. Line a getting ready sheet with cloth paper.
2. Spot loaf cuts onto the readied heating sheet. Shower with 2 Tbsp olive oil. Spot into broiler and heat for 8-10MIN, or until incredible earthy colored.
3. To make the balsamic lower, together with balsamic vinegar and earthy colored sugar to a bit pan over medium warm temperature. Bring to a slight bubble and reduce notably, round 6-8MIN; put in a secure spot and let cool.
4. In a substantial bowl, be a part of tomatoes, avocado, staying 2 Tbsp olive oil, salt, and pepper, to taste.
5. Top every roll cut with tomato blend, embellished with basil.
6. Serve fast, showered with balsamic lower.
- **Nutrition Info:** Calories 179, fat 6g, carbohydrate 12g, Protein 18g.

389.Bacon Bell Peppers

Servings: 16
Cooking Time: 5 Minutes
Ingredients:

- 1 pack bacon slices
- 12 bell peppers, sliced in half
- 8 oz. cream cheese

Directions:

1. Stuff bell pepper halves with cream cheese.
2. Wrap with bacon slices.
3. Preheat Ninja Foodi Grill to 500 degrees F.
4. Add bell peppers to the grill.
5. Grill for 3 to 5 minutes.

390.Puff Pastry Pizza Twists

Servings: 27
Cooking Time:15min
Ingredients:

- 2 - sheets puff pastry defrosted if frozen
- ¼ cup tomato sauce plus more for dipping
- ¾ cup mozzarella shredded low-moisture
- 1 egg yolk
- 1 teaspoon water
- ½ teaspoon dried oregano
- ¼ teaspoon garlic powder
- ¼ cup grated Parmesan cheese

Directions:

1. Preheat broiler to 400°F and fix two heating sheets with material or softly oil.
2. On a gently floured surface, roll the 2 sheets of puff cake into smooth, equivalent square shapes.
3. Brush the tomato sauce over the highest point of one of the puffs baked good sheets, leaving a½ inch outskirt around the edges. Sprinkle equally with the destroyed mozzarella. Top with the other sheet of puff baked well.
4. In a little bowl, beat together the egg yolk and water. Brush over the highest point of the puff baked well. Equally top with the oregano, garlic powder, and ground Parmesan cheddar.
5. Cut the sheet the long way into 9 equivalents long strips, at that point across twice to slice the strips into thirds to make 27 little sticks. Bend each stick tenderly while holding the two sheets together and place it on the readied heating sheet.
6. Heat in the preheated stove until puffed and brilliant, around 15-20MIN. Present with extra tomato sauce for plunging.
- **Nutrition Info:** Calories 123, fat 6g, carbohydrate 15g, Protein 3g.

391.Healthy Granola Bites

Servings: 4
Cooking Time: 20 Minutes
Ingredients:

- Salt and pepper to taste
- 1 tablespoon coriander
- A handful of thyme, diced
- ¼ cup of coconut milk
- 3 handful of cooked vegetables, your choice
- 3 ounce plain granola

Directions:

1. Preheat your Ninja Foodi to 352 degrees F in AIR CRISP mode, set a timer to 20 minutes
2. Take a bowl and add your cooked vegetables, granola
3. Use an immersion blender to blitz your granola until you have a nice breadcrumb-like consistency
4. Add coconut milk to the mix and mix until you have a nice firm texture
5. Use the mixture to make granola balls and transfer them to your Grill
6. Cook for 20 minutes
7. Serve and enjoy!

392. Air-fried Tomato Slices

Servings: 2
Cooking Time: 10 Mins
Ingredients:
- ½ cup flour
- 1 medium-sized egg
- ½ tsp salt
- 1 squashed garlic clove for seasoning
- 1 tbsp grated cheddar
- 1/8 cup milk
- 1/4 tbsp cilantro, ¼ rosemary
- 1/3 tsp pepper
- 2 tomatoes – the firmer, the better, cut into slices.
- 1/4 cup breadcrumbs

Directions:
1. Place your Ninja Foodi crisper basket in the unit and close the hood. Choose AIR FRY. Select START/STOP to start your pre-heating.
2. Beat the eggs, then add milk in a bowl with them.
3. Combine the salt and pepper with the flour in another bowl.
4. Put the herbs, squashed garlic, and breadcrumbs in a dish
5. Dip your slices into each bowl, starting with the egg
6. Lightly coat with oil
7. Place a few of the slices in the crisper basket and allow to cook for 2-3 mins until golden brown. Keep shaking the basket to enjoy an even crisp.
8. Allow cooling before serving
- **Nutrition Info:** Calories: 163 Fat: 3g Saturated Fat: 1g Trans Fat: 0g Carbohydrates: 27g Fiber: 2g Sodium: 250mg Protein: 5g

393. Grilled Tomato Salsa

Servings: 4 To 8
Cooking Time: 10 Minutes
Ingredients:
- 1 onion, sliced
- 1 jalapeño pepper, sliced in half
- 5 tomatoes, sliced
- 2 tablespoons oil
- Salt and pepper to taste
- 1 cup cilantro, trimmed and sliced
- 1 tablespoon lime juice
- 1 teaspoon lime zest
- 2 tablespoons ground cumin
- 3 cloves garlic, peeled and sliced

Directions:
1. Coat onion, jalapeño pepper and tomatoes with oil.
2. Season with salt and pepper.
3. Add grill grate to your Ninja Foodi Grill.
4. Press grill setting.
5. Choose max temperature and set it to 10 minutes.
6. Press start to preheat.
7. Add vegetables on the grill.
8. Cook for 5 minutes per side.
9. Transfer to a plate and let cool.
10. Add vegetable mixture to a food processor.
11. Stir in remaining ingredients.
12. Pulse until smooth.

394. Cheese Dredged Cauliflower Snack

Servings: 4
Cooking Time: 33 Minutes
Ingredients:
- 1 head cauliflower
- ¼ cup butter, cut into small pieces
- ½ cup parmesan cheese, grated
- 1 teaspoon avocado mayonnaise
- 1 tablespoon mustard

Directions:
1. Set your Ninja Foodi to Sauté mode and add butter and cauliflower.
2. Sauté for 3 minutes
3. Add rest of the ingredients
4. Give it a nice stir
5. Close the lid
6. Cook on HIGH pressure for 30 minutes
7. Release pressure naturally over 10 minutes
8. Serve and enjoy!

395. Tarragon Asparagus

Servings: 4
Cooking Time: 16 Minutes
Ingredients:
- 2 lbs. fresh asparagus, trimmed
- 1/2 teaspoon pepper
- 1/4 cup honey
- 2 tablespoons olive oil
- 1 teaspoon salt
- 4 tablespoons minced fresh tarragon

Directions:
1. Liberally season the asparagus by tossing with oil, salt, pepper, honey, and tarragon.
2. Prepare and preheat the Ninja Foodi Grill on the medium temperature setting.
3. Once it is preheated, open the lid and place the asparagus on the grill.
4. Cover the Ninja Foodi Grill's lid and grill on the "Grilling Mode" for 8 minutes per side, give them a toss after 4 minutes.
5. Serve warm.
- **Nutrition Info:** Calories 248, Total Fat 15.7 g, Saturated Fat 2.7 g, Cholesterol 75 mg, Sodium 94 mg, Total Carbs 31.4 g, Fiber 0.6 g, Sugar 15 g, Protein 14.1 g

396. Cob With Pepper Butter

Servings: 8
Cooking Time: 30 Minutes

Ingredients:
- 1 cup butter, softened
- 8 medium ears sweet corn
- 2 tablespoons lemon-pepper seasoning

Directions:
1. Season the corn cob with butter and lemon pepper liberally.
2. Prepare and preheat the Ninja Foodi Grill on a medium-temperature setting.
3. Once it is preheated, open the lid and place the corn cob in the grill.
4. Cover the Ninja Foodi Grill's lid and grill on the "Grilling Mode" for 15 minutes while rotating after every 5 minutes.
5. Grill the corn cobs in batches.
6. Serve warm.
- **Nutrition Info:** Calories 148, Total Fat 22.4 g, Saturated Fat 10.1 g, Cholesterol 320 mg, Sodium 350 mg, Total Carbs 32.2 g, Fiber 0.7 g, Sugar 0.7 g, Protein 4.3 g

397.Veggie Egg Rolls

Servings: 4
Cooking Time: 5 Mins
Ingredients:
- 1 diced eggplant
- ½ tomato chopped
- Vegetable oil for air frying
- Egg roll wrappers (pre-packaged)
- Juice of 1 lime
- 1 tbsp garlic powder
- 2 tbsp fresh chopped spinach
- ¼ cup diced red onion
- Salt and pepper to taste

Directions:
1. Place your Ninja Foodi crisper basket in the unit and close the hood. Choose AIR FRY. Select START/STOP to start your pre-heating.
2. Cook the eggplant for a few minutes in a hot skillet
3. Mash the warm eggplant in a bowl, then the rest of your ingredients and mix.
4. Spoon of the mixture into the center of each egg roll wrapper and roll according to directions.
5. Lightly coat in vegetable oil.
6. Place a small batch in the air fryer and cook for 2-3 mins until golden brown, shaking the basket for an even crisp.
7. Serve with a dip of your choice.
- **Nutrition Info:** Calories: 186 Fat: 12g Saturated Fat: 5g Trans Fat: 0g Carbohydrates: 16g Fiber: 4g Sodium: 78mg Protein: 2g

398.Crispy Rosemary Potatoes

Servings: 4
Cooking Time: 20-25 Minutes

Ingredients:
- 2 pounds baby red potatoes, quartered
- 2 tablespoons extra virgin olive oil
- 1/4 cup dried onion flakes
- 1/2 teaspoon onion powder
- 1/2 teaspoon garlic powder
- 1/4 teaspoon celery powder
- 1/4 teaspoon freshly ground black pepper
- 1/2 teaspoon dried parsley
- 1/2 teaspoon salt

Directions:
1. Take a large bowl and add all listed ingredients, toss well and coat them well
2. Preheat Ninja Foodi by squeezing the "AIR CRISP" alternative and setting it to "390 Degrees F" and clock to 20 minutes
3. Let it preheat until you hear a beep
4. Once preheated, add potatoes to the cooking basket
5. Lock and cook for 10 minutes, making sure to shake the basket and cook for 10 minutes more
6. Once done, check the crispiness, if it's alright, serve away.
7. If not, cook for 5 minutes more
8. Enjoy!

399.Crock Pot Margarita Chicken Dip

Servings: 12
Cooking Time: 1 Hr 10 Min
Ingredients:
- 12 - oz cream cheese, softened
- 1½ cups chicken, cooked and shredded
- 2½ cups Monterrey Jack cheese, shredded
- ¼ cup tequila
- ¼ cup lime juice
- 1 - tbsp lime zest
- 2 - tbsp fresh orange juice
- 1 - tsp kosher salt
- 1 - tsp cu MIN
- 2 - cloves garlic, Minced
- A small container of Pico de Gallo

Directions:
1. Cut the cream cheddar into little shapes and layer over the bottom of a medium-sized stewing pot.
2. Spread the destroyed chook over top of the cream cheddar and unfold with destroyed cheddar. Add the relaxation of the fixings to the sluggish cooker.
3. Turn the simmering pot on high, unfold, and heat for approximately an hour or till the plunge is warmed via. Mix the plunge some instances as its miles warfare Ming up to mix the fixings and protect the base from cooking.
4. Serve heat with tortilla chips and pinnacle with Pico de Gallo.

- **Nutrition Info:** Calories 186, fat 3g, carbohydrate 17g, Protein 24g.

400.Honey Glazed Bratwurst

Servings: 4
Cooking Time: 10 Minutes
Ingredients:
- 4 bratwurst links, uncooked
- 1/4 cup Dijon mustard
- 4 brat buns, split
- 2 tablespoons mayonnaise
- 1 teaspoon steak sauce
- 1/4 cup honey

Directions:
1. First, mix the mustard with steak sauce and mayonnaise in a bowl.
2. Prepare and preheat the Ninja Foodi Grill on a High-temperature setting.
3. Once it is preheated, open the lid and place the bratwurst on the grill.
4. Cover the Ninja Foodi Grill's lid and grill on the "Grilling Mode" for 10 minutes per side until their internal temperature reaches 320 degrees F.
5. Serve with buns and mustard sauce on top.
- **Nutrition Info:** Calories 213, Total Fat 14 g, Saturated Fat 8 g, Cholesterol 81 mg, Sodium 162 mg, Total Carbs 53 g, Fiber 0.7 g, Sugar 19 g, Protein 12 g

401.Bacon & Sausages

Servings: 4
Cooking Time: 20 Minutes
Ingredients:
- 4 sausages
- 8 bacon slices

Directions:
1. Add crisper plate to the air fryer basket inside the Ninja Foodi Grill.
2. Press air fry setting.
3. Preheat at 360 degrees F for 3 minutes.
4. Wrap 2 bacon slices around each sausage.
5. Add these to the crisper plate.
6. Cook for 10 minutes per side.

402.Chocolate Chip Cookie

Servings: 6
Cooking Time: 12 Minutes
Ingredients:
- 1/2 cup butter, softened
- 1/2 cup sugar
- 1/2 cup brown sugar
- 1 egg
- 1 tsp vanilla
- 1/2 tsp baking soda
- 1/4 tsp salt
- 1 1/2 cups flour, preferably all-purpose
- 1 cup of chocolate chips

Directions:

1. Grease the Ninja baking pan with cooking spray.
2. Beat butter with sugar and brown sugar in a mixing bowl.
3. Stir in vanilla, egg, salt, flour, and baking soda, then mix well.
4. Fold in chocolate chips then knead this dough a bit.
5. Spread the dough in the prepared baking pan evenly.
6. Transfer this pan to the Ninja oven and Close its lid.
7. Rotate the Ninja Foodi dial to select the "Bake" mode.
8. Press the Time button and again use the dial to set the cooking time to 12 minutes.
9. Now press the Temp button and rotate the dial to set the temperature at 400 degrees F.
10. Serve oven fresh.
- **Nutrition Info:** Calories 253 ; Fat 8.9 g ; Carbs 24.7 g ; Fiber 1.2 g ;Sugar 11.3 g ; Protein 5.3 g

403.Fried Garlic Pickles

Servings: 6
Cooking Time: 15 Minutes
Ingredients:
- 1/4 cup all-purpose flour
- Pinch baking powder
- 2 tablespoons water
- Salt to taste
- 20 dill pickle slices
- 2 tablespoons cornstarch
- 1 1/2 cups panko bread crumbs
- 2 teaspoons garlic powder
- 2 tablespoons canola oil

Directions:
1. In a bowl, combine flour, baking powder, water and salt.
2. Add more water if batter is too thick.
3. Put the cornstarch in a second bowl, and mix breadcrumbs and garlic powder in a third bowl.
4. Dip pickles in cornstarch, then in the batter and finally dredge with breadcrumb mixture.
5. Add crisper plate to the air fryer basket inside the Ninja Foodi Grill.
6. Press air fry setting.
7. Set it to 360 degrees F for 3 minutes.
8. Press start to preheat.
9. Add pickles to the crisper plate.
10. Brush with oil.
11. Air fry for 10 minutes.
12. Flip, brush with oil and cook for another 5 minutes.

404.Corn Fritters

Servings: 6
Cooking Time: 8 Minutes

Ingredients:
- ½ cup all-purpose flour
- 1 ½ cup corn kernels
- 1 teaspoon sugar
- ¼ cup milk
- 1 egg, beaten
- 2 stalks green onion, chopped
- ½ cup cheddar cheese, shredded
- Salt and pepper to taste
- Cooking spray

Directions:
1. Combine all the ingredients in a bowl.
2. Drop 2 to 3 tablespoons of the mixture onto the air crisp tray.
3. Spray with oil.
4. Select air crisp function.
5. Air fry at 350 degrees F for 3 minutes.
6. Flip and air fry for another 5 minutes.

405.Zucchini Strips With Marinara Dip

Servings: 8
Cooking Time: 30 Minutes
Ingredients:
- 2 zucchinis, sliced into strips
- Salt to taste
- 1 1/2 cups all-purpose flour
- 2 eggs, beaten
- 2 cups bread crumbs
- 2 teaspoons onion powder
- 1 tablespoon garlic powder
- 1/4 cup Parmesan cheese, grated
- 1/2 cup marinara sauce

Directions:
1. Season zucchini with salt.
2. Let sit for 15 minutes.
3. Pat dry with paper towels.
4. Add flour to a bowl.
5. Add eggs to another bowl.
6. Mix remaining ingredients except marinara sauce in a third bowl.
7. Dip zucchini strips in the first, second and third bowls.
8. Cover with foil and freeze for 45 minutes.
9. Add crisper plate to the air fryer basket inside the Ninja Foodi Grill.
10. Select air fry function.
11. Preheat to 360 degrees F for 3 minutes.
12. Add zucchini strips to the crisper plate.
13. Air fry for 20 minutes.
14. Flip and cook for another 10 minutes.
15. Serve with marinara dip.

406.Barbeque Chicken Egg Rolls

Servings: 6
Cooking Time: 5 Mins
Ingredients:
- 1 diced onion
- Vegetable oil for air frying
- 1 cup barbeque sauce

- ½ cup fresh spinach, finely chopped
- 1 chopped bell pepper
- Egg roll wrappers (pre-packed)
- 2 cups of cubed cooked chicken
- 1 cup sweetcorn
- 2 cups shredded cheese (any melting kind will do)
- ½ tsp salt
- ¼ tsp pepper

Directions:
1. Mix the chicken in the barbeque sauce until fully saturated. Leave to settle for an hour in the fridge.
2. Place your Ninja Foodi crisper basket in the unit and close the hood. Choose AIR FRY. Select START/STOP to start your pre-heating.
3. Combine herbs, vegetables, and chicken in a bowl. Add the rest of the ingredients and mix thoroughly.
4. Spoon two tbsp of mixture into the center of each egg roll wrapper and roll according to directions.
5. Lightly coat in vegetable oil.
6. Place a small batch in the air fryer and cook for 1-2 mins until golden brown, shaking the basket for an even crisp.
7. Serve with a dip of your choice.
- **Nutrition Info:** Calories: 130 Fat: 8g Saturated Fat: 3g Trans Fat: 0g Carbohydrates: 9g Fiber: 1g Sodium: 243mg Protein: 6g

407.Garlic Parmesan Fries

Servings: 4
Cooking Time: 20 Minutes
Ingredients:
- 3 potatoes, sliced into sticks
- 2 tablespoons vegetable oil, divided
- 1/4 cup Parmesan cheese, grated
- 2 cloves garlic, minced
- 1 teaspoon garlic powder
- Salt to taste

Directions:
1. Coat potato strips with half of oil.
2. Add crisper plate to the air fryer basket inside the Ninja Foodi Grill.
3. Select air fry function.
4. Preheat at 360 degrees F for 3 minutes.
5. Add fries to the crisper plate
6. Cook for 12 minutes.
7. Flip and cook for another 5 minutes.
8. Combine remaining ingredients in a bowl.
9. Toss fries in the mixture and serve.

408.Crispy Cheddar Onion Rings

Servings: 12
Cooking Time: 15 Mins
Ingredients:

- 4 cups breadcrumbs
- 4 large onions
- 4 medium eggs
- 2 tsp chili powder
- 2 ½ cup flour
- Vegetable oil to coat for air frying
- 2 cup grated cheddar
- 2 tsp of baking powder

Directions:
1. Place your Ninja Foodi crisper basket in the unit and close the hood. Choose AIR FRY. Select START/STOP to start your pre-heating.
2. Slice onions into rings
3. Put the flour and baking powder in one bowl, the whisked eggs in another, and the breadcrumbs and seasoning in a third.
4. Dip your onion slices in each bowl, starting with the eggs.
5. Lightly coat in vegetable oil
6. Place a few of the rings in the crisper basket and allow to cook for 2-3 mins until golden brown. Keep shaking the basket to enjoy an even crisp.
7. Serve immediately with dipping sauce
- **Nutrition Info:** Calories: 270 Fat: 4g Saturated Fat: 3g Trans Fat: 0g Carbohydrates: 42g Fiber: 2g Sodium: 311mg Protein: 11g

409.Chicken Bowls

Servings: 4
Cooking Time: 20 Minutes
Ingredients:
- 8 eggs, whisked
- 1 pound chicken breast, skinless, boneless and cut into strips
- 1 tablespoon olive oil
- 1 yellow onion, chopped
- 1 teaspoon chili powder
- 1 cup baby spinach
- 1 tablespoon parsley, chopped
- 2 tablespoons chives, chopped
- Salt and black pepper to the taste

Directions:
1. Heat up your air fryer with the oil at 360 degrees f, add the meat and onion and cook for 5 minutes.
2. Add the eggs mixed with the other ingredients, toss gently, cook for 15 minutes more, divide everything into bowls and serve for breakfast.
- **Nutrition Info:** calories 251, fat 8, fiber 4, carbs 15, protein 4

410.Air-fried Grilled Cheese

Servings: 2 Sandwiches
Cooking Time: 10 Mins Per Sandwich
Ingredients:

- 4 slices of bread
- 1 tbsp butter or your favorite light cooking spray
- An ounce and a half of your favorite melting cheese

Directions:
1. Place your Ninja Foodi crisper basket in the unit and close the hood. Choose AIR FRY. Select START/STOP to start your pre-heating.
2. Place the cheese on the bread and then butter the outside. Use toothpicks to keep it all together.
3. Air fry at 360 degrees for 3-5 mins.
4. Flip the sandwich, increase heat, and fry for longer to taste. Keep shaking the basket to enjoy an even crisp.
5. Allow cooling before serving. Don't forget to take out the toothpicks!
- **Nutrition Info:** Calories: 415 Fat: 22g Saturated Fat: 17g Trans Fat: 0g Carbohydrates: 27g Fiber: 1g Sodium: 1095mg Protein: 12g

411.Peanut Butter & Banana Snacks

Servings: 4
Cooking Time: 10 Minutes
Ingredients:
- 1 cup peanut butter
- 8 slices whole wheat bread
- 1 cup jam
- 2 bananas, sliced
- 2 teaspoons ground cinnamon
- 1/4 cup white sugar
- Cooking spray

Directions:
1. Spread peanut butter on 4 bread slices.
2. Spread jam on the remaining bread slices.
3. Add bananas and make 4 sandwiches.
4. In a bowl, mix cinnamon and sugar.
5. Select air fry function in your Ninja Foodi Grill.
6. Set it to 390 degrees F for 3 minutes.
7. Add crisper plate to the air fryer basket.
8. Spray sandwiches with oil and sprinkle with cinnamon mixture.
9. Air fry sandwiches for 6 minutes.
10. Flip and cook for 3 more minutes.

412.Grilled Eggplant

Servings: 4
Cooking Time: 10 Minutes
Ingredients:
- 2 small eggplants, half-inch slices
- 3 teaspoons Cajun seasoning
- 2 tablespoons lime juice
- 1/4 cup olive oil

Directions:

1. Liberally season the eggplant slices with oil, lemon juice, and Cajun seasoning.
2. Prepare and preheat the Ninja Foodi Grill on the medium temperature setting.
3. Once it is preheated, open the lid and place the eggplant slices in the grill.
4. Cover the Ninja Foodi Grill's lid and grill on the "Grilling Mode" for 5 minutes per side.
5. Serve.
- **Nutrition Info:** Calories 372, Total Fat 11.1 g, Saturated Fat 5.8 g, Cholesterol 610 mg, Sodium 749 mg, Total Carbs 16.9 g, Fiber 0.2 g, Sugar 0.2 g, Protein 13.5 g

413.Ninja Foodi Meatballs

Servings: 36
Cooking Time:45 Min
Ingredients:
- 8 - medium fresh shiitake mushrooms Minced
- 1 - medium shallot Minced
- ¾ - cup Minced sweet potato
- 2 - Tbsp Minced cilantro
- 2 - pounds ground beef
- 1½ - Tbsp Red Boat fish sauce
- 2 - Tbsp tomato paste
- Mushroom Powder
- Freshly-ground black pepper
- 2 - Tbsp melted fat

Directions:
1. Line two rimmed preparing sheets with material paper or foil, and preheat the stove to 375°F. Meanwhile, finely mince the mushrooms, shallot, yam, and cilantro.
2. In an enormous bowl, join the ground meat, fish sauce, tomato glue, and the Minced veggies and herbs. Sprinkle on Magic Mushroom Powder and pepper. In case you're uncertain of how much flavoring to utilize, start with ½ teaspoons Magic Mushroom Powder and a couple of drudgeries of newly ground dark pepper. Altogether consolidate the fixings yet don't exhaust the meat.
3. To check if your flavoring is right, structure, and fry a MIN patty. Chow it down and alter the meatball blend for extra salt and pepper if necessary.
4. Scoop out uniform balls with medium dishes and turn out three dozen meatballs. Every meatball ought to be about 1½ crawl in breadth.
5. Gap the meatballs onto the two lined heating sheets. Prepare every plate of meatballs for 15 to 20MIN, pivoting the plate at the midpoint to guarantee in any event, cooking.
6. Plate and serve promptly, or store in a water/air proof holder in the ice chest for as long as three days. You can likewise

freeze the concocted meatballs for a half year. Basically freeze them in a solitary layer and afterward place the strong spheres in a cooler pack or fixed compartment.
- **Nutrition Info:** Calories: 69 Carbohydrates: 1g Protein: 5g Fat: 5g Fiber: 1g

414.Brownie Bars

Servings: 8
Cooking Time: 28 Minutes
Ingredients:
- Brownie:
- 1/2 cup butter, cubed
- 1-oz. unsweetened chocolate
- 2 large eggs, beaten
- 1 tsp vanilla extract
- 1 cup of sugar
- 1 cup flour, preferably all-purpose
- 1 tsp baking powder
- 1 cup walnuts, chopped
- Filling:
- 6 oz. cream cheese softened
- 1/2 cup sugar
- 1/4 cup butter, softened
- 2 tbsp all-purpose flour
- 1 large egg, beaten
- 1/2 tsp vanilla extract
- Topping:
- 1 cup (6 oz.) chocolate chips
- 1 cup walnuts, chopped
- 2 cups mini marshmallows
- Frosting:
- 1/4 cup butter
- 1/4 cup milk
- 2 oz. cream cheese
- 1-oz. unsweetened chocolate
- 3 cups confectioners' sugar
- 1 tsp vanilla extract

Directions:
1. In a small bowl, add and whisk all the ingredients for filling until smooth.
2. Melt butter with chocolate in a large saucepan over medium heat.
3. Mix well, then remove the melted chocolate from the heat.
4. Now stir in vanilla, eggs, baking powder, flour, sugar, and nuts then mix well.
5. Spread this chocolate batter in the Ninja baking pan.
6. Drizzle nuts, marshmallows, and chocolate chips over the batter.
7. Place this baking pan in the Ninja oven and Close its lid.
8. Rotate the Ninja Foodi dial to select the "Air Fry" mode.
9. Press the Time button and again use the dial to set the cooking time to 28 minutes.

10. Now press the Temp button and rotate the dial to set the temperature at 350 degrees F.
11. Meanwhile, prepare the frosting by heating butter with cream cheese, chocolate and milk in a saucepan over medium heat.
12. Mix well, then remove it from the heat.
13. Stir in vanilla and sugar, then mix well.
14. Pour this frosting over the brownie.
15. Allow the brownie to cool then slice into bars.
16. Serve.
- **Nutrition Info:** Calories 271 ; Fat 15 g ; Carbs 33 g ; Fiber 1 g ; Sugar 26 g ; Protein 4 g

415.Lemon-garlic Shrimp Caesar Salad

Servings: 4
Cooking Time: 5 Minutes
Ingredients:
- 1-pound fresh jumbo shrimp
- 2 heads romaine lettuce, chopped
- 3/4 cup Caesar dressing
- 1/2 cup parmesan cheese, grated
- 1/2 lemon juice
- 3 garlic cloves, minced
- Sea salt
- Black pepper, grounded

Directions:
1. Besides, the flame broils mesh and closes the hood. Preheat Ninja Foodi by pressing the "GRILL" option at and setting it to "MAX" and timer to 5 minutes
2. Take a large bowl; toss the shrimp with the lemon juice, garlic, salt, and pepper
3. Let it marinate while the grill is preheating
4. Once it preheats until you hear a beep
5. Arrange the shrimp over the grill grate lock lid and cook for 5 minutes
6. Toss the romaine lettuce with the Caesar dressing
7. Once cooked completely, remove the shrimp from the grill
8. Sprinkle with parmesan cheese
9. Serve and enjoy!

416.Sweet Potato Wedges

Servings: 4
Cooking Time: 20 Minutes
Ingredients:
- 2 sweet potatoes, sliced into wedges
- 1 tablespoon vegetable oil
- 1 teaspoon smoked paprika
- 1 tablespoon honey
- Salt and pepper to taste

Directions:

1. Add air fryer basket to your Ninja Foodi Grill.
2. Choose air fry setting.
3. Preheat at 390 degrees for 25 minutes.
4. Add sweet potato wedges to the basket.
5. Cook for 10 minutes.
6. Stir and cook for another 10 minutes.
7. Toss in paprika and honey.
8. Sprinkle with salt and pepper.

417.Homemade Fries

Servings: 6
Cooking Time: 45 Minutes
Ingredients:
- 1 lb. large potatoes, sliced into strips
- 2 tablespoons vegetable oil
- Salt to taste

Directions:
1. Toss potato strips in oil.
2. Add crisper plate to the air fryer basket inside the Ninja Foodi Grill.
3. Choose air fry function. Set it to 390 degrees F for 3 minutes.
4. Press start to preheat.
5. Add potato strips to the crisper plate.
6. Cook for 25 minutes.
7. Stir and cook for another 20 minutes.

418.Healthy Onion Rings

Servings: 4
Cooking Time: 10 Minutes
Ingredients:
- 1/4 teaspoon salt
- 1 egg
- 3/4 cup milk
- 1 tablespoon baking powder
- 3/4 cup breadcrumbs
- 1 large onion
- 1 cup flour
- 1 teaspoon paprika

Directions:
1. Preheat Ninja Foodi by squeezing the "AIR CRISP" alternative and setting it to "340 Degrees F" and timer to 10 minutes
2. Let it preheat until you hear a beep
3. Take a bowl and whisk the egg, milk, salt, flour, paprika together
4. Slice the onion and separate into rings
5. Grease your Ninja Foodi Grill with cooking spray
6. Then dip the onion rings into batter and coat with breadcrumbs
7. Arrange them in Ninja Foodi Grill Cooking Basket
8. Cook for 10 minutes
9. Serve and enjoy!

DESSERTS RECIPES

419.Apple, Cream And Hazelnut Crumble

Servings: Up To 6 People
Cooking Time: 15 - 30
Ingredients:
- golden apples: 6
- water: 150 ml
- brown sugar: 75 gr
- sugar: 75 gr
- cinnamon: 1
- fresh cream: 300 ml
- chopped hazelnuts: q.b.

Directions:
1. In a bowl mix the peeled and diced apples, brown sugar, regular sugar and cinnamon.
2. Insert the mixing shovel into the bowl.
3. Pour the apples inside, add water, close the lid, select BAKE program, set 20min and press program start/stop key.
4. The cooking time may vary depending on the type of apple used and the size of the pieces. At the end, divide the apples into serving glasses, cover with the previously whipped cream and sprinkle with the hazelnut grain.

420.Simple Strawberry Cobbler

Servings: 4
Cooking Time: 25 Minutes
Ingredients:
- Heavy whipping cream, ¼ cup
- Cornstarch, 1 ½ tsp.
- White sugar, ¼ cup
- Water, ½ cup
- Salt, ¼ tsp.
- Butter, 2 tsp.
- Hulled strawberries, 1 ½ cup
- White sugar, 1 ½ tsp.
- Diced butter, 1 tbsp.
- Butter, 1 tbsp.
- All-purpose flour, ½ cup
- Baking powder, ¾ tsp.

Directions:
1. Lightly grease the baking pan of the air fryer with cooking spray. Add water, cornstarch, and sugar. Cook for 10 minutes 390 ºF or until hot and thick. Add strawberries and mix well. Dot the top with 1 tablespoon butter.
2. In a bowl, mix well salt, baking powder, sugar, and flour. Cut in 1 tablespoon and 2 teaspoons butter. Mix in cream. Spoon on top of berries.
3. Cook for 15 minutes at 390°F, until the top is lightly browned.
4. Serve and enjoy.

- **Nutrition Info:** Calories: 255; Protein: 2.4 g; Fat: 13.0 g; Carbs: 32.0 g

421.Glazed Carrots

Servings:8
Cooking Time: 15 Minutes
Ingredients:
- ¼ cup of butter
- ¼ cup of packed brown sugar
- 2 pounds of carrots, should be peeled and cut into steaks
- ¼ teaspoon of salt
- 1/8 teaspoon of ground white pepper

Directions:
1. Place the carrots into a large saucepan, pour water to reach 1-inch depth, and bring to a boil. Reduce the heat to low, cover, and simmer the carrots until they become tender in about 8-10 minutes. Drain and transfer to a neat bowl.
2. Melt butter in the same saucepan, stir salt, brown sugar, and white pepper into the butter until the salt and sugar have dissolved. Transfer the carrots into brown sugar sauce; cook and keep stirring until the carrots are glazed with the sauce in about 5 minutes.

- **Nutrition Info:** Calories 123.6, Carbohydrates 17.6 grams 6% DV, Protein 1.1 grams 2% DV, Fat 6 grams 9% DV, Cholesterol 15.3 mg 5% DV, Sodium 193.8 mg 8% DV

422.Original French Pineapple Toast

Servings: 4
Cooking Time: 16 Minutes
Ingredients:
- 10 bread slices
- ¼ cup of sugar
- ¼ cup milk
- 3 large whole eggs
- 1 cup of coconut milk
- 10 slices pineapple, peeled
- ½ cup coconut flakes
- Cooking spray as needed

Directions:
1. Take a mixing bowl and whisk in coconut milk, sugar, eggs, milk and stir well
2. Dup breads in the mixture and keep the mon the side for 2 minutes
3. Preheat Ninja Foodi by pressing the "GRILL" option and setting it to "MED" and timer to 16 minutes
4. Let it preheat until you hear a beep
5. Arrange bread slices over the grill grate, lock lid, and cook for 2 minutes. Flip and cook for 2 minutes more, let them cook until the timer reads 0

6. Repeat with remaining slices, serve, and enjoy!

423.Ninja Foodi Grilled-banana Splits

Servings: 4
Cooking Time: 9 Min
Ingredients:
- 4 - bananas
- 4 - tbsp. butter
- 1 - pt. vanilla ice cream
- ½ c. chocolate syrup
- 1 - Butterfinger or Heath candy bar
- whipped cream

Directions:
1. Preheat Ninja Foodi oven broil. Brush cut sides of bananas with liquefied spread, at that point, laid them on hot Ninja Foodi oven broil grind. Cook over medium-high warmth until bananas are brilliant earthy colored and Ninja Foodi oven broil marks appear, about 2MIN. Turn, skin side down; barbecue until delicate, 2MIN more.
2. To gather the parfaits, remove the bananas from their skins and mastermind two parts in every one of 4 dishes. Scoop some dessert into each bowl. Shower with chocolate sauce and sprinkle with hacked treats. Enhancement with whipped cream, on the off chance that you wish.
- **Nutrition Info:** Calories 155, fat 3g, carbohydrate 34g, Protein 2g.

424.Coffee Flavored Doughnuts

Servings: 6
Cooking Time: 6 Minutes
Ingredients:
- Baking powder 1 tsp.
- Salt ½ tsp.
- Sunflower oil 1 tbsp.
- Coffee ¼ cup
- Coconut sugar ¼ cup
- White all-purpose flour 1 cup
- Aquafaba 2 tbsp

Directions:
1. Combine sugar, flour, baking powder, salt in a mixing bowl.
2. In another bowl, combine the aquafaba, sunflower oil, and coffee.
3. Mix to form a dough.
4. Let the dough rest inside the fridge.
5. Preheat the air fryer to 400°F.
6. Knead the dough and create doughnuts.
7. Arrange inside the air fryer in a single layer and cook for 6 minutes.
8. Do not shake so that the donut maintains its shape.
- **Nutrition Info:** Calories: 113; Protein: 2.16 g; Fat: 2.54 g; Carbs: 20.45 g

425.Grilled Angel Food Cake With Strawberries In Balsamic

Servings: 6
Cooking Time: 15 Min
Ingredients:
- 1½ lb. strawberries
- 2 - tbsp. balsamic vinegar
- 1 - tbsp. sugar
- 1 - store-bought angel food cake
- Whipped cream (optional)

Directions:
1. In a medium bowl, sling strawberries with balsamic vinegar and sugar. Let remain at room temperature until sugar breaks down, at any rate, 30MIN, mixing at times.
2. In the interim, get ready outside Ninja Foodi oven broil for direct barbecuing on medium. Cut light, fluffy cake into 6 wedges.
3. Spot cake on the hot Ninja Foodi oven broil rack and cook 3 to 4MIN or until daintily toasted on the two sides, turning over once. Spoon strawberries with their juice onto 6 sweet plates. Spot Ninja Foodi oven-broiled cake on plates with strawberries; present with whipped cream in the event that you like.
- **Nutrition Info:** Calories 150, fat 1g, carbohydrate 33g, Protein 3g.

426.Rois Crackers

Servings: Up To 8 People
Cooking Time: 30 - 45
Ingredients:
- Puff pastry: n.2
- Almond flour: 100g
- Egg: n.1
- Sugar: 75g
- Butter: 50g
- Almond flavor: n.1 vial
- Porcelain bean: n.1

Directions:
1. First prepare the filling:
2. Mix the flour, egg, sugar, butter at room temperature and almond extract in a bowl.
3. Remove the mixing paddle from the bowl.
4. Roll out a sheet of pastry with baking paper underneath the bowl; prick it with a fork and stuff with the filling; roll out well.
5. Place the bean inside, choosing an external position for the cake.
6. Cover with the second roll of pastry and seal the edges well; brush the surface with a yolk diluted with milk and make decorative incisions.
7. Close the cover, select BAKE program, power level 2, set 35min and press program start/stop button.

8. Tradition has it that whoever happens to have the object hidden in his piece of cake, is considered the king of the day.

427.French Brioches

Servings: Up To 4 People
Cooking Time: 15 - 30
Ingredients:
- frozen brioches: 4 pcs

Directions:
1. Remove the mixing shovel from the pot.
2. Place the brioches on top of the baking paper inside the pan.
3. Close the lid, select the BAKE program, set 30 minutes and press the START key.

428.Cheesy Cauliflower Steak

Servings: 4
Cooking Time: 30 Minutes
Ingredients:
- 1 tablespoon mustard
- 1 head cauliflower
- 1 teaspoon avocado mayonnaise
- ½ cup parmesan cheese, grated
- ¼ cup butter, cut into small pieces

Directions:
1. Set your Ninja Foodi to Sauté mode, and add butter and cauliflower.
2. Sauté for 3 minutes.
3. Add remaining ingredients and stir.
4. Lock the lid and cook on High pressure for 30 minutes.
5. Release pressure naturally over 10 minutes.
6. Serve and enjoy!
- **Nutrition Info:** Calories: 155 Fat: 13g Saturated Fat: 2 g Carbohydrates: 4 g Fiber: 2 g Sodium: 162 mg Protein: 6 g

429.The Original Pot-de-crème

Servings: 4
Cooking Time: 12 Minutes
Ingredients:
- 6 egg yolks
- 2 cups heavy whip cream
- 1/3 cup cocoa powder
- 1 tablespoon pure vanilla extract
- ½ teaspoon liquid stevia
- Whipped coconut cream as needed for garnish
- Shaved dark chocolate, for garnish

Directions:
1. Take a medium bowl and whisk in yolks, heavy cream, cocoa powder, vanilla, and stevia
2. Pour the mixture into 1 and ½ quart baking dish and place the dish in your multi-cooker insert
3. Add enough water to reach about halfway up the sides of the baking dish

4. Lock lid and cook on HIGH pressure for 12 minutes
5. Quick-release pressure once the cycle is complete
6. Remove the baking dish from the insert and let it cool
7. Chill the dessert in the refrigerator and serve with a garnish of whipped coconut cream and shaved dark chocolate
8. Enjoy!

430.Easter Tsoureki

Servings: Up To 8 People
Cooking Time: 30 - 45
Ingredients:
- flour 0: 500 gr
- fresh yeast: 20 gr
- milk: 125 ml
- eggs: 2
- sugar: 50 gr
- oranges: 2
- butter at room temperature: 75 gr
- mahlepi: 2 spoons
- warm water: 100 ml
- Red colored boiled eggs: 3

Directions:
1. Pour the flour into a bowl, form a hole in the center and add all the other ingredients (keep only the boiled eggs aside).
2. Knead well with your hands until you get a smooth and soft dough with which you will form a ball that you will leave to rise in a bowl sprinkled with flour on the bottom. Cover with a clean cloth and store in a warm place away from drafts.
3. In the meantime cook the eggs in water for 9 min from the moment of boiling and once cooled color them red following the instructions on the color pack.
4. Remove the stirrer blade from the tank.
5. After about 1 h of leavening take the dough and divide it into 3 pieces; roll each piece into a cylinder of about 45 cm and start to form a braid. Then join the ends to form a crown that will be placed inside the previously buttered tank.
6. Place the 3 cooled eggs on top of the crown and brush the dough with egg yolk.
7. Close the lid, select the BAKE program, power level 2, set 35min and press the program start/stop button.
8. After baking, cool the bread and serve with butter.

431.Jam Tart

Servings: Up To 10 People
Cooking Time: 45 -60
Ingredients:
- flour: 250 gr

- butter: 125 gr
- sugar: 110 gr
- eggs (1 whole and 1 yolk): 2
- salt: q.b.
- jam: 170gr

Directions:
1. Put in the mixer the flour, sugar, eggs, butter just removed from the refrigerator and cut into chunks and a pinch of salt.
2. Blend everything until the dough is compact and elastic enough. Put everything to rest in the refrigerator for at least half an hour.
3. Remove the mixer blade from the bowl.
4. Butter and flour the bottom well. Spread 2/3 of the shortcrust pastry at a thickness of 3-4 mm and place it in the bottom of the pot cutting out the edge carefully.
5. Punch the bottom of the pan with the tines of a fork and spread the jam over it, levelling it out with a spoon.
6. With the advanced dough create strips to be placed crossed over the jam.
7. Close the lid, select the program BAKE, set 50min and press the program start/stop button.
8. Once it has cooled well turn it into a dish and serve.

432.Lovely Rum Sundae

Servings: 4
Cooking Time: 8 Minutes
Ingredients:
- Vanilla ice cream for serving
- 1 pineapple, cored and sliced
- 1 teaspoon cinnamon, ground
- ½ cup brown sugar, packed
- ½ cup dark rum

Directions:
1. Take a large deep bowl and add sugar, cinnamon, and rum
2. Add the pineapple in the layer, dredge them properly and make sure that they are coated well
3. Pre-heat your Foodi in "GRILL" mode with "MAX" settings, setting the timer to 8 minutes
4. Once you hear the beep, strain any additional rum from the pineapple slices and transfer them to the grill rate of your appliance
5. Press them down and grill for 6- 8 minutes. Make sure to not overcrowd the grill grate, cook in batches if needed
6. Top each of the ring with a scoop of your favorite ice cream, sprinkle a bit of cinnamon on top
7. Enjoy!
- **Nutrition Info:** Calories: 240 Fat: 4 g Saturated Fat: 1 g Carbohydrates: 43 g Fiber: 8 g Sodium: 85 mg Protein: 2 g

433.Chocolate Chip Cookies

Servings: 12
Cooking Time: 15 Minutes
Ingredients:
- 15 oz. yellow cake mix
- ¼ cup butter, melted
- 2 eggs, beaten
- 1 cup chocolate chips

Directions:
1. Combine all the ingredients in a bowl.
2. Form cookies from the mixture.
3. Add the cookies to the air crisp tray.
4. Select bake function.
5. Bake at 330 degrees F for 15 minutes.

434.Cinnamon Apple Chips

Servings: 4
Cooking Time: 12 Minutes
Ingredients:
- 1 apple, sliced thinly
- 2 teaspoons vegetable oil
- 1 teaspoon ground cinnamon
- Cooking spray

Directions:
1. Coat the apples slices in oil and sprinkle with cinnamon.
2. Spray the air fryer basket with oil.
3. Choose air fry setting in the Ninja Foodi Grill.
4. Air fry the apples at 375 degrees F for 12 minutes, flipping once or twice.

435.A Fruit Salad To Die For

Servings: 4
Cooking Time: 4 Minutes
Ingredients:
- 2 peaches, pitted and sliced
- 1 can (9 ounces) pineapple chunks, drained, juice reserved
- ½ pound strawberries washed, hulled, and halved
- 1 tablespoon freshly squeezed lime juice
- 6 tablespoons honey, divided

Directions:
1. Add pineapple, peaches, strawberries, and ½ of honey, toss well
2. Preheat your Ninja Foodi by pressing the "GRILL" option and setting it to "MAX."
3. Set the timer to 4 minutes
4. Allow it to preheat until it beeps
5. Transfer fruits to Grill Grate and close the lid
6. Cook for 4 minutes
7. Add remaining 3 tablespoons of honey, lime juice, 1 tablespoon reserved pineapple juice into a small-sized bowl
8. Once cooked, place fruits in a large-sized bowl and toss with honey mixture
9. Serve and enjoy!

436.Peanut Butter Cups

Servings: 4
Cooking Time: 5 Minutes
Ingredients:
- 4 graham crackers
- 4 peanut butter cups
- 4 marshmallows

Directions:
1. Add crisper plate to the air fryer basket of your Ninja Foodi Grill.
2. Choose air fry function.
3. Preheat at 360 degrees F for 3 minutes.
4. Break the crackers in half.
5. Add crackers to the crisper plate.
6. Top with the peanut butter cups.
7. Cook for 2 minutes.
8. Sprinkle mushrooms on top and cook for another 1 minute.
9. Top with the remaining crackers and serve.

437.Cinnamon Bun

Servings: 8
Cooking Time: 15 Minutes
Ingredients:
- 1 cup almond flour
- ½ teaspoon baking powder
- 3 tablespoon Erythritol
- 2 tablespoon ground cinnamon
- ½ teaspoon vanilla extract
- 1 tablespoon butter
- 1 egg, whisked
- ¾ teaspoon salt
- ¼ cup almond milk

Directions:
1. Mix up together the almond flour, baking powder, vanilla extract, egg, salt, and almond milk.
2. Knead the soft and non-sticky dough.
3. Roll up the dough with the help of the rolling pin
4. Sprinkle dough with the butter, cinnamon, and Erythritol.
5. Roll the dough into the log.
6. Cut the roll into 7 pieces.
7. Spray multi-cooker basket with cooking spray.
8. Place the cinnamon buns in the basket and close the lid.
9. Set the Bake mode and cook the buns for 15 minutes at 355F
10. Check if the buns are cooked with the help of the toothpick.
11. Chill the buns well and serve!

438.Caramelized Pineapple Sundaes With Coconut

Servings: 10
Cooking Time: 30 Min
Ingredients:
- 1 - pineapple
- 2 tsp. vegetable oil
- ½ c. sweetened shredded coconut
- 2½ pt. fat-free vanilla frozen yogurt
- Mint sprigs

Directions:
1. Switch on Ninja Foodi broil. Brush the pineapple jewelry with the vegetable oil. Ninja Foodi oven broil over modestly high warm temperature, turning every so often till the pineapple is daintily roasted and mollified, approximately 8MIN. Move the jewelry to a work surface and reduce into reduced down portions.
2. In a medium skillet, toast the coconut over slight warmth until awesome, about 2MIN. Move to a plate to chill.
3. Scoop the yogurt into dessert glasses or bowls. Top with the Ninja Foodi oven-broiled pineapple, sprinkles with the coconut, adorn with the Mint twigs, and serve at once.
- **Nutrition Info:** Calories 214, fat 9g, carbohydrate 31g, Protein 3g.

439.Grilled Apple Pie

Servings: 8
Cooking Time: 30 Minutes
Ingredients:
- 8 cups cold water
- 1 tablespoon lemon juice
- 8 apples, diced
- 1/2 cup brown sugar
- 1/2 teaspoon ground cinnamon
- 1/2 teaspoon ground ginger
- 3 tablespoons all-purpose flour
- 1/2 cup applesauce
- 1 frozen pie crust

Directions:
1. In a bowl, mix water, lemon juice and apples.
2. Let sit for 10 minutes.
3. Drain and pat dry.
4. Add grill grate to Ninja Foodi Grill.
5. Press grill setting.
6. Set it to max and preheat for 8 minutes.
7. Coat apples with sugar.
8. Grill for 8 minutes without flipping.
9. In a bowl, combine the remaining ingredients.
10. Stir in grilled apples.
11. Pour the mixture into a small baking pan.
12. Top with the pie crust.
13. Select bake setting.
14. Cook pie at 350 degrees F for 20 minutes.

440.Oatmeal With Apples And Cinnamon

Servings: Up To 4 People
Cooking Time:x
Ingredients:

- Oat flakes: 100 gr.
- Water: 650ml
- Butter: 30 gr
- Walnuts: 20 gr.
- Sugar: 2 spoons
- Cinnamon: 1/2 teaspoon
- Apples: 2
- Honey: 1 tablespoon

Directions:
1. Peel the apples, cut them into cubes of about 0.7x0.7 mm; Cut the nuts into small pieces.
2. Remove the mixing shovel from the tank.
3. Grease the tub with butter and insert the apples, then sprinkle with cinnamon and sugar. Close the lid, select AIRGRILL program, power level 3, set 15 minutes and press program start/stop key.
4. At the end of cooking, pour the cereals and water into the tank. Close the lid, select the program BAKE, power level 4, set 15 minutes and press the program start/stop key.
5. At the end of cooking add butter, honey and sprinkle with walnuts.
6. The cooking time varies depending on the size of the flakes.

441.Sponge Cake

Servings: Up To 10 People
Cooking Time: 30 - 45
Ingredients:
- eggs: 6
- sugar: 190 gr
- flour 00: 150 gr
- potato starch: 75 gr
- vanillin: 2 gr

Directions:
1. In a bowl beat the eggs with sugar until frothy and puffy. At this point add the flour, starch and vanillin sieved and mix with a whisk until you get a homogeneous mixture, taking care not to dismantle it.
2. Remove the mixer blade from the bowl.
3. Butter and flour the bowl and pour the dough into the center, leveling it well.
4. Close the lid, select the program "BAKE", power level 2, set 40 minutes and press the START key.

442.Peanut Butter Banana Melties

Servings:4
Cooking Time: 15 Minutes
Ingredients:
- ½ cup of peanut butter
- ½ cup of chocolate chips
- 4 large bananas

Directions:

1. Without peeling the bananas, slice each of them vertically. Smear the inside of each of them with peanut butter and sprinkle with chocolate chips. Place the 2 halves back together and wrap each banana individually in aluminum foil.
2. Now cook in the hot coal of a campfire until the banana becomes hot, and the chocolate has melted in about 10-15 minutes (this depends on the level of heat from the coals).
- **Nutrition Info:** Calories 411.3, Carbohydrates 50.6 grams 16% DV, Protein 10.5 grams 21% DV, Fat 23 grams 35% DV, Sodium 151.7 mg 6% DV.

443.Strawberry Crumble

Servings: 5
Cooking Time: 2 Hours
Ingredients:
- 1 cup almond flour
- 2 tablespoons butter, melted
- 8-10 drops liquid Stevia
- 3-4 cups fresh strawberries, hulled and sliced
- 1 tablespoon butter, chopped

Directions:
1. Lightly, grease the pot of Ninja Foodi.
2. In a bowl, add the flour, melted butter, and Stevia and mix until a crumbly mixture form.
3. In the pot of the prepared Ninja Foodi, place the strawberry slices and dot with chopped butter.
4. Spread the flour mixture on top evenly.
5. Close the Ninja Foodi with the crisping lid and select Slow Cooker.
6. Set on Low for 2 hours.
7. Press Start/Stop to begin cooking.
8. Place the pan onto a wire rack to cool slightly.
- **Nutrition Info:** Calories: 233 g Fats: 19.2 g Net Carbs: 6.6 g Carbs: 10.7 g Fiber: 4.1 g Sugar: 5 g Proteins: 0.7 g Sodium: 50 mg

444.Blackberry Cake

Servings: 4
Cooking Time: 20 Minutes
Ingredients:
- 4 tablespoons butter
- 3 tablespoon Erythritol
- 1 oz blackberries
- 1 cup almond flour
- ½ teaspoon baking powder

Directions:
1. Combine all the liquid ingredients.
2. Then add baking powder, almond flour, and Erythritol.
3. Stir the mixture until smooth.
4. Add blackberries and stir the batter gently with the help of the spoon.

5. Take the non-stick springform pan and transfer the batter inside.
6. Place the springform pan in the pot and lower the air fryer lid.
7. Cook the cake for 20 minutes at 365 F.
8. Chill it little and serve!

445.Baked Apples

Servings: 4
Cooking Time: 45 Minutes
Ingredients:
- 2 apples, sliced in half
- 1 tablespoon lemon juice
- 4 teaspoons brown sugar
- ¼ cup butter, sliced into small cubes

Directions:
1. Add the crisper plate to the air fryer basket inside the Ninja Foodi Grill.
2. Choose the Air Fry function.
3. Preheat it to 325°F for 3 minutes.
4. Add apples to the crisper plate.
5. Drizzle with lemon juice and sprinkle with brown sugar.
6. Place butter cubes on top.
7. Air fry for 45 minutes.
8. serving Suggestionss: Top with caramel syrup or crushed graham crackers.
9. preparation/Cooking Tips: Poke apples with a fork before cooking.
- **Nutrition Info:** Calories: 234 Fat: 17 g Carbohydrates: 4 g Protein: 21 g

446.Foil Pack Chocolate Marshmallow Banana

Servings: 1
Cooking Time: 10 Min
Ingredients:
- 1 - banana
- 1 - handful chocolate chips
- 1 - handful MIN marshmallows

Directions:
1. Tear a square bit of foil that is round 12-inch with the aid of 12-inch.
2. Spot stripped banana on foil and reduce it longwise approximately ¾ of the course through. Spread it separated and load up with marshmallows and chocolate chips. Firmly enclose banana by way of foil.
3. At the factor whilst organized to prepare dinner, place wrapped banana on hot Ninja Foodi oven broil or over the hearth for approximately 5MIN.
4. Take out from the barbecue, open up, and respect!
- **Nutrition Info:** Calories 228, fat 12g, carbohydrate 31g, Protein 5g.

447.Poached Pears

Servings:4

Cooking Time: 45 Minutes
Ingredients:
- 1 cup of orange juice
- 4 slices of orange
- 1 teaspoon of vanilla extract
- ½ (750 milliliters) bottle of champagne
- 1 cup of white sugar
- 2/3 cup of semisweet chocolate chips
- 4 eaches of whole cloves
- 4 medium pear (approximately 2-1/2 per lbs.) pears, to be peeled but the stems intact.

Directions:
1. Get a saucepan and place on medium heat, then combine orange juice, champagne, and sugar inside. Add cloves, orange slices, and vanilla. Then, let it get to a boil and stir until the sugar is dissolved. Place pears inside the saucepan and reduce the heat. Cover it up and allow it to simmer for approximately 15 minutes. Then, the next thing is to remove the cover and let it simmer for an extra 30 minutes, remove the pears from the liquid, and cool down.
2. Heat the chocolate in a bowl over hot water and keep stirring until it completely melts. Then pour the chocolate over the pears and serve.
- **Nutrition Info:** calories 542.2, Carbohydrates 104.7 grams 34% DV, Protein 2.5 grams 5% DV, Fat 8.8 grams 14% DV, Sodium 12.8 mg 1% DV.

448.Fried Oreos

Servings: 8
Cooking Time: 5 Minutes
Ingredients:
- 8 oz. crescent rolls (refrigerated)
- 16 Oreos
- 3 tablespoons peanut butter

Directions:
1. Spread dough onto a working surface.
2. Slice into 8 rectangles.
3. Slice each rectangle into 2.
4. Add cookie on top of the dough.
5. Spread with peanut butter.
6. Wrap the dough around the Oreos.
7. Place these in the air fryer basket inside the Ninja Foodi Grill.
8. Choose air fry setting.
9. Air fry at 320 degrees F for 5 minutes.

449.Butter Cake

Servings: 6
Cooking Time: 12 Minutes
Ingredients:
- 14 oz. cookie butter
- 3 eggs, beaten
- ¼ cup granulated sugar
- Cooking spray

Directions:

1. Microwave cookie butter for 90 seconds, stirring every 30 seconds.
2. In a bowl, add the cookie butter, eggs and sugar.
3. Spray a small baking pan with oil.
4. Pour the batter onto the baking pan.
5. Air fry at 320 degrees F for 10 minutes.

450.Cauliflower Steaks — Roasted

Servings:4
Cooking Time: 30 Minutes
Ingredients:

- 1 pinch of red pepper flakes
- 2 cloves of garlic, minced
- 1 pinch of salt and ground black pepper
- 1 tbsp. of lemon juice (fresh)
- 1 cauliflower (large head), sliced vertically into four.
- ¼ cup of olive oil

Directions:

1. Preheat the oven to 400 ºF (200 ºC). Get a parchment paper to line your baking sheet.
2. Next is to put cauliflower steaks on the already prepared sheet.
3. Whisk lemon juice, olive oil, red pepper flakes, garlic, black pepper, and salt inside a small bowl. Then, apply about half quantity of the olive oil you've already mixed on the cauliflower steaks.
4. Then, in the already preheated oven, you will need to put the cauliflower steaks and roast it for about 15 minutes. Each steak should be turn to the other side and you will then apply the leftover olive oil on it as you did earlier. You will need to roast for about 15-20 minutes when the steaks would become tender with golden color.
- **Nutrition Info:** calories 175.8, Carbohydrates 12.1 grams 4% DV, Protein 4.3 grams 9% DV, Fat 13.8 grams 21% DV, Sodium 63.6 mg 3% DV.

451.Warm Glazed Up Carrots

Servings: 4
Cooking Time: 5 Minutes
Ingredients:

- 2 pounds carrots
- Pepper as needed
- 1 cup of water
- 1 tablespoon coconut butter

Directions:

1. Wash carrots thoroughly and peel then, slice the carrots.
2. Add carrots, water to the Ninja Foodi.
3. Lock pressure lid and cook for 4 minutes on High pressure.
4. Release pressure naturally.
5. Strain carrots and strain carrots.

6. Mix with coconut butter, enjoy with a bit of pepper.
- **Nutrition Info:** Calories: 228 Fat: 8 g Saturated Fat: 2 g Carbohydrates: 36 g Fiber: 2 g Sodium: 123 mg Protein: 4 g

452.Cashew Cream

Servings: 10
Cooking Time: 10 Minutes
Ingredients:

- 3 cups cashews
- 2 cups chicken stock
- 1 teaspoon salt
- 1 tablespoon butter
- 2 tablespoons ricotta cheese

Directions:

1. Combine the cashews with the chicken stock in the Multicooker.
2. Add salt and close the multicooker lid. Cook the dish on Pressure mode for 10 minutes.
3. Remove the cashews from the multicooker and drain the nuts from the water. Transfer the cashews to a blender and add the ricotta cheese and butter.
4. Blend the mixture until it is smooth. When you get the texture you want, remove it from a blender. Serve it immediately or keep the cashew butter in the refrigerator.
- **Nutrition Info:** Calories: 252 Fat: 20.6 g Carbs: 13.8 g Protein: 6.8 g

453.Ginger Cheesecake

Servings: 6
Cooking Time: 20 Minutes
Ingredients:

- Ground nutmeg ½ tsp.
- Soft cream cheese 16 oz.
- Rum 1 tsp.
- Crumbled ginger cookies ½ cup
- Vanilla extract ½ tsp.
- Melted butter 2 tsp.
- Eggs 2.
- Sugar ½ cup

Directions:

1. Grease a pan with butter and spread cookie crumbs on the bottom.
2. In a bowl, beat cream cheese, eggs, rum, vanilla, and nutmeg. Whisk well and spread over the cookie crumbs.
3. Place in the air fryer and cook at 340°F for 20 minutes.
4. Cool and keep in the refrigerator.
5. Slice and serve.
- **Nutrition Info:** Calories: 412; Fat: 12 g; Protein: 6 g; Carbs: 20 g

454.Marshmallow Banana Boat

Servings: 4
Cooking Time: 6 Minutes

Ingredients:
- ½ cup peanut butter chips
- 1/3 cup chocolate chips
- 1 cup mini marshmallow
- 4 ripe bananas

Directions:
1. Take the banana and slice them gently, keeping the peel
2. Make sure to not cut it all the way through
3. Use your hands to carefully peel the banana skin like a book, revealing the banana flesh
4. Divide your marshmallow, peanut butter, chocolate chips among the prepared bananas, stuff them well
5. Preheat your Grill in "MEDIUM" mode, with the timer set to 6 minutes
6. Once you hear a beep, transfer your prepared bananas to the grill grate, cook for 6 minutes until the chocolate melts well
7. Serve and enjoy!

455.The Healthy Granola Bites

Servings: 4
Cooking Time: 15-20 Minutes
Ingredients:
- Salt and pepper to taste
- 1 tablespoon coriander
- A handful of thyme, diced
- ¼ cup of coconut milk
- 3 handful of cooked vegetables, your choice
- 3-ounce plain granola

Directions:
1. Preheat your Ninja Foodi to 352°F in Air Crisp mode, set a timer to 20 minutes.
2. Take a bowl and add your cooked vegetables, granola.
3. Use an immersion blender to blitz your granola until you have a nice breadcrumb-like consistency.
4. Add coconut milk to the mix and mix until you have a nice firm texture.
5. Use the mixture to make granola balls and transfer them to your Grill.
6. Cook for 20 minutes.
7. Serve and enjoy!
- **Nutrition Info:** Calories: 140 Fat: 10 g Saturated Fat: 3 g Carbohydrates: 14 g Fiber: 4 g Sodium: 215 mg Protein: 2 g

456.Chocolate Fudge

Servings: 24
Cooking Time: 6 Hours
Ingredients:
- ½ teaspoon organic vanilla extract
- 1 cup heavy whipping cream
- 2 ounces butter softened
- 2 ounces 70% dark chocolate, finely chopped

Directions:

1. Select Sauté and Md: Hi on Ninja Foodi, and add vanilla and heavy cream. Sauté for 5 minutes at Low.
2. Sauté for 10 minutes, and add butter and chocolate.
3. Sauté for 2 minutes and pour this mixture into a serving dish.
4. Refrigerate it for some hours and serve.
- **Nutrition Info:** Calories: 292 Total Fat: 26.2 g Saturated Fat: 16.3 g Cholesterol: 100 mg Sodium: 86 mg Total Carbs: 8.2 g Fiber: 0 g Sugar: 6.6 g Protein: 5.2 g

457.Apple Tart

Servings: 8
Cooking Time: 12 Minutes
Ingredients:
- 8 teaspoons brown sugar
- 4 tablespoons granulated sugar
- 2 teaspoons ground cinnamon
- 1 ½ teaspoons lemon juice
- 4 apples, sliced thinly
- Pinch salt
- 1 package biscuit dough
- Cooking spray

Directions:
1. Mix sugars and cinnamon in a bowl.
2. Take 1 ½ tablespoons of this mixture and transfer to another bowl.
3. Stir in lemon juice, apples and salt.
4. Mix until fully combined.
5. Roll out the dough and separate into smaller pieces.
6. Top each piece with apple mixture.
7. Top with another piece and press the edges to seal.
8. Add to the grill grate.
9. Choose grill setting.
10. Set it to low.
11. Set time to 9 minutes.
12. Press start to preheat.
13. Grill for 6 minutes per side.

458.Cookies

Servings: 2
Cooking Time: 10 Minutes
Ingredients:
- 4 oz. cookie dough

Directions:
1. Choose air fry setting in your Ninja Foodi Grill.
2. Set it to 350 degrees F.
3. Preheat it for 1 minute.
4. Line air fryer basket with parchment paper.
5. Create 6 cookies from the dough.
6. Add these to the air fryer basket.
7. Place air fryer basket inside the unit.
8. Cook for 8 to 10 minutes.

459.Chocolate Brownies

Servings: 4
Cooking Time: 15 Minutes
Ingredients:
- ½ cup all-purpose flour
- ¾ cup sugar
- 6 tablespoons unsweetened cocoa powder
- ¼ teaspoon baking powder
- ¼ teaspoon salt
- ¼ cup unsalted butter, melted
- 2 large eggs
- 1 tablespoon vegetable oil
- ½ teaspoon vanilla extract

Directions:
1. Grease a 7-inch baking pan generously. Set aside.
2. In a bowl, add all the ingredients and mix until well combined.
3. Place the mixture into the prepared baking pan, and with the back of a spoon, smooth the top surface.
4. Arrange the drip pan at the bottom of the Instant Ninja Foodi Plus Air Fryer Oven cooking chamber.
5. Select "Air Fry" and then adjust the temperature to 330 degrees F.
6. Set the timer for 15 minutes and press the "Start."
7. When the display shows "Add Food," place the baking pan over the drip pan.
8. When the display shows "Turn Food," do nothing.
9. When cooking time is complete, remove the pan from the Ninja Foodi and place onto a wire rack to cool completely before cutting.
10. Cut the brownie into desired-sized squares and serve.

460.Stuffed Baked Apples

Servings: 4
Cooking Time: 12 Minutes
Ingredients:
- 4 tbsps. honey
- ¼ c. brown sugar
- ½ c. raisins
- ½ c. crushed walnuts
- 4 large apples

Directions:
1. Preheat the Air Fryer to a temperature of 350°F (180°C).
2. Cut the apples from the stem and remove the inner using a spoon.
3. Now fill each apple with raisins, walnuts, honey, and brown sugar.
4. Transfer apples in a pan and place in an Air Fryer basket, cook for 12 minutes.
5. Serve.

461.Crusted Mozzarella Sticks

Servings: 12
Cooking Time: 5 Minutes
Ingredients:
- Italian seasoning, 1 tsp.
- Beaten large eggs, 2.
- Garlic salt, ½ tsp.
- Halved mozzarella sticks string cheese, 12.
- Parmesan cheese, ½ cup
- Almond flour, ½ cup

Directions:
1. Mix almond flour with Italian seasoning, garlic salt, and parmesan cheese.
2. Whisk eggs in a separate bowl and keep them aside.
3. Dip the mozzarella sticks in eggs then coat with cheese mixture.
4. Arrange them on a well-lined baking tray with wax paper.
5. Freeze the sticks for 30 minutes, then place them in the air fryer basket.
6. Ground ginger, ½ tsp.
7. Egg whites, 4.
8. Let your air fryer preheat to 400°F.
9. Meanwhile, toss the chicken cubes with sesame oil and salt.
10. Mix coconut flour with ground ginger in a Ziploc bag then place the chicken in it.
11. Zip the bag and shake well to coat the chicken well.
12. Whisk egg whites in a bowl, then dip the coated chicken in egg whites.
13. Coat them with sesame seeds and shake off the excess.
14. Place the nuggets in the air fryer basket and return the basket to the fryer.
15. Air fry the nuggets for 6 minutes, then flip them.
16. Spray the nuggets with cooking oil and cook for another 6 minutes.
17. Serve fresh.
- **Nutrition Info:** Calories: 130; Fat: 10.3 g; Carbs: 9 g; Protein: 74.7 g

462.Apple Cake

Servings: 6
Cooking Time: 20 Minutes
Ingredients:
- 1 cup brown sugar
- 3 eggs, beaten
- 1 cup apples, diced
- 1 cup all-purpose flour
- Cooking spray

Directions:
1. Mix eggs and sugar in a bowl.
2. Fold in the flour and mix well.
3. Stir in the apples.
4. Spray your pie pan with oil.
5. Pour the mixture into the pie pan.

6. Place inside the unit.
7. Set it to bake.
8. Cook at 320 degrees F for 15 to 20 minutes.

463.Great Mac And Cheese Bowl

Servings: 4
Cooking Time: 10 Minutes
Ingredients:
- 1 tablespoon parmesan cheese, grated
- Salt and pepper to taste
- 1½ cup cheddar cheese, grated
- ½ cup warm milk
- ½ cup broccoli
- 1 cup elbow macaroni

Directions:
1. Preheat your Ninja Foodi to 400°F in Air Crisp mode, set a timer to 10 minutes.
2. Once you hear the beep, it is preheated.
3. Take a pot and add water, bring the water to a boil.
4. Add macaroni and veggies, boil for 10 minutes until cooked.
5. Drain pasta and veggies, toss pasta and veggies with cheese and sauce.
6. Season well with salt and pepper and transfer to Ninja Foodi.
7. Sprinkle more cheese on top and cook for 15 minutes.
8. Take it out and let it cool for 10 minutes.
9. Serve and enjoy!
- **Nutrition Info:** Calories: 180 Fat: 11 g Saturated Fat: 3 g Carbohydrates: 14 g Fiber: 3 g Sodium: 287 mg Protein: 6 g

464.Almond Cherry Bars

Servings: 12
Cooking Time: 35 Minutes
Ingredients:
- Xanthan gum, 1 tbsp.
- Almond flour, 1 ½ cup
- Salt, ½ tsp
- Pitted fresh cherries, 1 cup
- Softened butter, ½ cup
- Eggs, 2
- Water, ¼ cup
- Vanilla, ½ tsp
- Erythritol, 1 cup

Directions:
1. Combine almond flour, softened butter, salt, vanilla, eggs, and erythritol in a large bowl until you form a dough.
2. Press the dough in a baking dish that will fit in the air fryer.
3. Set in the air fryer and bake for 10 minutes at 375°F.
4. Meanwhile, mix the cherries, water, and xanthan gum in a bowl.
5. Take the dough out and pour over the cherry mixture.

6. Cook again for 25 minutes more at 375°F in the air fryer.
- **Nutrition Info:** Calories: 99; Carbs: 2.1 g; Fat: 9.3 g; Protein: 1.8 g

465.Chocolate Muffins

Servings: Up To 10 People
Cooking Time: 15 - 30
Ingredients:
- flour 00: 300gr
- sugar: 300gr
- butter: 150gr
- bitter cocoa powder: 70gr
- chemical yeast: 6gr
- fresh whole milk: 180ml
- salt: 1gr
- eggs: 4
- bicarbonate: 2gr
- dark chocolate: 100gr
- vanilla berry: 1

Directions:
1. In a food processor beat the softened butter with the sugar; also add the seeds of a vanilla berry.
2. When the mixture is clear and frothy, add the eggs at room temperature one at a time. Work all the ingredients for a few minutes and then add the flour, bitter cocoa, yeast, bicarbonate of soda and salt all sieved alternating them with milk at room temperature.
3. Add the grated dark chocolate last.
4. Remove the mixer blade from the bowl.
5. Fill the little cups with the dough and place them inside the tank (7/8 per baking).
6. Close the lid, select the BAKE program, power level 2, set 25min and press the on/off key.
7. At the end let it cool down; if desired, you can sprinkle it with icing sugar.

466.Lemon Cheesecake

Servings: 12
Cooking Time: 4 Hours
Ingredients:
- For the Crust:
- 1½ cups almond flour
- 4 tablespoons butter, melted
- 3 tablespoons sugar-free peanut butter
- 3 tablespoons Erythritol
- 1 large organic egg, beaten
- For Filling:
- 1 cup ricotta cheese
- 24 ounces cream cheese, softened
- 1½ cups Erythritol
- 2 teaspoons liquid Stevia
- 1/3 cup heavy cream
- 2 large organic eggs
- 3 large organic egg yolks

- 1 tablespoon fresh lemon juice
- 1 tablespoon organic vanilla extract

Directions:
1. Grease the pot of Ninja Foodi.
2. For the crust: in a bowl, add all the ingredients and mix until well combined.
3. In the pot of prepared of Ninja Foodi, place the crust mixture and press to smooth the top surface.
4. With a fork, prick the crust at many places.
5. For the filling: in a food processor, add the ricotta cheese and pulse until smooth.
6. In a large bowl, add the ricotta, cream cheese, Erythritol, and Stevia, and with an electric mixer, beat over medium speed until smooth.
7. In another bowl, add the heavy cream, eggs, egg yolks, lemon juice, and vanilla extract and beat until well combined.
8. Add the egg mixture into cream cheese mixture and beat over medium speed until just combined.
9. Place the filling mixture over the crust evenly.
10. Close the Ninja Foodi with the crisping lid and select Slow Cooker.
11. Set on Low for 3-4 hours.
12. Press Start/Stop to begin cooking.
13. Place the pan onto a wire rack to cool.
14. Refrigerate to chill for at least 6-8 hours before serving.
- **Nutrition Info:** Calories: 410 Fats: 37.9 g Net Carbs: 5.1 g Carbs: 6.9 g Fiber: 1.8 g Sugar: 1.3 g Proteins: 13 g Sodium: 260 mg

467.Easy Blueberry Cobbler

Servings:8
Cooking Time: 1 Hour 5 Minutes
Ingredients:
- 1 cup of self-rising flour
- 1 cup of white sugar
- 4 cups of fresh blueberries
- 1 cup of milk
- ½ cup of butter

Directions:
1. Preheat your oven to 350 ºF (175 ºC) and put butter to use in an 8-inch square baking dish
2. Then, melt the butter in the preheating oven for like 5 minutes and then remove it from the oven.
3. Mix sugar, flour, and milk in a bowl until they all combine. Then pour batter over the melted butter and scatter the blueberries over the batter.
4. Bake in the already preheated oven until you insert a toothpick at the center, and it comes out clean in approximately 1 hour.
- **Nutrition Info:** Calories 310.4, Carbohydrates 48.5 grams 16% DV, Protein

3.2 grams 6% DV, Fat 12.5 grams 19% DV, Cholesterol 32.9 mg 11% DV, Sodium 293.4 mg 12% DV.

468.Strawberry & Cake Kebabs

Servings: 5
Cooking Time: 6 Minutes
Ingredients:
- 1 pack white cake mix
- 2 cups strawberries, sliced in half
- 2 tablespoons honey
- ¼ cup sugar
- Cooking spray

Directions:
1. Cook cake mix according to the directions in the box.
2. Insert the grill grate in the Ninja Foodi Grill.
3. Choose the Grill setting.
4. Preheat at 325°F for 15 minutes.
5. While waiting, slice the cake into cubes.
6. Toss strawberries in honey and sugar.
7. Thread cake cubes and strawberries alternately onto skewers.
8. Grill for 3 minutes per side.
9. serving Suggestionss: Serve with vanilla ice cream.
10. preparation/Cooking Tips: When preparing the cake mix, you can replace water with pudding to make the cake thicker.
- **Nutrition Info:** Calories: 234 Fat: 17 g Carbohydrates: 5 g Protein: 28 g

469.Lime Cheesecake

Servings: 6
Cooking Time: 30 Minutes
Ingredients:
- ¼ cup plus 1 teaspoon Erythritol
- 8 ounces cream cheese, softened
- 1/3 cup Ricotta cheese
- 1 teaspoon fresh lime zest, grated
- 2 tablespoons fresh lime juice
- ½ teaspoon organic vanilla extract
- 2 organic eggs
- 2 tablespoons sour cream

Directions:
1. In a bowl, add ¼ cup of Erythritol and remaining ingredients except for eggs and sour cream. With a hand mixer, beat on high speed until smooth.
2. Add the eggs and beat on low speed until well combined.
3. Transfer the mixture into a 6-inch greased springform pan evenly.
4. With a piece of foil, cover the pan.
5. In the pot of the Ninja Foodi, place 2 cups of water.
6. Arrange a reversible rack in the pot of Ninja Foodi.

7. Place the springform pan over the reversible rack.
8. Close the Ninja Foodi with the pressure lid and place the pressure valve to the Seal position.
9. Select Pressure and set it to High for 30 minutes.
10. Press Start/Stop to begin cooking.
11. Switch the valve to Vent and do a Natural release.
12. Place the pan onto a wire rack to cool slightly.
13. Meanwhile, in a small bowl, add the sour cream and remaining Truvia and beat until well combined.
14. Spread the cream mixture on the warm cake evenly.
15. Refrigerate for about 6-8 hours before serving.
- **Nutrition Info:** Calories: 182 Fats: 16.6 g Net Carbs: 2.1 g Carbs: 2.1 g Fiber: 0 g Sugar: 0.3 g Proteins: 6.4 g Sodium: 152 mg

470.Caramelized Pineapple With Ice Cream

Servings: Up To 4 People
Cooking Time: 15 - 30
Ingredients:
- pineapple: 4 slices
- butter: 20 gr
- cane sugar: 50 gr
- vanilla ice cream

Directions:
1. Clean and slice the pineapple into 1 cm slices.
2. Remove the mixer blade from the tank
3. Insert the butter inside. Close the cover, select program BAKE, set 15min and press program start/stop key.
4. As soon as the butter becomes "sparkling" (about 3-4min) add the pineapple slices and brown them 2/3 minutes per side.
5. Sprinkle them with brown sugar and continue cooking for another 10 min. turning them halfway through cooking (lower the cooking power level if necessary).
6. Serve the caramelized pineapple on plates, decorating each one with a scoop of vanilla or cream ice cream.

471.Cream And Pine Nuts Tart

Servings: Up To 10 People
Cooking Time: 45 -60
Ingredients:
- flour: 250 gr
- butter: 125 gr
- sugar: 110 gr
- eggs (1 whole and 1 yolk): 2

- salt: q.b.
- custard cream: 500m

Directions:
1. Put in the mixer the flour, sugar, eggs, butter just removed from the refrigerator and cut into chunks and a pinch of salt.
2. Blend everything until the dough is compact and elastic enough. Put everything to rest in the refrigerator for at least half an hour.
3. Remove the mixer blade from the bowl.
4. Butter and flour the bottom well. Spread the shortcrust pastry at a thickness of 3-4 mm and place it in the bottom of the tank covering the edge well.
5. Prick the bottom with the tines of a fork and spread the custard over it, leveling it with a spoon.
6. Finish the tart by covering it all with pine nuts.
7. Close the lid, select the BAKE program, set 55min and press the program start/stop button.
8. Let the pie cool well before turning it upside down.

472.Strawberry Pop Tarts

Servings: 6
Cooking Time: 20 Minutes
Ingredients:
- 8 oz. strawberries
- 1/4 cup granulated sugar
- 1 refrigerated pie crust
- Cooking spray

Directions:
1. Combine strawberries and sugar in a pan over medium heat.
2. Cook while stirring for 10 minutes.
3. Let cool.
4. Spread pie crust on your kitchen table.
5. Slice into rectangles.
6. Add strawberries on top of the rectangles.
7. Brush edges with water.
8. Wrap and seal.
9. Spray tarts with oil.
10. Add tarts to the air fryer basket.
11. Choose air fry setting in your Ninja Foodi Grill.
12. Air fry at 350 degrees F for 10 minutes.
13. Let cool before serving.

473.Blueberry Mint Smoothie

Servings:2
Cooking Time: 40 Minutes
Ingredients:
- 1 cup of water
- 1 avocado, to be peeled and pitted
- 2 teaspoons of lemon juice
- 2 cups of frozen blueberries
- 1 cup of fresh mint leaves

- ½ cup of orange juice

Directions:
1. Blend blueberries, mint leaves, water, avocado, lemon juice, and orange juice in a blender until they become smooth.
- **Nutrition Info:** Calories 273.2, Carbohydrates 35 grams 11% DV, Protein 3.5 grams 7% DV, Fat 15.9 grams 25% DV, Sodium 13.1 mg 1% DV

474.Gingerbread

Servings: Up To 10 People
Cooking Time: 0 - 15
Ingredients:
- flour 00: 350 gr
- sugar: 160 gr
- butter: 150 gr
- egg: 1
- salt: 1 pinch
- honey: 150 gr
- cinnamon: 2 teaspoons
- nutmeg: 1/4 teaspoon
- ginger: 2 teaspoons
- cloves (powder): 1/2 teaspoon

Directions:
1. Put all the ingredients in a mixer (the butter must be cold as soon as it is taken out of the fridge).
2. Blend everything until you get a compact and quite elastic dough. Put everything to rest in the refrigerator for about 2 hours.
3. Remove the mixer blade from the tank.
4. After the necessary time, roll out with the rolling pin a sheet of dough 4 mm thick. Cut out shapes with cookie cutters of different Christmas shapes, and place them inside the tub over the baking paper.
5. Close the lid, select the program BAKE, power level 4, set 15min and press the program start/stop key.
6. After about 7min, turn the baking paper 180° and finish cooking. Once cooled, decorate as desired.

475.Fried Cream

Servings: Up To 8 People
Cooking Time: 15 - 30
Ingredients:
- Whole milk: 500mL
- Egg yolks: n.3
- Sugar: 150g
- Flour: 50g
- Vanillin: n.1 sachet
- Eggs: n.2
- Breadcrumbs: q.b.
- Oil: liv.4

Directions:
1. First prepare the custard; once cooked, pour it into a baking pan previously covered with transparent film and level it well; let it cool at room temperature for about 2 hours.
2. Remove the mixing paddle from the bowl.
3. Pour the oil into the tank and distribute it well over the entire bottom.
4. When the cream is cold, transfer it to a chopping board and cut it into cubes; pass each piece of cream first in the breadcrumbs, covering it well on all sides, then in the beaten egg and finally in the breadcrumbs.
5. Place each piece inside the tub, select the BAKE program, set 12min and press the program start/stop key.
6. Rotate the cream 1-2 times during cooking to even out the external browning.
7. With the doses of this cream you will have to do 2/3 cooking in sequence.

476.Chantal's New York Cheesecake

Servings: 12
Cooking Time: 1 Hour
Ingredients:
- 2 tablespoons of butter, to be melted
- 1 ½ cups of white sugar
- 4 (8 ounce) packages cream cheese
- 4 large eggs
- ¾ cup of milk
- 1 cup of sour cream
- 15 large rectangular piece or either 2 squares or 4 small rectangular pieces of graham crackers, to be crushed
- 4 large eggs
- ¼ cup of all-purpose flour
- 1 tablespoon of vanilla extract

Directions:
1. Preheat the oven to 350 ºF (175 ºC). Then grease a 9-inch springform pan.
2. Get a medium bowl and mix melted butter with graham cracker crumbs. Then, press on the bottom of the springform pan.
3. Get a large bowl and mix sugar with cream cheese until they become smooth. Blend in milk, and after that, mix the eggs one after the other and let it incorporate. Then mix in vanilla, sour cream, and flour until they become smooth. Then pour filling into the prepared crust.
4. Bake in the already preheated oven for like 1 hour. Turn off the oven and leave the cake to cool in it while the oven door is closed for about 5-6 hours; this is necessary to prevent cracking. Then chill in the refrigerator until you are ready to serve.
- **Nutrition Info:** Calories 533.4, Carbohydrates 44.2 grams 14% DV, Protein 10.3 grams 21% DV, Fat 35.7 grams 55% DV, Cholesterol 158.9 mg 53%, Sodium 380.4 mg 15% DV.

477.Mozzarella Sticks And Grilled Eggplant

Servings: 4
Cooking Time: 14 Minutes
Ingredients:

- Salt as needed
- ½ pound buffalo mozzarella, sliced into ¼-inch thick
- 12 large basil leaves
- 2 heirloom tomatoes, sliced into ¼ inch thickness
- 2 tablespoon canola oil
- 1 eggplant, ¼-inch thick

Directions:

1. Take a large bowl and add the eggplant, add oil and toss well until coated well.
2. Preheat your Ninja Foodi to MAX and set the timer to 15 minutes.
3. Once you hear the beeping sound, transfer the prepared eggplants to your Grill and cook for 8-12 minutes until the surface is charred.
4. Top with cheese slice, tomato, and mozzarella.
5. Cook for 2 minutes, letting the cheese melt.
6. Remove from grill and place 2-3 basil leaves on top of half stack.
7. Place remaining eggplant stack on top alongside basil.
8. Season well with salt and the rest of the basil.
9. Enjoy!
- **Nutrition Info:** Calories: Fat: 19 g Saturated Fat: 19 g Carbohydrates: 11 g Fiber: 4 g Sodium: 1555 mg Protein: 32 g

478.Grilled Pineapple Butterscotch Sundaes

Servings: 12
Cooking Time: 25 Minutes
Ingredients:

- 2 tablespoons of white sugar
- 2 eaches of fresh pineapples, to be peeled, cored, and cut into 6 spears
- 1 cup of packed brown sugar
- 6 tablespoons of butter
- ¼ teaspoon of ground nutmeg
- ½ cup of butter
- ½ cup of heavy whipping cream
- 1 pinch of salt
- 1 teaspoon vanilla extract
- 3 cups of vanilla ice cream

Directions:

1. Preheat the grill with medium heat and lightly oil the grate
2. Heat 6 tablespoons of butter, nutmeg, and white sugar in a saucepan on medium heat and stir until the sugar dissolves in about 5 minutes. Then brush the pineapple spears with butter mixture.
3. Arrange pineapple on the already preheated grill and cover, grill until it becomes lightly brown, turning frequently; this should last between 7 to 10 minutes. Then transfer the pineapple to a platter.
4. Get another saucepan and melt the remaining ½ cup of butter using medium heat. Stir in heavy cream and brown sugar, then bring to a boil, stirring as frequently as possible. Remove from the heat and add salt and vanilla extract. Serve the pineapple topped with ice cream and cream sauce.
- **Nutrition Info:** Calories 388.2, Carbohydrates 51.9 grams 17% DV, Protein 2.7 grams 6% DV, Fat 21 grams 32% DV, Cholesterol 63.7 mg 21% DV, Sodium 131.2 mg 5% DV.

OTHER FAVORITE RECIPES

479.Chive Scones

Servings: 6 Serves
Cooking Time: 17 Minutes
Ingredients:
- 40 g cheddar mature – grated
- 6 g powder baking.
- 1/2 teaspoon salt.
- 1 teaspoon cabbage – cut.
- 1 egg & 1 teaspoon of brushing milk
- 270 g flat meal (TYP 405)
- 1 ovum.
- 100 g of butter – soft
- 40 g cheddar mature – grated
- 60 g fresh cream.

Directions:
1. Add flour, baking powder, salt, chives, and cheddar in a large bowl. Mix well and add egg, cream fraiche, and softened butter. Combine as much as you can, place it on a clean surface and knead until you have cut into the dough all the loose meals. The pudding should not be overworked because the scones should be fluffy and buttery
2. Using a cooking pot without a mounted grill or crisper container. Close the lid. Close the lid. Choose bake, set the temp to 170 ° C, and set the time to 17 minutes. To start preheating, press start/stop.
3. During preheating, roll the dough about 3 cm thick. Using a biscuit cutter, cut out the dough.
4. Add egg and milk in a small bowl and combine well. Brush the top of the egg and mix scones.
5. Once it has been preheated, spray the pot lightly with cooking spray and add scones. Close cap to start cooking
6. When the cooking is finished, remove the scones and cool down. Serve with butter, chutney or soup, and stews side by side.

480.Grinders Sauce And Peppers

Servings: 6 Serves
Cooking Time: 26 Minutes
Ingredients:
- 6 cheap sausages, like hot Italian or Bratwurst, four ounces each
- 1 white onion, peeled, 1-inch rings cut.
- As desired, kosher salt
- Black pepper ground, as desired.
- 2 bell peppers, seeds, and ribs removed in sections.
- 2 tablespoons of canola oil, split.
- 6 hot dogs.
- Terms, as requested.

Directions:

1. Add the grill to the machine and remove the hood. Set temperature to low, pick grill and set time to 26 minutes. To start preheating, select start/stop.
2. Toss bell peppers and onions with butter, salt, and black pepper while the machine is preheating.
3. If the device shows that it is preheated, place peppers and onions on the grill. Open the hood and cook without flipping for 12 minutes.
4. Move peppers and onions to a medium mixing bowl after 12 minutes. Close the hood and cook for 6 minutes on a grill grate.
5. Flip sausages after 6 minutes. Close the hood and cook 6 minutes longer.
6. Split the grilled onions into single rings and blend with the peppers.
7. Pull sausages from the grill after 6 minutes. Place the buns on the grill, cut-sided down. Close the hood and cook for 2 minutes.
8. When the cooking is done, spread the seasonings onto the buns, then put the sausages into the buns. Top each with peppers and onions liberally and serve.

481.Margarita Pineapple

Servings: 2 Serves
Cooking Time: 5 Minutes
Ingredients:
- 1 1/4 cup of frozen bananas chunks
- 1/4 cup of bananas juice.
- 1/4 cup three times dry.
- 1 cubicle lime juice.
- 1/2 cup of tequila red.

Directions:
1. Place all ingredients in the order listed in the 20-ounce single-serve blending cup.
2. Choose frozen drink.
3. Attach a sealed spout lid for convenience on-the-go.

482.Grilled Lamb Chops With Salad Parsley

Servings: 4 Serves
Cooking Time: 10 Minutes
Ingredients:
- 1 full-milk cup of yogurt (not Greek).
- 1 teaspoon Black pepper freshly made.
- 1 teaspoon Field cumin.
- 1 teaspoon Paprika.
- 5 teaspoons ground cinnamon.
- 2 teaspoon sumac.
- 5 teaspoons ground nutmeg.
- 12 untrimmed lamb rib chops (approximately 3 lb.), painted white.
- Kosher salt.

- 1 small, very thinly sliced red onion.
- 1 cup of chopped parsley grossly.
- 1 teaspoon fresh citrus juice.
- 1/2 teaspoon Farm cardamom. Farm cardamom.
- 1 teaspoon ground coriander.
- More Ingredient
- Sumac, a sweet, citrus spice usually sold in ground form, is available on markets in the Middle East, in specialty food stores and online.

Directions:
1. In a big bowl, mix yogurt, black pepper, cumin, cardamom, cinnamon, and nutmeg.
2. Season both sides of the lamb chop with salt generously and add the marinade to the bowl. Shift lamb to coat in marinade; cover and chill up to 12 hours and a minimum of three hours.
3. Let lamb sit 1 hour before grilling at room temperature.
4. Prepare a medium-high heat grill lamb for desired doneness, medium-rare approximately 3 minutes per side. Leave for 5–10 minutes to rest.
5. Meanwhile, throw onion, parsley, lemon juice, and sumac in a medium bowl with a pinch of salt.

483.Hazelnut Cookies Lave

Servings: 7 Serves
Cooking Time: 15 Minutes
Ingredients:
- 280 g flat meal.
- Unsalted butter 125 g.
- Spread 5-6 teaspoon hazelnut.
- 1 big duck.
- Refined 185 g brown sugar.nd
- Extract 2 teaspoons of vanilla.

Directions:
1. Start by preheating the oven to 180°c.
2. In the microwave, melt the butter and the brown sugar for 30 seconds, remove the butter from the microwave, and mix.
3. Attach melted butter with brown sugar and the whole egg, meal, and vanilla extract with the bowl and plastic blade of your Ninja Kitchen Machine.
4. Pick low before the ingredients are combined in a cookie paste.
5. Scoop 2 cookie dough tablespoons and flatten your hand palm. Put 1 spoon of hazelnut in the middle on the baking tray and spoon. Roll in a ball to ensure that the distribution is in the center. Repeat until all the cookie dough is used.
6. Bake the cookies in the oven for about 12 minutes, allow the cookies to cool before kept in a container

484.Sausage And Pepper Calzones

Servings: 4 Serves
Cooking Time: 33 Minutes
Ingredients:
- 2 extra virgin olive oil tablespoons, divided.
- 1 large Italian sausage (6 ounces) uncooked, removed from the case.
- 1 bell pepper with thin slices and removed stems and seeds
- 1 small, peeled, sliced onion
- 1/2 cup of sauce pizza.
- 4 for all purposes, including dusting
- Store pizza dough 1 pound, room temperature
- 1/2 kosher salt teaspoon.
- Mozzarella cheese, cut in 1/2 inch cubes, 1/2 cup (4 ounces)

Directions:
1. Cut the pizza dough in half and let it sit until necessary.
2. Choose sear/sauté and set MD: HI temperature. To start, select start/stop. Put 1 tablespoon of oil in the pot and heat for about 3 minutes until shimmering.
3. Add the pepper, onion, and salt to the pot and cook for about 5 minutes till the onions are translucent. Add sausage and cook about five minutes until it has stopped being pink, breaking into small pieces with a wooden spoon. To turn off sear/sauté, select start/stop, and let the mixture cool slightly.
4. Roll every dough on a slightly blurred surface into a 9-inch circle. Spread 1/4 cup pizza sauces on half of each circle and spread half of the sausage mixture over sauce. Fold the dough over and pinch it tightly to stick to it. Cut 2 small slits on each calzone with a knife to release steam.
5. Select bake/roast, set the temperature to 375 ° F, and set the time to 3 minutes to preheat it. To start, select start/stop.
6. Cut a piece of parchment paper to 12 x 17 cm and fold it halfway through 12 x 8 1/2 cm. Place the plywood on the reversible rack, ensuring the rack is in the lower position—transfer calzones to a rack facing each other with straight edges (they can touch).
7. Lower rack into the pot after 3 minutes and brush on tops of calzones with 1 tablespoon oil remaining. Close crooked deck. Set the temperature to 375 degrees F and set the time to 20 minutes. To start, select start/stop.
8. After 10 minutes, open the lid and remove the rack from the pot carefully. Pull parchment paper carefully to slip off the rack and the calzones. Unfold the

parchment under the calzones and place the uncooked side over the other half of the perch. To move calzones back to rack, return the rack to bowl, and close the lid to resume cooking, use parchment as a sling.

9. Cooking is completed when the calzones on the other hand are well browned. Enable 5 minutes to cool before serving.

485.Patties Sweet Potato

Servings: 6 Serves
Cooking Time: 15 Minutes
Ingredients:
- 1/2 teaspoon flakes of chilli.
- 100 g gluten-free meal.
- New parsley 6 g.
- 1 teaspoon of pepper.
- 2 garlic cloves.
- Salt and potatoes.
- 500 g of sweet potato – Cut into cubes and peeled.
- 1 inch of olive oil.

Directions:
1. Bring a cup of water to boil. Add sweet potato chunks and cook for 12-15 minutes or until tender enough to pick with a knife easily.
2. Drain the sweet potato once cooked and cool.
3. Fill your food processor with cooled sweet potato and mix with the puree.
4. In addition to olive oil, add the remaining ingredients to the food processor. Blend well together. Add more meals if the mix still looks a little wet.
5. In a frying pan, add the olive oil over medium heat and heat.
6. Shape the sweet potato mixture into patties with your hands. Put the patties in the pot.
7. Cook on the other side for 3-4 minutes before turning and frying.
8. Serve straight away or keep in the refrigerator and eat within 2 days. It can also be consumed cold or reheated!

486.Bread Quick Sourdough

Servings: 1 Serve
Cooking Time: 40 Minutes
Ingredients:
- Instant or active 1 1/2 teaspoons of dry yeast
- 2 kosher salt teaspoons.
- 1 charcoal of sugar.
- 3 all-purpose cups of rice.
- 1 cup of Greek plain yogurt
- 1 1/2 cups of water, split up.

Directions:
1. Warm 1/2 pot water to 110 ° F, mix in the bowl with yeast and sugar and leave to sit

for about 5 minutes until the mixture becomes spumous.

2. Add rice, yogurt, and salt to the yeast mixture and fasten bowl with a dough hook attachment to stand mixer. Mix at medium-low speed, around 2 minutes, until the dough gets together. Rub the sides of the bowl with a rubber spatula, then increase to medium speed for 5 minutes.
3. Choose the bake/roast machine to warm up, set the temperature to 250 ° F, and set the time to 1 minute. To begin, click start/stop.
4. Shape dough into a smooth ball, put it in a warm spot, and cover with a towel for the kitchen. Allow the dough to rest until it doubles in size for approximately 2 hours.
5. Cut a circle of parchment paper into the reversible rack. Put it in the lower position on the rack and grease with a kitchen spray.
6. Once the dough is finished, move to a smooth ball and mold it to a slightly blurred surface. Place on the round parchment shelf, cover with a kitchen towel and let stand for 15 minutes. Then use a sharp knife to cut the middle of the dough into a 4-inch line 1/2-inch deep down.
7. Put the remaining 1 cup of water in the pot and put rack with ough in the tub. Choose roast, set the temperature at 325 ° F, set the time to 40 minutes. To begin, click start/stop.
8. Cooking is complete when browned and baked at the bottom. Remove the pot and parchment paper and put it on the cooling rack at least 2 hours until it is cooled to room temperature.

487.Mexican Adobo Grilled Tenderloin

Servings: 4 Serves
Cooking Time: 33 Minutes
Ingredients:
- Olive oil 1 teaspoon.
- 18 oz tenderloin pork.
- Aaron's Adobo 3 teaspoon.
- To taste, kosher salt.

Directions:
1. Rub the tenderloin olive oil and a pat on the adobo. Set aside for approximately 30 minutes.
2. Preheat the grill or preheat the broiler. Season pork generously with salt.
3. Grill until 145 ° F, shout take about 20 to 22 minutes. Make sure 145°F is read instantly before inserting in the centre.
4. Let the pork rest approximately 5 minutes before slicing.

488.Cookie Chocolate Skillet Chip

Servings: 6 Serves
Cooking Time: 25 Minutes

Ingredients:

- 1/2 teaspoon soda baking.
- 1/2 cup, whenever desired, cut walnuts, pecans, or almonds.
- 1/2 kosher salt tablespoon.
- 1 cup of chocolate semi-sweet.
- 1 stick (1/2 cup) unsalted, smoothed butter, plus more to grate
- 1 cup + 2 all-purpose tablespoons of flour.
- 6 tablespoons of granular sugar.
- 6 tablespoons of brown sugar packed.
- Extract 1/2 teaspoon of vanilla.
- 1 big egg.

Directions:

1. Close crooked deck. Choose bake/roast, set temperature to 325 ° F, and set the time to 5 minutes. Preheat the unit. To start, select start/stop.
2. During preheating, whisk flour, baking soda, and salt in a mixing bowl together.
3. Beat the butter, sugars, and vanilla in a separate mixing bowl until creamy. Attach egg and beat until fully incorporated and smooth.
4. Add dry ingredients slowly, about 1/3 at a time, to the egg blend. Use a rubber spatula to clean off the sides and add all the dry ingredients. Make sure that the cookie is not over-mixed or dense when baked.
5. Layer chocolate chips and nuts into the cookie dough until distributed uniformly.
6. Grasp the bottom of the Ninja Multifunctional Pan (or 8-inch baking pan) generously. Attach the cookie dough to the pot and ensure that it is distributed evenly.
7. Place the pan on the reversible rack once the machine is preheated, and make sure the rack is in the lower position. Place the rack in the pot with the pan. Close crooked deck. Set temperature to 325 ° F, and set time to 23 minutes, select bake/roast. To start, select start/stop.
8. Allow cookies to cool for 5 minutes after cooking is complete. Then serve warm with your choice of toppings.

489.Pear Fritters

Servings: 6
Cooking Time: 20 Mins
Ingredients:

- ½ tsp salt
- ⅓ cup milk
- ½ tsp ground cinnamon
- ½ cup honey
- 1 tbsp brown sugar
- 2 washed, peeled pears
- A little vegetable oil
- 1 large egg
- ½ cup of flour

Directions:

1. Place your Ninja Foodi crisper basket in the unit and close the hood. Choose AIR FRY. Select START/STOP to start your pre-heating.
2. In a large bowl, sift together the flour and dry ingredients except for peas.
3. Mix the eggs and honey then fold with the flour mixture
4. Add milk and continue to fold.
5. Combine with the pears, chopped finely
6. Lightly coat with vegetable oil if you wish for a nice crisp
7. Place ¼ of the batter into the crisper basket and allow it to cook. Keep shaking the basket to enjoy an even crisp.
8. Dip the tops of the fritters into the glaze, then allow to set before serving immediately
- **Nutrition Info:** Calories: 276 Fat: 14g Saturated Fat: 12g Trans Fat: 0g Carbohydrates: 14g Fiber: 1g Sodium: 102g Protein: 1.5g

490.Tropical Smooth Berry

Servings: 4 Serves
Cooking Time: 5 Minutes
Ingredients:

- 1 taste of ice.
- 1 cup of water.
- 1 cup of spinach for baby.
- 1 cup of fresh fruit, hulled.
- 1 cup of blueberry.
- 2 cups of chunks of mango.

Directions:

1. Put the high-speed blade in the jar and then add all ingredients in the order.
2. Pulse 3 times, then proceed for 60 seconds or until you reach the desired consistency.

491.Watermelon Grilled

Servings: 6 Serves
Cooking Time: 2 Minutes
Ingredients:

- 6 slices of watermelon, each measuring 3 inches in size and 1 inch thick
- 2 tablespoons of sweetheart.

Directions:

1. Place the grill in the unit and close the hood. Select grill, set max, and set time to 2 minutes. To start preheating, click start/stop.
2. While the unit is preheating, the brush slices watermelon with sweet melon on both sides.
3. If the unit is used to indicate it is preheated, put watermelon on the grill. Push gently to increase grate touch. Open the hood and grill without flipping for 2 minutes.

4. When cooking is complete, serve immediately.

492.Brussels And Free Bacon

Servings: 4 Serves
Cooking Time: 26 Minutes
Ingredients:
- 1 small, peeled, thinly sliced red onion
- Heavy cream for 1/2 cup.
- 2 cubic meters of olive oil
- 1 kosher salt teaspoon.
- 1 tea cubicle fine ground black pepper
- 1 cup of cheddar cheese shredded.
- 3 bacon strips, slimly thin
- 1/2 cup of Parmesan cheese shredded, divided
- 1/4 cup of seasoned crumbs of bread
- Brussels sprouts 1 pound, trimmed, cut in quarters.
- Fresh, chopped parsley, to be served.

Directions:
1. Remove basket crisper plate. Choose the air roast for the preheat unit and set the temperature to 400 ° F and set the time to 3 minutes. To start preheating, click start/stop.
2. When the Ninja grill is preheated, combine Brussels sprouts in a large mixing bowl with red onion, bacon, 1/4 cup Parmesan, olive oil, salt, and pepper.
3. Put the mixture in the basket once the machine is preheated; insert the container.
4. Set the temperature to 400 ° F, set the time to 24 minutes, and pick air roast. To start cooking, click start/stop.
5. Remove the basket after 8 minutes and stir the mixture, then reinsert the basket.
6. In the meantime, mix in a bowl 1/4 cup of Parmesan, cheddar, and bread crumbs.
7. After 16 minutes, pour the basket and heavy cream into the mixture of sprout in Brussels. Fill with the mixture of bread crumb. To resume cooking, reinsert the pot.
8. Remove gratin from the basket when cooking is complete. Top the parsley and serve as soon as possible.

493.Fried Green Beans

Servings: 4
Cooking Time: 10 Minutes
Ingredients:
- 1 cup green beans
- 1 tablespoon avocado oil
- 2 tablespoons bread crumbs
- Salt and pepper to taste

Directions:
1. Toss the green beans in oil.
2. Season with the salt and pepper.
3. Coat with the bread crumbs.

4. Cook at 390 degrees F for 8 minutes.
5. Flip and cook for 2 more minutes.

494.Noodle Chicken Soup

Servings: 4 Serves
Cooking Time: 15 Minutes
Ingredients:
- 1 cup of dry noodles of the egg.
- 1/4 of a teaspoon of thyme crushed.
- 2 celery stalks, cut into 1-inch pieces.
- The stock of 3 1/2 cups of chicken.
- 1/2 kosher salt tablespoon.
- 1 little onion, peeled, cut into pieces of 1 inch.
- 1/4 of a tea cubicle ground black pepper.
- 2 carrots, peeled, cut in pieces of 1 inch.
- 1 cup of chicken uncooked, cut into 1-inch pieces.

Directions:
1. In the order listed, place all ingredients, except noodles, in the blender pitcher.
2. Choose hearty Broth.
3. Add egg noodles with 6 minutes left on the schedule. Serve immediately.

495.Peanut Butter Crunchy Flapjacks

Servings: 12 Serves
Cooking Time: 15 Minutes
Ingredients:
- Cocoa powder 35 g.
- 15 g almonds.
- Gluten-free oats 250 g.
- 90 g smooth butter of peanut.
- Maple syrup of 105ml.
- 90 g of coconut oil melted.
- Pumpkin seeds 15 g.
- Cocoa 10 g nibs.
- 80 g of coconut oil melted.
- 45ml maple juice.
- 30 g smooth butter of peanut.

Directions:
1. Preheat the oven to 160° and cut into 7 bis.
2. centimetres with paper that are greaseproof.
3. Attach the oats and almonds to the food processor and pulse 3-4 times, before they break down.
4. Remove it to a bowl and add the rest of the ingredients.
5. Press the flapjack blend into the tin.
6. Bake 15 minutes, cool in the tin.
7. Place the flapjacks once cool in the fridge for an hour to make cutting easier.
8. Combine the ingredients in your blender and combine until the combine is smooth for a few seconds.
9. Cut the bottle in bars and dip into the chocolate mixture.

10. For added texture sprinkle the top of each one, I used grated cocoa and some pumpkin seed.

496.Sweet Potato Air-crisped Wedges

Servings: 4 Serves
Cooking Time: 24 Minutes
Ingredients:
- 1/2 tea cubicle ground black pepper
- 1 tablespoon sweetheart, plus more for garnish
- 1 teaspoon of paprika smoked, plus more for garnishing.
- 1 coarse tea cubicle kosher salt
- 2 sweet potatoes or yams (about 1 pound each)
- 1 charcoal canola oil.
- Sauce of convenience dipping.

Directions:
1. Rinse and clean in cold water sweet potatoes and yams, and then pat dry. Cut each half longitudinally, then split every half into four or five wedges.
2. Mix the remaining ingredients in a wide bowl and then remove the potato wedges to cover.
3. Install crisper in Ninja grill. Set the temperature to 390 ° F and set the time to 24 minutes; pick air crisp. To start preheating, click start/stop.
4. If the cooker preheated, layout the wedges uniformly in the bowl, pinch the hood and cook for 10 minutes.
5. Throw or stir wedges after 10 minutes with rubber-tipped tongs. Close hood for 10 more minutes to resume cooking.
6. Check wedges for doneness after 10 minutes. Cook up to 4 more minutes, if necessary, until the wedges achieve their desired degree of liability.
7. When cooking is complete, add extra honey and paprika, if desired, and serve with the choice of dipping sauce.

497.Pear, Dark Chocolate And Blondes Mocha

Servings: 12 Serves
Cooking Time: 20 Minutes
Ingredients:
- Instant coffee 3 tea cubes + 6 tea cubes boiling water.
- 150 g of cocoa or date sugar
- Dark chocolate 75 g, cut.
- 100 g of cocoa oil.
- 1 teaspoon powder baking.
- Extract 1 teaspoon of vanilla.

Directions:
1. Preheat the oven to 180°C and grate and baked in a 9x9 in the bakery.

2. Melt the cocoon oil and set aside for a little cooling. In the meantime, dissolve the coffee in a small bowl with boiling water and leave to cool.
3. Nutri Ninja adds all the ingredients other than pear and chocolate and blends until a batter formed in your Ninja Kitchen.
4. Fold the diced pear and chocolate into the prepared tin and evenly smooth out. Bake until firm and skewer gets clean for 25-30 minutes (you want the blonde still a little squishy).
5. Let the tin cool and cut into 9-12 pieces. Love!

498.Grilled Flatbread Vegetable

Servings: 16 Serves
Cooking Time: 20 Minutes
Ingredients:
- 1 cup of fresh mixed herbs (e.g., pink flakes, tiny mint foliage and chopped chives)
- 1 1/2 cup plus 1/3 cup extra virgin olive oil, divided and brushing more.
- 3 pounds (for example cabbage, turquoise, red onion, and baby bell peppers) of mixed vegetables
- 4 kosher salt teaspoons, divided, more to taste.
- 6 new lemon juice tablespoons, split.
- Aleppo pepper or sweet paprika 1 1/2 tablespoon
- Split 6 cloves of garlic, smashed.
- Divided 1 (30-x 14-inch) lava blossom (for example: Ara-Z) or 4 (11 1/2-x 8 1/4-inch) lava blossom (for example, for Joseph's).
- 1 1/4 cups of smoked almonds (6 1/2 ounces approximately)
- 6 to 9 tablespoons of water divided.
- 2 1/2 teaspoons of grenade molasses split.
- Flaky separated sea salt, to compare.
- 3 (1/3-inch) deaf slices of bread (approximately 3 ounces)

Directions:
1. Preheat a medium-high (450 ° F to 500 ° F) carbon or gas grill. Drizzle with 2 tablespoons of oil. Unoiled grills place bread and pepper, and grill uncovered and sometimes switched to the toast, for about 2 to 3 minutes, and peppers on all sides, for about 18 to 20 minutes. Move to a medium bowl bell peppers and cover tightly with plastic wrap, allow 10 minutes to stand. Cut the peppers in half and cut the peppers and leave in the bowl some juice. Remove skin, stalks, and seeds. Place peeled peppers and toasted sourdough aside.
2. Cut squash and courgettes into 1/2 inch slices. Cut in 1 inch wedges the onion, leaving the root end untouched. Split half of

the baby bell peppers. Toss vegetables in a large bowl with 3 tablespoons of olive oil. Grill vegetables until tender and slightly charred (see cook time note). Remove the grill and put in an even layer in a baking dish of 13-x 9-inch; sprinkle with 2 teaspoons of kosher salt. Stir in 1 cup of butter, 2 slippers of lemon juice, 1/2 tablespoon of Aleppo pepper and 3 cloves of garlic in a medium bowl. Cover and let stand for at least 30 minutes or up to 3 hours at room temperature.

3. Reduce the gas grill temperature to low (250 ° F to 300 ° F), or allow low burning of carbon. Set sangak on grills (brush both sides lightly with olive oil if using lavash). Grill flatbread, fried, often rotating and tossing, for 6 to 10 minutes, until slightly toasted. Set aside. Set aside.

4. Place the bread with sourdough into small pieces in a food processor. Attach bell peppers, 1/3 cup of oil, 3/4 cup of almonds, 6 tablespoons of sugar, 11/2 tablespoons of molasses of granite, 1/4 cup of lemon juice remaining, 1 tablespoon of Aleppo, 2 teaspoons of salt, and 3 cloves of garlic remaining, and process around 45 seconds, until smooth. Let the blend stand for 10 minutes. If necessary, add 3 tablespoons of water remaining 1 tablespoon per table until a thick but spreadable consistency is achieved—season to taste with kosher salt. Chop the remaining 1/2 cup of almonds roughly; reserve.

5. Move by Move

6. Disseminate the muhammara onto flatbread. Arrange marinated flatbread vegetable mixture. Drizzle with 3 tablespoons of dish marinade and 1 tablespoon pomegranate molasses left. Sprinkle with almonds chopped. Taste the season with flaccid sea salt. Just before eating, sprinkle with remaining 3 tablespoons of olive oil.

499.Bowl Strawberry Acai

Servings: 2 Serves
Cooking Time: 5 Minutes
Ingredients:
- 1/4 of a cup of bananas sliced.
- 2 spoonfuls of agave nectar.
- 1 tablespoon of coconut shredded.
- 1 1/4 cup almond milk vanilla
- 8 new leaves of mint.
- 1 pack (3.5 oz) frozen acai, thawed.
- Sliced strawberries of 1/4 cup.
- 1 teaspoon of almonds slivered.
- 2 cubes of citrus juice.
- 1 tea cubicle chia seeds.
- 2 1/2 cups of frozen fragrances

Directions:

1. In the order listed, place all ingredients in the 72-ounce pitcher.
2. Choose ice cream.
3. Fill in garnishes.

500.Tacos Air Grill Salmon

Servings: 4 Serves
Cooking Time: 10 Minutes
Ingredients:
- Tomatoes – chopped finely
- 1 garlic clove – gritty
- 1/2 teaspoon new chili pepper – chopped finely.
- Limestone zest.
- 1/2 limestone juice.
- 1 Olive oil teaspoon.
- To taste salt and pepper.
- The guacamole
- 2 salmon pieces.
- 1/2 little onion – sliced finely
- Tomato 1/2 – finely cut
- 1 clove of garlic – hairy
- 1/2 teaspoon new chili pepper – chopped finely.
- To taste salt and pepper.
- 4 pancakes.
- Salad.
- 1 teaspoon cilantro.
- Coriander & garnish cheese

Directions:

1. Mix garlic, pepper, lemon zest, olive oil, salt, and pepper with salmon, remove and marinate.
2. Choose grill and set a high temperature. To start preheating, click start/stop.
3. While the unit is preheating, prepare the guacamole with all ingredients in a blender and lightning to combine but leave small pieces—season to taste with salt and pepper.
4. When the unit beeps to indicate that it is preheated, spray the barbecue with cooking spray and skin the salmon. To start, press start/stop. Close the lid for five minutes and cook.
5. After 5 minutes, flip the fish over to ensure even cooking on both sides. Close the lid and cook 5 minutes more.
6. When the cooking process finishes, flake salmon up and serve with salad, tomatoes, and guacamole in a tortilla hot, garnish with cool coriander, lime juice, and/or cheese.

501.Cocoa Frozen

Servings: 2 Serves
Cooking Time: 10 Minutes
Ingredients:
- Whipped Topping Chocolate Dairy.
- 2 dining spoons of hot water.

- 3/4 cup of fat milk free.
- 1-1/2 tablespoons of ice.
- Diet Hot Cocoa Mix is enveloped in 3 envelopes (0.29 oz each).

Directions:
1. In a small cup, add the mixture of cocoa and hot water. Put the cocoa mixture, milk, and ice in the mixer and blend. Pour into chilled cups or chilled glasses and top each one (2 tablespoons) of a serving Reddi-Wip. Serve immediately.

502.Milkshake Unicorn

Servings: 2 Serves
Cooking Time: 5 Minutes
Ingredients:
- Cookies for the wafer.
- 2 cups of ice cream vanilla.
- 1 cup of milk.
- 1/4 cup of frosting coffee.
- 1/4 cup of hard colorful sweets.
- 1 cup of frozen fragrances.
- Whipped cream.
- 1/2 cup of marshmallow miniature, plus more to garnish.

Directions:
1. Place a complete blade of crush & power in the pot, then add strawberries, ice cream, and milk.
2. Run for 45 seconds continuously or until the desired consistency is reached.
3. Place in each glass 1/4 cup of mini marshmallows. Then, rim the glasses with frosting with a spoon.
4. Put milkshake in a saucepan. Stick candies carefully on the frosty rims of the glasses.
5. Garnish with toppings desired.

503.Tenderloin Rouben Stuffed Pork

Servings: 4 Serves
Cooking Time: 35 Minutes
Ingredients:
- 50 of a cup of sauerkraut, well-drained.
- 1/4 tea cucumber caraway kernels.
- 3 teaspoon 1000 Island dressing.
- 2 oz thinly sliced pastrami turkey.
- Fat Swiss cheese reduced by 2 oz.
- 18 ounce of tenderloin trimmed pork.
- Olive oil 1/2 teaspoon.
- 1 teaspoon of powdered garlic.
- 1 teaspoon gross salt.

Directions:
1. Preheat oven to 425 degrees F.
2. Cut the middle of the tenderloin into a length split in 1/2 "(not to be cut all the way). Open the tenderloin, and it's flat. On each half, split the centre lengthwise to a depth of 1/2-inch; cover with a plastic wrap.
3. Apply to 1/4-in—thickness with a suitcase.

4. Remove the plastic wrap; spread pork on one side of the Thousand Islands. Place the pastrami on top, then the Swiss cheese and the pork sauerkraut.
5. Roll up the pork jelly-roll style from a long side. At 2-inch intervals, tie the roast with a 12-inch kitchen string, then freeze the pork with the olive oil.
6. In a small bowl, add garlic powder, salt, and caraway seeds; rub over the pork.
7. Bake uncovered on a pan, 425 ° until a meat thermometer reads 160 °, about 35 minutes.
8. Move to a moveable plate or cutting board. Let it stand 10 minutes before string and slice are removed. Cut into eight pieces.

504.Steak Salad Southwest

Servings: 4 Serves
Cooking Time: 1 Hour, 10 Minutes
Ingredients:
- 1 large pepper jalapeno.
- 1 little lettuce iceberg head, chopped coarsely
- 2 big red bell peppers.
- 4 ears of young, sweet maize with husks (water-soaked)
- 1/4 cup of new cilantro chopped.
- Top sirloin steak with 1 pound of boneless beef
- Wish-Bone Cup Italian dressing, split.

Directions:
1. Place 1/2 cup of the dressing in large, shallow glass baking dish or plastic bag over steak and peppers; turn to cover. Close or cover bag and occasionally marinate in the refrigerator for 30 minutes up to three hours.
2. Remove maize from water and leave the husks on. Grill maize, occasionally turning, until finished; set aside and stay warm.
3. Remove marinade steak and peppers, discard marinade. Grill the steak and peppers, turn the steak once and brush the dressing for 1/4 cup, 10 minutes or till the steak is needed, and tender vegetables. Slice steak thinly.
4. Remove the maize kernels from the sharp knife cobs. Peel from peppers any burnt skin; seed and chop. In a medium bowl, threw in corn, peppers, coriander, and the remaining 1 tablespoon dressing.
5. Arrange the lettuce on the dish. Top with steak and then mix with maize, just before eating, drizzle, covering.

505.Gazpacho Grilled-vegetable

Servings: 10 Serves
Cooking Time: 30 Minutes
Ingredients:
- 2 corn paws, husked.

- Unpeeled 2 big, cored, and quartered red bell peppers.
- 1/2 teaspoon of red pepper crushed.
- 2 big, cored, and quartered yellow bell peppers.
- 2 cups of tomato juice.
- 2 medium zucchini, by longitudinally cut.
- 1/2 centimeter thick, 1 large white onion, cut into 1/2 centimeter dome.
- 4 large cloves of garlic.
- 1 thinly sliced English cucumber.
- 2 cups vegetable oil. 2 cubs.
- Salt kosher and pepper freshly ground.
- 2 tablespoons of vinegar red wine.
- 1 1/2 tea cubes ground cumin.
- Clean orange juice 1/2 cup.
- 3 cups of citrus juice.
- 1/4 cup of coriander chopped.

Directions:
1. Power a barbecue. Place the cloves of garlic on a skewer. Clean the garlic gently, bell pepper, courgette, onion, and maize with vegetable oil and add salt and pepper to the season. Grill the vegetables over moderately high heat and regularly rotate for about ten minutes until they are lightly charred and crisp. Place the peppers in a pot, plastic cover, and let it steam for 10 minutes.
2. Remove the garlic cloves from the sprouts, peel, and transfer to a large cup. Split the charred corn kernels into the bowl with a large clamped knife. Peel and put in a bowl the peppers with courgette, onion, cumin, red pepper crushed, tomato juice, orange juice, lemon juice, and vinegar.
3. Puree the vegetable mixture in the blender or food processor for batches. In a clean tub, pour the gazpacho and season with salt and pepper. Cover and refrigerate for about 2 hours until chilled.
4. Remove the cilantro into the gazpacho just before serving. Place the soup in cups, add the cucumber and eat.

506.Salmon In Salt Crust

Servings: Up To 2 People
Cooking Time: 15 - 30
Ingredients:
- salmon fillet: 500g
- Coarse salt: 1kg

Directions:
1. Remove the mixer blade from the tank.
2. Place the baking paper on the bottom of the tank with the salmon skin facing upwards; cover with coarse salt.
3. Close the cover, select GRILL program, power level MEDIUM, set 30min and press the start/stop button.
4. When finished, remove the salt from the fish and serve with a drizzle of oil on top.

507.Peanut Dressing

Servings: 2 Serves
Cooking Time: 3 Minutes
Ingredients:
- 1 cup of butter or almond.
- 1/2 tablespoon of soy sauce.
- 1/2 cup of rice vinegar wine.
- 8 garlic cloves, peeled.
- Seeds of sesame, for garnishing.
- 1/2 tablespoon of agave nectar.

Directions:
1. Put the High-Speed Blade in the jar and then add all of the ingredients in the order shown.
2. Pulse 3 times and run continuously for 30 seconds or until you reach the desired consistency.
3. Garnish, if desired, with sesame seeds.
4. Serve chopped salad with Spicy Peanut.

508.Roasted Italian Style Peppers

Servings:12 Serves
Cooking Time:1 Hour, 30 Minutes
Ingredients:
- 1/8 tea cubicle ground black pepper.
- 1 cup of Italian Wish-Bone ® dressing.
- 1/4 cup fresh, chopped or thinly sliced, basil leaves.
- 6 large bell peppers, red, green and/or yellow.

Directions:
1. Place the peppers in the large baked aluminum foil or on the broiler pan. Broil, occasionally turn, 20 minutes or almost completely black until peppers turn. Place immediately in a paper bag; close the bag, and allow it to cool for about 30 minutes. Remove the springs and seeds from the skin under cold running water, slice into long and thick strips.
2. Combine bell peppers, basil, and black pepper in a large bowl with Italian seasoning. Refrigerate and marinate, occasionally stirring for a minimum of 2 hours.
3. Serve peppers at room temperature for the best taste.

509.Chicken Breasts Frozen Barbecue

Servings: 4 Serves
Cooking Time: 22 Minutes
Ingredients:
- Ground, as desired, black pepper.
- 2 tablespoons of canola oil, split.
- As desired, kosher salt

- 4 frozen, skinless chicken breasts (each 8 ounces)
- 1 cup of barbecue sauce prepared.

Directions:
1. Place the grill in the unit and close the hood. Choose grill, set medium temperature, and set time to 25 minutes. To start preheating, select start/stop.
2. During preheating, brush with 1/2 tablespoon canola oil each chicken breast evenly. Then season as needed with salt and pepper.
3. When the device is preheated, place the chicken breasts on the grill. Steam the hood for 10 minutes.
4. Flip chicken after 10 minutes. Cover the hood for 5 minutes to finish cooking.
5. After five minutes, mix chicken with grilled sauce and then flip over and baste liberally on the other side. Cover the hood for 5 minutes to continue cooking.
6. Repeat step 5 after 5 minutes. Close the cap and cook 2 minutes longer.
7. If required, grind chicken again and cook until the centre of the chicken reaches 165 ° F internal temperature for up to 3 minutes.
8. Remove the chicken from the unit when cooking is complete and let it stand 5 minutes before serving.

510.Tortilla Spanish

Servings: 8 Serves
Cooking Time: 13 Minutes
Ingredients:
- 1 onion, 1/4-inch thick, peeled.
- 8 large eggs.
- Extra virgin olive oil 1/4 cup
- 1 1/2 kosher salt teaspoons, split.
- Gold potatoes 1 1/2 pounds Yukon, peeled, thinly cut in 1/4 inch rounds.
- 1/2 tea cubicle ground, pepper black
- 1/2 cup of water.

Directions:
1. Combine potted potatoes, onion, water, olive oil, and 1/2 teaspoon of salt.
2. Assemble the pressure cover to ensure that the pressure release valve is in place Lock. Choose pressure and set high. Set 1 minute time and choose start/stop to start.
3. When pressurized cooking is complete, pressurize quickly by turning the pressure release valve to the vent position. When the device has finished releasing strain, carefully remove the cap.
4. Choose and set sear/sauté to high. To start, select start/stop. Cook, without mixing, for about 5 minutes to evaporate and start browning.
5. In a large bowl, whisk eggs, one teaspoon of salt and pepper until frothy.

6. Choose start/stop to disable sear/sauté after 5 minutes. Add the egg blend to the bowl.
7. Set the temperature to 400 ° F and set time to 7 minutes. To start, select start/stop.
8. Cooking is complete when eggs are easily set and removed from the pot side. Place a large dish upside down over the pot and cover the pot on top with the plate with the oven mitts or with the dishtowel. Invert the tortilla and the pot onto the plate. Remove the bowl, place another broad plate over the tortilla, and turn it upright. Remove the top layer. Remove ground. Let the tortilla stay, slice into wedges, and eat for 3 minutes.

511.Black-olive Burger With Japanese Vinegar Grilled

Servings: 5 Serves
Cooking Time: 25 Minutes
Ingredients:
- 4 slices of Swiss cheese.
- 2 tablespoons (30ml) of Chinese Chinkiang vinegar (kurozu)
- Kosher salt.
- 2 mayonnaise tablespoons (30ml)
- 2 tablespoons of black olives (about 15 pitted olives), chopped roughly.
- 12 ounces of freshly ground (340 g) beef, ideally 20% fat
- 2 brioche hamburger buns.

Directions:
1. In a medium bowl, mix beef gently and vinegar, only mix as long as it is necessary to combine them (overmixing the meat will make it to form a tighter and more meatloaf-like texture, so do not do it as necessary). Shape 2 patties slightly wider than the bun's width, press a dimple in the centre of each thumb and sauté with salt all over. Cool for a minimum of 30 minutes and up to 1 hour.
2. Meanwhile, whisk together olives and mayonnaise in a small bowl. Cool until ready to use.
3. Light one charcoal-filled chimney. When all the coal is lit and filled with grey ash, pour it out and disperse more than half the carbon grill equally. Alternatively, put half the gas grill burners in high heat. Set the grate in place, cover the grill, and allow 5 minutes of preheating. Wash the grilling grill and grease.
4. Place the patties directly over warm coals and cook, turning periodically on an instant-reading thermometer for about 7 minutes, until well charred and burgers centre register at 43 ° C (110 ° F). Continue to cook 2 slices of cheese until cheese is melted and burgers record 125 ° F for a medium-rare or

135 ° F (57 ° C) for a medium, 1 to 2 minutes longer. Move burgers to a large plate and leave for 5 minutes to rest. (Move burgers anytime to the cooler side of the grill if they start to fire, but are not yet in final internal temperature.)

5. Toast coals with buns. Spread the mayonnaise olive on top and bottom of each bowl. Place pads on lower buns, close burgers, and serve immediately.

512.Loaded Greek Style Tater Tots

Servings: 6 Serves
Cooking Time: 25 Minutes
Ingredients:
- 3 garlic cloves, sliced, hacked.
- 3 fresh dill tablespoons, chopped, plus more to garnish.
- 1/2 cup of feta cheese crumbled.
- Tomato 1/2 cup, diced.
- Sliced 1/4 cup of black olives.
- New dill, garnish. Fresh dill.
- 2 pounds of tater frozen tots.
- 1 cup of pure Greek milk yogurt
- 1 grated English cucumber.
- 2 cups fresh citrus juice.
- 1/4 of a cup of red onion, peeled, diced.
- 1 kosher salt tablespoon.
- 1 teaspoon of black pepper cracked.

Directions:
1. Choose air fry and set it to 450 ° F and set it to 25 minutes. To start preheating, press start/pause.
2. Place the tater tots in an air fry basket in a single layer.
3. Slide the basket into the top rails of the oven when the machine is preheated.
4. Press start/pause to pause the machine after 15 minutes, take the basket out of the oven, and transfer to a large bowl. Toss with feta, tomatoes, olives, and red onion. Disseminate the mixture on the Ninja ® Sheet Tray. Put the pan in the oven and press start/pause for 10 more minutes to resume cooking.
5. While cooking tots, whisk in a medium bowl all the sauce ingredients of tzatziki together. Set aside.
6. When the kitchen is full, remove the pot from the oven and switch to a bowl. Garnish with tzatziki sauce and fresh dill.

513.Grilled Squash Red Onion With Feta

Servings: 4 Serves
Cooking Time: 10 Minutes
Ingredients:
- 4 Jar of banana peppers, thinly sliced crosswise.
- 1 Clove of garlic, finely grated.
- 4 Medium squash and/or zucchini in season, 1/4 "thick in a lengthwise break.
- 2 Leaves on the sea.
- Kosher salt, the pepper freshly ground.
- 1/2, and 3 tablespoons. Extra virgin olive oil, plus grill.
- Feta, 8 oz., crumbled into large bits.
- 1 Medium red onion, cut into 8 wedges by root end.
- The pinch of crushed red pepper flakes is generous.

Directions:
1. Prepare a grill from medium-high heat; lightly grease foil. Combine garlic, vinegar, and 1/2 cup oil in a small bowl; set aside marinade.
2. On a rimmed baking sheet, mix squash, onion, and bay leaves with the remaining 3 3 tablespoons of oil to coat; season generously with salt and black pepper.
3. Grill squash, untreated, until grill marks appear, should take around 3 minutes. Turnover and grill on the second side until tender and start releasing liquid, should take around 2 minutes. Transfer squash back to the baking sheet. Grill onion, turning periodically, until tender and charred around edges, should take around 10 minutes. Transfer back to the baking sheet.
4. Arrange squash, onion, bay leaves, and feta on a rimmed plate and pour over the reserved marinade. Scatter banana peppers on top and sprinkle with red pepper flakes. Rest at least 15 minutes before serving for up to 1 hour.

514.Sweet And Almon Specy

Servings: 3 Serves
Cooking Time: 45 Minutes
Ingredients:
- 2 tablespoon citrus.
- 1/2 tablespoon water.
- 4 garlic cloves, crushed.
- 1 tablespoon of powdered cumin.
- 1/2 tablespoon red powder chili.
- 1/4 tablespoon of peat.
- 2 tablespoon of olive oil.
- Tamarind 1/2 teaspoon.
- 3 fillets of salmon (200 g each).
- Soft light brown sugar for 1 tablespoon.

Directions:
1. Mix all the ingredients, except salmon, to make a marinade.
2. Marinade the salmon for 1 hour in the mixture.
3. The Ninja Grill is preheated.
4. Put the fillets on the grill, put them up, and close the lid.

5. Cook for ten to twelve minutes, check midway and adjust temperature and time if the grilling is too fast.

515.Rice And Berries Pudding

Servings: 4
Cooking Time: 20 Minutes
Ingredients:
- 1 cup white rice
- 3 cups almond milk
- 1 cup blackberries
- 2 tablespoons sugar
- 2 tablespoons butter, soft
- 1 teaspoon vanilla extract

Directions:
1. In your air fryer's pan, combine the rice with the almond milk and the other ingredients, toss and cook at 370 degrees f for 20 minutes.
2. Divide the rice pudding into bowls and serve.
- **Nutrition Info:** calories 202, fat 12, fiber 4, carbs 7, protein 2

516.Almond & Pesto Kale

Servings: 4 Serves
Cooking Time: 10 Minutes
Ingredients:
- 1 handful of fresh leaves of basil.
- 2 garlic cloves.
- Olive oil 6 teaspoon.
- 6 teaspoons of water.
- 1 lemon juice.
- Almonds 100 g.
- 30 g kale.
- Salt and potatoes.

Directions:
1. Before heating the oven to 180 ° C
2. Put almonds and peeled garlic cloves on the bakery tray, roast about 10 minutes in the oven, or until they are much browned. Take care not to burn them! Enable cooling.
3. Connect your food processor olive oil, tea, lemon juice, kale, and basil. Blend in 30 seconds with high power.
4. Add almonds, garlic, salt and pepper, and lightning to the food processor until all is well mixed. If the pesto looks too thick, add a little more olive oil or water.
5. Use immediately or hold in a tub in the refrigerator and eat in a week.

517.Navy Beans With Ham

Servings: 4
Cooking Time: 18 Minutes
Ingredients:
- 1 tablespoon olive oil
- 1 onion, chopped
- 2 carrot, shredded
- 2 tablespoons garlic, minced
- 2 stalks celery, chopped
- 6 cups chicken stock
- 24 oz. dried navy beans
- 1 teaspoon ground thyme
- 1 teaspoon paprika
- 1 lb. cooked ham, sliced into small cubes
- 14 oz. canned diced tomatoes
- Salt and pepper to taste

Directions:
1. Set the Ninja Foodi to sauté. Pour in the oil.
2. Cook the onion and carrot for 2 minutes.
3. Add the garlic and celery. Cook for 3 minutes.
4. Stir in the rest of the ingredients except the ham and tomatoes.
5. Cover the pot.
6. Set it to pressure.
7. Cook at high pressure for 10 minutes.
8. Release the pressure naturally. Stir in the tomatoes and ham.
9. Simmer for 5 minutes by pressing the sauté function.

518.Air Grill Snails Pizza

Servings: 4 Serves
Cooking Time: 15 Minutes
Ingredients:
- 5 slices of bacon.
- 1 teaspoon oil.
- Mozzarella 170 g – polished
- 200 g of passata tomato.
- 1 teaspoon orange
- 1 Ready to dough with pizza.
- 1 teaspoon basil.
- Salt and pepper.

Directions:
1. Combine pasta, oregano, basil, sugar, salt, and pepper in a pot. Remove well before well combined.
2. Ensure that pot has been installed. Set the temperature to 200 ° C, select bake, and set the timer up to 10 minutes. To start preheating, select start/stop.
3. Place pizza dough and spread tomato sauce evenly on the dough surface, leaving only 2 cm of edge.
4. Cover the dough with 1/2 of the mozzarella and sprinkle it with ham and remaining cheese again. This means that the dough holds tightly together.
5. Form the dough tightly into a circle, leaving the transparent edge with its toppings. Brush the edge gently with water to ensure that it holds well and completes the roll. Cut the roll of pizza into 2 cm slices wide.
6. Once the unit has been replaced to indicate that it was preheated, place the crisper basket and baking paper in half of the pizza.

Open the deck, add the crisper to the unit and close the deck to cook.

7. Once the cooking is done, remove the snails from the pizza and repeat steps 2 and 6.
8. Serve hot with chives garnished with sour cream.

519.Honeyed Grilled Peaches

Servings: 4
Cooking Time: 6 Mins
Ingredients:
- 2 peaches
- 2 tbsp honey
- 1 tsp cinnamon
- ¼ teaspoon salt
- ½ tbsp vegetable oil

Directions:
1. Place your Ninja Foodi grill grate in the unit and close the hood. Choose GRILL, set temperature to MAX, and set time to 6 minutes. Select START/STOP to start your pre-heating.
2. Mix the honey, cinnamon, salt, and oil
3. Half the peaches and dip in the mixture
4. When the pre-heating timer goes off, place the peaches cut side down on the grill, close the hood, and cook for 4 mins
5. Serve immediately
- **Nutrition Info:** Calories: 49 Fat: 2g Saturated Fat: 1.5g Trans Fat: 0g Carbohydrates: 4g Fiber: 2g Sodium: 76mg Protein: 1.5g

520.Good Grill And Air Fryer Lasagne Vegetable

Servings: 9 Serves
Cooking Time: 1 Hour
Ingredients:
- To taste salt and pepper.
- Heavy cream 250ml.
- 1 squash – finely diced.
- Broccoli 140 g – thinly diced.
- 1 red pepper bell – smooth diced.
- 1 pack of dried pasta leaves.
- Cheese layer.
- Hard 140 g grated cheese.
- 140 g mozzarella grated.
- 1 bell pepper yellow – fine diced.
- 2 slices of olive oil.
- Oregan 1 tablespoon.
- 1 tablespoon of basil.
- 2 garlic cloves – gritty.
- Thyme 1/2 teaspoon.
- Mushroom 140 g – finely diced.
- 500 g of passata tomato.
- 100ml water.
- Rosemary 1/2 teaspoon.
- Nutmeg grab.

- Salt and pepper.

Directions:
1. Put 400 g of tomato passata, garlic, oregano, basil, thyme, rosemary, salt, and pepper into a big cup. Combine well. Combine well.
2. In the tomato sauce, add all chopped vegetables and mix well.
3. Combine hard cheese, mozzarella, heavy cream, nutmeg, salt, and pepper in a medium bowl.
4. Combine the remainder of the tomato passata with water and spread half the mixture on the bottom of the bowl.
5. Cover the base of the cooking pot with lasagne sheets and spread evenly over 1/4 of the vegetable mixture. Spread 1/3 of the cheese mixture with more pasta sheets, Repeat until all the vegetables and cheese mix is used.
6. When done, add the remaining tomato water mix to your lasagne. Cover with a bakery and aluminum foil layer to prevent the baker from drying out.
7. In the oven, pick BAKE, set the temperature to 170 ° C and set the time to 45 minutes. To start preheating, select start/stop once the device has beeped to show that the cooking has been preheated, opened, and closed.
8. Remove pot from the unit when cooking is done and allow to rest for 10 minutes.
9. Serve hot with parmesan and basil freshly grated.

521.Cod Meatballs With Tartar Sauce

Servings: Up To 6 People
Cooking Time: 15 - 30
Ingredients:
- cod heart: 350 gr
- bread crumb: 50 gr
- parsley: 1 tuft
- thyme: q.b.
- eggs: 1
- garlic: 1 clove
- Grana cheese: 40 gr
- salt, pepper, flour: q.b.
- tartar sauce: q.b.

Directions:
1. To prepare the meatballs start by blending the bread crumbs in a food processor, then add the fish, thyme, chopped parsley, garlic, grated cheese, eggs and salt and pepper to taste.
2. Mix well to amalgamate everything and with your hands form small balls. Flour each meatball and put them in a skewer (3 meatballs per skewer).
3. Remove the mixing shovel from the bowl.
4. Place the skewers on the bottom of the tank, close the lid, select the ROAST program, set

20min and press the start/stop program key.
5. After 10min turn the skewers on themselves and finish cooking.
6. Serve accompanied with tartar sauce.

522.Cheeseburgers Grilled Juicy

Servings: 4 Serves
Cooking Time: 35 Minutes
Ingredients:
- 2 Worcestershire teaspoons of sauce.
- 1 garlic clove.
- 1 cubicle shallot.
- 2 ketchup cubicles.
- 1 cubicle of salt.
- A minimum of 1 lb of ground beef 15 percent fat
- 1 cubicle of pepper.
- 1 tablespoon grain Dijon mustard course

Directions:
1. Simple the shallot and garlic. Don't ask why I have prepared 3 shallots in this picture. I don't know myself!
2. Add garlic, shallots, mustard, ketchup, salt, pepper, and Worcestershire sauce to the ground beef in a mixing bowl.
3. Mix the ingredients, but don't mix them over. It's just going to make mushy burgers over mixing.
4. Take a palm in your hand full. Place it flat in your hand and use your hand to make it a round patty.
5. Let it rest while being preheated on your grill.
6. During the preheating process, get your garnishes ready. Oh, how I wished I recalled the grocery store's avocados and bacon.
7. Put your patties over direct heat and cover the grill with the grill nice and hot. Cook them for 3 minutes.
8. Roll out the burgers and cook for 5 (medium) 6 (medium) or 7 (good) minutes, respectively. Put cheese on top in the last 2-3 minutes on the grill to let cook. Keep the grill to the fullest extent possible.
9. Add buns on the top of the rack face down when the cheese are placed, if it is toast.
10. Once the burgers are done, let them rest for about 5 minutes.
11. Get on your bun, serve, and enjoy with your garnishes!!

523.Cornbread Cheddar

Servings: 8 Serves
Cooking Time: 25 Minutes
Ingredients:
- 2 teaspoons powder baking.
- 3/4 cup of maize meal.
- 1/4 of a cup of canola oil
- 1/4 taste of sugar.
- 2 kosher salt teaspoons.
- 1 egg.
- 1 cup of whole milk.
- 1 1/4 cups of the all-purpose meal
- 1 cup of cheddar cheese shredded.

Directions:
1. On the reversible rack, place the Ninja ® multi-purpose saucepan * (or 8-inch baking pan) to make sure the rack is in the lower position. In the pot, place the rack—close crooked deck. Choose BROIL and set the time at 10 minutes to preheat the unit and pot. To start, click start/stop.
2. Whisk flour, cornmeal, sugar, baking powder, and salt together in a medium bowl.
3. To combine dry ingredients, add egg, milk, and oil. Add the cheese and add it to the mixture.
4. When the device and pot are preheated, open the lid and spray with the spray for 10 minutes. Pour batter into pan. Pour into pan.
5. Close crooked deck. Set the temperature to 350 ° F and set the time to 25 minutes. Select bake / roast. To start, click start/stop. Bake at least 20 minutes until golden brown cornbread and clean the wooden toothpick inserted in the middle.
6. When cooked, remove the rack from the unit with a pot and allow a cooling rack to cool for 5 minutes before serving. Toast thick slices of maize bread in butter if desired with the sear / sauté (MD: H.I.) configuration.

524.Sausage & Beans

Servings: 4
Cooking Time: 48 Minutes
Ingredients:
- 1 onion, chopped
- 3 stalks celery, chopped
- 1 bay leaf
- 4 carrot, chopped
- 1 sprig fresh rosemary
- 4 sprigs fresh thyme
- 4 cloves garlic, minced
- 1/4 teaspoon oregano, dried
- 1/2 teaspoon pepper
- 6 cups chicken broth
- 1 lb. white beans
- 1-pound chopped sausage roll

Directions:
1. Cook for 3 minutes.
2. Add the rosemary, thyme, garlic, and oregano.
3. Add the sausage and stir-cook to brown evenly.
4. Cook for 1 minute.
5. Add the pepper and stir in broth.

6. Simmer for 5 minutes.
7. Stir in the white beans.
8. Lock the lid in place.
9. Set it to pressure.
10. Cook at high pressure for 40 minutes. Release the pressure naturally.
11. Cook at high pressure for 40 minutes.
12. Release the pressure naturally.

525.Balsamic Marinade Maple

Servings: 4 Serves
Cooking Time: 55 Minutes
Ingredients:
- 2 teaspoons of fresh thyme finely chopped.
- Wish-Bone ® 3/4 cup balsamic sauce
- 1/3 cup of pure maple jar
- 8 boneless chicken thighs without skin

Directions:
1. For a small cup, mix balsamic dressing, maple syrup, and thyme. Pour in a large, shallow glass baker's bag or plastic bag 1/2 cup marinade over chicken. Bag cover or close. Bag cover or close.
2. Marinate chicken, occasionally turning, and 30 minutes to 3 hours in the refrigerator. Remove marinade chicken, discard marinade.
3. Barbeque or broil chicken, turn once and burn with remaining marinade frequently until chicken is thoroughly cooked for about 15 minutes.

526.Peas Bake

Servings: 4
Cooking Time: 20 Minutes
Ingredients:
- ½ pound baby peas
- 1 tablespoon avocado oil
- 8 eggs, whisked
- 1 cup cheddar cheese, shredded
- 1 red onion, chopped
- 1 cup bacon, cooked and chopped
- Salt and black pepper to the taste

Directions:
1. Heat up the air fryer with the oil at 360 degrees f, add the onion and cook for 5 minutes.
2. Add the peas and the other ingredients except the cheese and toss.
3. Sprinkle the cheese on top, cook the mix for 15 minutes more, divide between plates and serve.
- **Nutrition Info:** calories 212, fat 9, fiber 4, carbs 13, protein 7

527.Stuffed Cuttlefish

Servings: Up To 4 People
Cooking Time: 15 - 30
Ingredients:

- small cuttlefish: 8
- breadcrumbs: 50 gr
- garlic: q.b.
- parsley: q.b.
- egg: 1
- salt: q.b.
- pepper: q.b.

Directions:
1. Clean the cuttlefish, cut and separate the tentacles; in a mixer pour the breadcrumbs, the parsley without stalks, the egg, the salt a drizzle of olive oil and the cuttlefish tentacles.
2. Blend until the mixture is more or less dense; fill the cuttlefish with the mixture obtained.
3. Remove the mixing shovel from the tank.
4. Place the cuttlefish inside, close the lid, select the GRILL program, power level MEDIUM, set 20min and press the program start/stop key.
5. The cooking time may vary depending on the size of the cuttlefish.

528.Coconut Mango Working

Servings: 4 Serves
Cooking Time: 10 Minutes
Ingredients:
- 8 fresh leaves of mint.
- 1/2 taste of ice.
- 4 cups of cocoa tea.
- 1 1/2 cups of chunks of frozen mangoes.

Directions:
1. Put the high-speed blade in the jar and then add all ingredients in the order.
2. Pulse 3 times, then run for 45 seconds or until you reach the desired consistency.

529.Tenderloin Filets Bacon-wrapped

Servings: 4 Serves
Cooking Time: 12 Minutes
Ingredients:
- Black pepper ground, as needed.
- 4 center-cut beef filets tenderloin (each 8 ounces)
- Toothpicks, if required.
- 2 tablespoons of canola oil, split.
- As desired, kosher salt
- 8 slices of bacon uncooked.

Directions:
1. Wrap 2 strips of bacon out of each filet all around. To secure the bacon, use toothpicks.
2. Stir wrapped fillets on all sides using canola oil, then season with salt and pepper as desired (using 1/2 tablespoon oil per fillet).
3. Install the grill in the unit and close the hood. Choose grill, set high temperature, and set time to 12 minutes. To start preheating, select start/stop.

4. If the unit indicates that it has preheated, the filets are placed on the grill. Press them down so that grill marks are maximized, and then close the hood and cook 6 minutes.
5. Flip filets after 6 minutes. Close the lid to continue cooking on a food temperature level for 6 minutes or until the internal temperature of the filets is 130 ° F. Delete device filets. They continue to cook as they rest at a food-safe temperature.
6. Allow filets to rest for 10 minutes before serving, allowing juices to be evenly redistributed via filets.

530. Crispy Letters

Servings: 4 Serves
Cooking Time: 14 Minutes
Ingredients:
- 1 charcoal canola oil.
- 2 pounds of chicken wings uncooked.
- 1 kosher salt tablespoon.
- 1 charcoal black pepper.

Directions:
1. Insert the crisper plate in the unit of the basket and the basket. Choose air fry to preheat, set temperature to 390 ° F, and set the time to 3 minutes. To start preheating, click start/stop.
2. During preheating, throw wings into a bowl of butter, salt, and pepper.
3. If the device is preheated, growing wings on the crisper tray. Set temperature to 390 ° F and set time to 24 minutes. Select air fry. To start cooking, select start/stop.
4. Toss wings after 12 minutes with silicone tongs, reinsert the cooking basket to resume.
5. Toss wings with the desired flavorings and serve when cooking is complete.

531. Salt Focaccia Be

Servings: 8 Serves
Cooking Time: 55 Minutes
Ingredients:
- Strong 350 g flat flour.
- 1 1/4 tea cubicles of fine salt.
- 60 ml (or use all the water) of white wine
- Water 225ml.
- 1 tea cubicle dried yeast.
- Sea salt flaked, brushed.
- 3 extra virgin olive oil tablespoons, split, plus a little extra greasing.

Directions:
1. Insert in a bowl meal, yeast, and fine sea salt, 2 tablespoons of olive oil, water, and wine. Mix it approximately with a single hand kneading action for about one to two minutes to make sure all is well combined. The dough is going to be sticky.

2. Clog the bowl and put it in the fridge to freeze for at least 8 hours or up to 24 hours. (Prove at room temperature for about 2 hours or till the size of the quick method was doubled.)
3. Remove the dough from the refrigerator about 2 hours before the focaccia is baked.
4. Line up the crooked basket with a bakery parchment approx. 5 cm on the sides. It doesn't have to be perfect and clean. Lightly oil the parchment with your hands. Take the dough into the crisping basket and spread it to the corners. (It is going to spread and fill the basket as it is proved).
5. Cover the crisping basket with the cling film and prove it for a minimum of 2-2 1/2 hours at room temperature. (If you've chosen the fastest proof method, the second proof is about half an hour or till the volume is doubled).
6. When the focaccia is ready to bake, mix the remaining 1 tablespoon of olive oil with 1 tablespoon of water and drain over the focaccia surface. Use both hands to scratch the dough across the surface by grabbing the fingertips. Sprinkle with sea salt flakes and any other toppings.
7. Check that the pot is inserted and close the deck. Set the temperature to 190 ° C and set the time to 25 minutes. Select bake. To start preheating, click start/stop.
8. If the unit beeps to indicate that it has preheated, put the punching basket in the pot and close the deck. After about 18 minutes, test the focaccia. When tapped, it sounds hollow and should be nicely browned. When the focus is cooked, remove the cropping basket carefully from the unit and focus on the bakery parchment. Transfer the focus to a cooling rack and remove the parchment. Let it cool before you eat.

532. Scallops With Butter

Servings: Up To 4 People
Cooking Time: 15 - 30
Ingredients:
- scallops (pulp): 400gr
- butter: 20gr
- garlic: 1 clove
- salt: q.b.
- pepper: q.b.
- parsley: q.b.
- lemon juice: 1/2

Directions:
1. Insert the mixer blade into the tank.
2. Peel the scallops, clean them and put them to dry well with absorbent paper.

3. Put the butter inside the pan, chopped garlic, close the lid, select program ROAST, set 15min and press program start/stop key.
4. Melt the butter for about 2-3 minutes.
5. Add scallops, salt, pepper and cook for 8 minutes.
6. Finally add the lemon juice, parsley and finish cooking.
7. Excellent as an appetizer to serve inside your shells.

533.Cheeseburgers Pimento-jalapeño

Servings: 4 Serves
Cooking Time: 25 Minutes
Ingredients:
- 4 slices of tomato ripe.
- 3/4 cup sliced jalapeño pickled peppers.
- Cut into a 1-inch cube (see note) 1 1/2 pounds beef chuck.
- Kosher salt and black pepper freshly ground.
- 4 soft buns.
- 1 1/2 cups of iceberg shredded salad
- 1/2 small, thinly sliced, white or yellow onion
- 1 cup of Cheese Pimento.

Directions:
1. In the food processor, place pimento cheese. Pulse 6 to 8 short pulses until finely chopped. Move to a small bowl with a spatula and, if used for molding meat, wash the food processor bowl.
2. Grind with a meat grinder: Place a grinding pipe, feeding tube, frame, die, and dust a meat grinder with a large blender in the freezer. Spread the beef chunks uniformly over a large platform or rimmed bakery in one sheet. Place meat in a freezer and freeze until the edges become firm, but still meltable for about 20 minutes. Set up a 3/8-inch meat grinder. In the cold bowl, grind beef. Fast working, grind meat with 1/4 inch plate. When grinder or meat gets too hot during grinding, return to freezer for 10 minutes before grinding.
3. To grind with a food processor, Spread beef chunks on a large platform or rimmed baking sheet evenly in a single layer. Place in a freezer and freeze until it gets solid, but still going, for approximately 20 minutes. Place meat cubes in a food processor's work bowl in three batches. Pulse, around 15 to 20 short pulses, until finely chopped. Transfer to a bowl with the remainder of the beef and repeat.
4. Former beef into four patties roughly 1/2 "wider than burger buns with moderate depression in the middle to cover the bulging when cooking. Apply salt and pepper generously and cool until ready to cook.
5. Light one charcoal-filled chimney. When the entire charcoal is lit and coated with grey ash, stretch the charcoal uniformly on one side. Instead, position half the gas grill burners at high temperatures. Put the cooking grill in place and cover with the grill and allow for 5 minutes to preheat. Wash the grilling grill and grease. Place burgers directly over hot coals, cover with open wind, and cook until well charred and centre of burgers record 110 ° F in instant thermometer read, approximately 5 minutes.

534.Crumble Blondes Apple

Servings: 8 Serves
Cooking Time: 10 Minutes
Ingredients:
- 2 cored and diced apples.
- 1 tablespoon powder baking.
- Extract 1 teaspoon of vanilla.
- 2 cinnamon tea cubes.
- 1/2 tea Kuchar nutmeg.
- 100 g of cocoa sugar.
- 1 ovum.
- Maple syrup of 80ml.
- 150 g flour of choice.
- 1 charcoal citrus juice.
- 125 ml of selecting oil.

Directions:
1. Preheat the oven to 180°C and grate the baking tin to 9x9 inches.
2. Place meal, baker powder, cinnamon, musk, olive oil, coconut sugar, eggs, maple syrup, and vanilla in the mixer and whizz into your Ninja Kitchen Nutri Ninja until you have a batter.
3. In the lemon juice, swirl the diced apples, then drag them into the mixture and fold in. Spoon in the tin and smooth out uniformly.

535.Pep In Your Book

Servings: 3 Serves
Cooking Time: 15 Minutes
Ingredients:
- 6 of a cup of white wine.
- 1/4 of Italian parsley bunch, trimmed.
- 1/4 cup of tomatoes sundried.
- 2 garlic cloves, peeled.
- 1 cup of low-sodium sprout.
- To try, salt and pepper.
- 3 roasted, peeled and cooled bell peppers.
- Vinegar balsamic, to be garnished.

Directions:
1. In the order specified, place all ingredients, except balsamic vinegar, in the 64-ounce Precision Processor.

2. Choose puree.
3. Switch soup to a medium saucepan and cook for about 10 minutes until heated. Serve hot in bowls with balsamic vinegar splash.

536.Bbq Chicken Drumsticks Fried

Servings: 6 Serves
Cooking Time: 1 Hour, 30 Minutes
Ingredients:
- 1/4 cayenne pepper teaspoon, optional.
- 5 kosher salt tablespoons, divided.
- 2 cups of hot water.
- 2 cold cups of water.
- 2 tablespoons of sugar granulated.
- 12 pickles (3-1/2 to 4 pounds).
- 1 teaspoon of peppers.
- 1/2 tea cubicle ground black pepper.
- 1/4 teaspoon of powdered onion.
- 1/4 tea cubicle powder garlic.

Directions:
1. Pour hot water into a deep container, add 4 tablespoons of salt and sugar, and stir until salt and sugar have dissolved; pour into cold water. Add chicken to salt, cover, and cool for 30 to 1 hour.
2. Spray cold gas grilles with grilling spray; preheat them for indirect heat by turning the grill on one side to high and leaving one side at very low temperatures.
3. In a small bowl, combine the rest of 1 tablespoon of salt, paprika, pepper, onion powder, garlic powder, and cayenne pepper. Drain and dry chicken with towels of paper. Season chicken with a mixture of spices. Place the chicken on a cool side of the grill, cover, and cook for 30-40 minutes until it is no longer pink (180 ° F).
4. Bake the BBQ sauce with the chicken, switch to the hot side of the grill and cook 2 minutes. Watch carefully for burning avoidance. Serve, if desired, with additional sauce.

537.Marinade Italian Marsale

Servings: 6 Serves
Cooking Time: 50 Minutes
Ingredients:
- 6 chicken breasts without bones.
- 3/4 cup coating
- 1 tablespoon of fresh rosemary finely chopped.
- 1/4 cup of wine from Marsala.

Directions:
1. In a medium bowl, combine the Italian dress, Marsala wine and rosemary.
2. Pour 1/2 cup of marinade into a large shallow glass bakery or plastic bag with chicken. Close the bag.

3. In refrigeration, marinate chicken, occasionally turning for 30 minutes to 3 hours.
4. Remove marinade chicken and discard marinade.
5. Grill or fry chicken, turning once and regularly burn until the chicken is thoroughly cooked around 12 minutes.

538.Grilled Cumin Tenderloin Spiced

Servings: 6 Serves
Cooking Time: 25 Minutes
Ingredients:
- 1/4 tea cubicle black pepper.
- 1 teaspoon of powdered garlic.
- 1 teaspoon of powdered chili.
- 1/2 square meters of cumin.
- 1 kosher salt tablespoon.
- 1/2 teaspoon of peppers.
- 1 pork tenderloin, approximately 18 oz.

Directions:
1. Combine the spices and season all over the tenderloin.
2. Preheat up the grill or preheat up the broiler.
3. Grill the grill or fried tenderloin, covered on each side for 5 minutes, then switch to indirect warmth while grilling, cover the grill and simmer for 10 to 12 minutes, turning halfway, to 145 ° F * (total approximately 22 to 25 minutes) in an instant-read thermometer mounted in the central position. Add more time for a thicker tenderloin.
4. Let the pork rest approximately 5 minutes before slicing.

539.Home Ground Grilled Cheeseburgers Thick And Juicy

Servings: 4 Serves
Cooking Time: 35 Minutes
Ingredients:
- 4 buns of hamburgers.
- Kosher salt and black pepper freshly made.
- 4 cheese slices.
- Cut into 1-inch cubes (see note) 1 1/2 pounds of chuck for beef.
- As needed, toppings.

Directions:
1. To grind with a meat grinder: place in the fridge grinding pipe, filling tube, pan, die and screw a meat grinder. Place beef chunks on a large plate or rimmed baking sheet uniformly into one layer. Put in the freezer and freeze for around 20 minutes before you get tightly around the edges but still meltable. Set up a 3/8ths inch meat grinder. Into a cold bowl grind beef. Grind meat easily with 1/4-inch plate again. If the meat

gets too warm during grinding, return to the freezer for 10 minutes before grinding again.

2. To be ground by a food processor: spread the beef chunks evenly over a large plate or rimmed baking sheet in one layer. Place in the freezer and freeze until it gets solid, but still malty, about 20 minutes. Place meat cubes in a food processor's work bowl in three batches. Pulse, about 15 to 20 short pulses until finely chopped. Take the remaining beef and rinse it in a bowl.

3. Beef forms approximately 1/2 centimetres wider in four patties than burger buns, the centre of which has a slight depression when cooking. Apply salt and pepper generously and cool until ready to cook.

4. Light one charcoal-filled chimney. When all of the fuel is lit and coated with grey ash, scatter it uniformly on one side of the energy grid. Alternatively, put half the gas grill burners in high heat. Set the grill in place, cover the grill, and allow for 5 minutes to preheat. Wash the grilling grill and grease.

5. Place burgers directly over hot coals, cover with winds and cook, occasionally turning until well charred and 110 ° F on an instant-read thermometer, approximately 5 minutes. Place the cheese on top of the burgers and cook until the cheese melted, and the burgers have 125 ° F medium-rare and 135 ° F regular, 1 to 2 minutes longer. Take the burgers to a large plate.

6. Carry buns over the middle of the grill to cook golden brown. Top burgers, put in buns, and serve as desired.

540.Carob, Raspberry, Raspberry And Chocolate

Servings: 6 Serves
Cooking Time: 30 Minutes
Ingredients:
- Cut 50 g of dark chocolate into pieces.
- 100 g of cocoa sugar.
- 1 tablespoon powder baking.
- 150 g flour of choice.
- A hundred ml of milk.
- 1 ovum.
- Extract 1 teaspoon of vanilla.
- 75 g of frozen frosts.
- 30 g paste of carob.

Directions:
1. Preheat the oven to 180°C and grass the pudding tins 4-6 x 150 ml.
2. Into the Ninja Kitchen Nutri ninja blender and whizz until smooth, place the meal, sugar, carob, baking powder, milk, egg, and

vanilla. Remove the chocolate and the raspberries.

3. Spread the mixture between the tins to the top. Place the pudding tins onto a baking tray and bake in the oven for about 30 minutes.

4. Let the tins cool down for 10 minutes, then take a knife and put out the puddings. You may enjoy them warmly – but let them cool if you want the yogurt topping.

5. Beat the yogurt, carob powder, and maple syrup with each cooled pudding. Disperse over cocoa nibs and freeze-dried raspberries and enjoy!

541.Marinated Chicken Sweet

Servings: 4 Serves
Cooking Time: 15 Minutes
Ingredients:
- Halves 1 pound skinless chicken breast
- 2 new thyme cubes.
- Original Syrup is 1/4 cup.
- Extra virgin olive oil 1/4 cup
- 2 tablespoons of vinegar balsamic.
- 1/4 tea cubicle oil.
- 1/8 tea cubicle ground black pepper

Directions:
1. In a medium bowl, combine syrup, olive oil, balsamic vinegar, herbs, salt, and pepper. Pour in a big, shallower, non-aluminum baker or plastic bag 1/2 cup of marinade over chicken. Cover or close bag and marinate regularly 15 to 30 minutes in the refrigerator.
2. Remove marinade chicken and discard marinade. Grill or brown chicken, turning once and often brush until chicken is thoroughly cooked (165 ° F) with remaining marinade (12 minutes).

542.Salmon Fillet In Salad

Servings:x
Cooking Time:x
Ingredients:
- salmon fillet: 600gr
- coarse salt: 1/2 teaspoon
- cayenne chili powder: 1 pinch
- lemon juice: 1 teaspoon
- extra virgin olive oil: liv 5
- water: 200ml

Directions:
1. Remove the mixer blade from the tank and insert the grid accessory.
2. Pour the water into the bottom of the tank to avoid unpleasant odours during cooking.
3. Season both sides of the fillet with coarse salt and chilli pepper, then add a few drops of lemon juice and olive oil.

4. Place the salmon directly above the grill, close the lid, select the GRILL program, power level MEDIUM, set 30min and press the program start/stop button.
5. Once cooked, serve the hot salmon; ideal served with fresh seasonal salad.

543.Salmon Teriyaki-marinated

Servings: 4 Serves
Cooking Time: 9 Minutes
Ingredients:
- 1 cup of marinade teriyaki.
- 4 uncooked fillets of skinless salmon (6 ounces each)

Directions:
1. In a large resealable plastic bag or container, place the fish fillets and the teriyaki sauce. Move nets around to coat sauce evenly. Chill for at least 1 hour and up to 12 hours.
2. Please insert the grill in the unit and the hood close. Choose grill, set the max temperature, and set the time to 8 minutes. To start preheating, select start/stop.
3. When the unit indicates that it has preheated, position the fillets on the grill and press them so that grill marks can be maximized. Cook the hood for 6 minutes. The fish do not have to flip during cooking.
4. Check filets for doneness after 6 minutes; the internal temperature should be 140 ° F. Close the hood and continue cooking for up to 2 minutes if necessary.
5. Serve fillets immediately when cooking is complete.

544.Kebabs Steak And Vegetable

Servings: 4 Serves
Cooking Time: 12 Minutes
Ingredients:
- Black pepper ground, as desired.
- 1 bell pepper, cut into two pieces (green, yellow, or red).
- 8 mushrooms, cut in half, cut out stems.
- 1 little white onion, peeled, quartered, 2-inch petals cut.
- As desired, kosher salt
- 2 New York strip steaks, cut into 2-inch cubes (10-12 units each).
- Seasoning steak, as needed.

Directions:
1. Add the grill to the machine and remove the hood. Select grill, set a high temperature, set the time to 12 minutes. To start preheating, select start/stop.
2. During the preheating time, assemble the skewers to almost full order – steak, mushroom, bell pepper, onion. Make sure the ingredients almost entirely forced down to the end of the sprouts.

3. Season sprouts with salt, pepper, and steak liberally.
4. If the device bites to show that it is preheated, put skewers on the grill. Open the hood and cook without flipping for 8 minutes.
5. Check the steak for the desired doneness after 8 minutes and cook up to 4 more minutes if desired.
6. Serve immediately when cooking is complete.

545.Cheesy Cauliflower

Servings: 4 Serves
Cooking Time: 20 Minutes
Ingredients:
- 1 single cubicle flour.
- 250ml beer.
- 65 g Italian crumbs of bread
- 2 tea cubicles are oil.
- 1 pinch ground muscle. 1 pinch ground.
- 40 g of dried currants or grapes
- 1 cauliflower ear, trimmed, cut into flowers.
- Parmesan 65 g grated cheese.
- 125ml twin cream.
- Cooking spray.

Directions:
1. Put the beer in the pot. Add chocolate, salt, mustache, and currants. Assemble the pressure cover to ensure that the pressure release valve is in place Lock.
2. Choose pressure and set high. Set 2 minutes to set time. To start, select start/stop.
3. Stir together the breadcrumbs and cheese while the cooling flower mixture is cooking; set aside. For a separate dish, whisk together the milk and flour.
4. After pressurizing is complete, release the pressure quickly by moving the release valve to the vent position. When the device has finished releasing strain, carefully remove the cap.
5. Add the meal blend to the pot. Choose sear/saute and set it to Medium. To start, select start/stop. Carry a bowl of sauce. Press the Power button to turn off sear/sauté after boiling.
6. Sprinkle the mixture of bread crumbs over the cauliflower. Spray with spray cooking.
7. Close crooked deck. Set the temperature to 200 ° C and set the time to 10 minutes. Select air crisp. To start, select start/stop. Cook until golden brown is the tip.

546.Dipping Donuts

Servings: 10
Cooking Time: 5 Mins
Ingredients:
- 1 cup flour

- 1/2 tsp baking powder
- 1/4 tsp baking soda
- 1/4 tsp salt
- 4 tbsp butter unsalted butter, softened
- 1 cup honey
- 2 large eggs
- 1 cup milk
- Vegetable oil for coating

Directions:
1. Set your Ninja Foodi appliance to AIR FRY. Select START/STOP to start your pre-heating.
2. Mix your wet ingredients and your dry ingredients separately then combine and mix until a dough is formed
3. Shape into small donuts and coat lightly with vegetable oil
4. Drop into the crisper basket and cook until golden brown
5. Serve
- **Nutrition Info:** Calories: 200 Fat: 17g Saturated Fat: 6g Trans Fat: 0g Carbohydrates: 42g Fiber: 1g Sodium: 122mg Protein: 3g

547.Granola Homemade Bars

Servings: 18 Serves
Cooking Time: 15 Minutes
Ingredients:
- 1/4 cup of chocolate semisweet chips
- 1/2 cup of pistachio shelled.
- 1/4 cup sweetheart.
- 1 cup of grain.
- 1/2 cup of crispy cereal rice.
- For a more tart taste, 1/4 cup of dried cranberries.

Directions:
1. Line an 8x8-inch plastic-wrapped bakery; set aside.
2. In the order specified, place all ingredients in the Nutri BowlTM.
3. Choose BOOSTTM Auto-iQ NO FUSION Blend.
4. Spread the mixture into a prepared bakery platter.
5. Cover the plastic wrap mixture and cool for 30 minutes.
6. Pre-serve cut into 1 1/2-inch square.

548.Strip Steak Grilled Ny With Asparagus

Servings: 4 Serves
Cooking Time: 12 Minutes
Ingredients:
- Black pepper ground, as desired.
- 2 spoonful of canola oil, divided.
- As needed, kosher salt.
- 2 New York strip steaks not cooked (14-16 ounces).
- 1 asparagus bunch, trimmed.

Directions:
1. Brush each steak in a 1/2 tablespoon of canola oil on each side and season as desired with salt and pepper. Place the remaining canola oil on the asparagus and season with the salt and pepper as desired.
2. Install a grill in the device and close the hood grill. Use GRILL set HIGH temperature and set time to 12 minutes. To start preheating, click start/stop.
3. If the device indicates that it has preheated, put steaks on the grill and press them down to maximize grill marks. Open the hood for 4 minutes and cook.
4. Flip steaks after 4 minutes. Open the cap and continue to cook until the internal temperature exceeds 125 ° F for 4 more minutes.
5. Remove steaks from the grill and let stand for 5 minutes, and start cooking while resting at a food-safe temperature. To ensure a healthy food temperature, using a cooking thermometer.
6. While the steaks rest, grill the asparagus. Steam the hood for 4 minutes.
7. Slice steaks and serve with asparagus when cooking and rest are full.

549.Sensational Carrot Puree

Servings: 4
Cooking Time: 4 Minutes
Ingredients:
- 1 and 1/2-pound carrots, chopped
- 1 tablespoon of butter at room temperature
- 1 tablespoon of agave nectar
- 1/4 teaspoon of sea salt
- 1 cup of water

Directions:
1. Clean and peel your carrots properly. Roughly chop up them into small pieces
2. Add 1 cup of water to your Pot
3. Place the carrots in a steamer basket and place the basket in the Ninja Foodi
4. Lock up the lid and cook on HIGH pressure for 4 minutes.
5. Perform a quick release
6. Transfer the carrots to a deep bowl and use an immersion blender to blend the carrots
7. Add butter, nectar, salt, and puree.
8. Taste the puree and season more if needed. Enjoy!

550.Korean Bulgogi Burgers With Kimchi Mayo And Pickled Daikon Grilled

Servings: 4 Serves
Cooking Time: 25 Minutes
Ingredients:
- For the Mayo Kimchi:
- 2 cups (approximately 200 g) of fine quartered, cored red chalk

- 2 cubs (30ml) kimchi water
- 1/2 cup drained kimchi finely diced (100 g).
- 4 sesame buns of seed, cut.
- 1 tablespoon (15ml) of sésame oil toasted.
- 1 cucharco (4 g) of sugar
- 1 small garlic clove, grated or hacked
- Two scallions, only white and light green, finely chopped (approximately 40 g).
- For the Sauce of Bulgaria:
- 2 teaspoons (10ml) of sésame oil toasted.
- 1/4 cup (50 g) brown sugar
- 1 1/2 cubic cubes (20 ml) gochujang (spicy red pepper paste)
- 1 tablespoon of grated fresh ginger (about 1 2-inch button)
- 1 cucharco (15ml) of rice vinegar.
- 3 big garlic, rubbed or hacked cloves.
- 1/2 cup of soy sauce (120 ml).

Directions:

1. Blend soy sauce, gochujang, garlic, ginger, vinegar, and brown sugar in a medium saucepan. Bring the mixture to a boil over medium-high heat, reduce to steam, and steam for 5 to 7 minutes until thick enough to cover the spoon. Remove from heat, add sésame oil and cool down. Use immediately or cool for up to 1 week in an airtight container.
2. For Kimchi Mayo: whisk the mayonnaise, kimchi sage, kimchi, sugar, sesame oils, garlic, and scallions until they are well mixed into a medium mixing cup. Hot until ready to use.
3. For Burgers: Shape 4 patties of beef, about a one-half inch wider than burger buns. Push a depression in the middle of any patty with your thumb to avoid bulging.
4. Light one charcoal-filled chimney. Once all the charcoal is lit and filled with grey ash, pour the coal over half the charcoal grate and scatter it evenly. Fire up to half the gas grill burners. Place grill in place, cover with grill and allow to preheat for 5 minutes. Wash the grilling grill, and grease.
5. Set patties over hot coals directly, cover with open winds and cook, turning periodically. When the paints are charred, and the centres record 110 ° F on an instant-reading thermometer, brush them on both sides with bulgogi. Continue to cook burgers, flip and sauce occasionally until 120 ° F or 130 ° F are registered as medium-rare or 130 ° F.
6. Remove the grill and spray with more sauce on both sides until they are well glazed and coated. Sprinkle with sesame seeds all over and leave for 5 minutes to rest.
7. In the meantime, the burger toast buns on a grill over moderate heat to light golden brown. Spread kimchi mayonnaise with top and bottom buns. Layer bottom buns, followed by the Danmuji with half the cob and patties. Brush the top of the patties with the bulgogi sauce again, then apply the rest of the col, close the top buns and serve.

Lightning Source UK Ltd.
Milton Keynes UK
UKHW030015230422
401922UK00007B/1423

9 781801 247788